THE ADMINISTRATION OF
MENTAL HEALTH SERVICES

The Administration of Mental Health Services

Edited by

SAUL FELDMAN, D.P.A.

National Institute of Mental Health
Rockville, Maryland

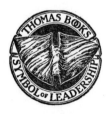

CHARLES C THOMAS · PUBLISHER
Springfield · Illinois · U.S.A.

Published and Distributed Throughout the World by
CHARLES C THOMAS • PUBLISHER
BANNERSTONE HOUSE
301-327 East Lawrence Avenue, Springfield, Illinois, U.S.A.

© *1973, by* CHARLES C THOMAS • PUBLISHER
ISBN 0-398-02804-4
Library of Congress Catalog Card Number: 72-11611

With THOMAS BOOKS *careful attention is given to all details of manufacturing and design. It is the Publisher's desire to present books that are satisfactory as to their physical qualities and artistic possibilities and appropriate for their particular use.* THOMAS BOOKS *will be true to those laws of quality that assure a good name and good will.*

Printed in the United States of America
N-1

CONTRIBUTORS

PAUL R. BINNER, Ph.D.
Chief of Research
Fort Logan Mental Health Center
Denver, Colorado

ROBERT H. CONNERY, Ph.D.
Professor of Government
Columbia University
President of the Academy of Political Science
New York, New York

HOWARD R. DAVIS, Ph.D.
Chief, Mental Health Services Development Branch
Division of Mental Health Service Programs
National Institute of Mental Health
Rockville, Maryland

SAUL FELDMAN, D.P.A.
Associate Director for Community Mental Health Services
Division of Mental Health Service Programs
National Institute of Mental Health
Rockville, Maryland

ERNEST C. HARVEY, Ph.D.
Senior Economist
Stanford Research Institute
Menlo Park, California

SEYMOUR R. KAPLAN, M.D.
Associate Professor of Psychiatry
Director, Residency and Fellowship Programs in
Administrative Psychiatry and Mental Health Planning
Albert Einstein College of Medicine
Bronx, New York

RALPH LITTLESTONE
Chief, Planning Branch
Office of Program Planning and Evaluation
National Institute of Mental Health
Rockville, Maryland

v

DAVID MECHANIC, Ph.D.
Professor of Sociology and Director,
Center for Medical Sociology and Health Services Research
University of Wisconsin
Madison, Wisconsin

SUTHERLAND MILLER, Ph.D.
Assistant Professor
Department of Psychiatry and Department of Community Health
Albert Einstein College of Medicine
New York, New York

JOHN A. MORGAN, JR., Ph.D.
Associate Professor
Political Science and Public Affairs
The George Washington University
Washington, D. C.

GREGORY M. ST. L. O'BRIEN, Ph.D.
Director and Associate Professor
Human Services Design Laboratory
School of Applied Social Sciences
Case Western Reserve University
Cleveland, Ohio

H. G. WHITTINGTON, M.D.
Director of Psychiatric Services and the
Comprehensive Community Mental Health Center
Denver General Hospital
Department of Health and Hospitals
Denver, Colorado

JACK F. WILDER, M.D.
Associate Professor
Department of Psychiatry
Albert Einstein College of Medicine
Acting Director and Acting Chairman, Department of Psychiatry
Bronx Municipal Hospital Center
Bronx, New York

TO

GLORIA

of course!

PREFACE

I T WOULD BE PRESUMPTUOUS to classify administration in mental health as either a field of knowledge or a professional discipline at this stage of development. The benchmarks ordinarily associated with such a classification (an organized body of research, recognized professional credentials, academic visibility, etc.), do not yet exist. At the same time, expenditures for mental health services now exceed $5 billion annually and are growing. Clearly, the need to accelerate our understanding of the practice and processes of administration in the mental health services setting is urgent.

This volume represents one such effort. Its content reflects my judgment about the critical issues and priorities at this time. Hard decisions were necessary to select out from so vast and yet so amorphous a subject matter the topical areas to be included. Some may be considered unconventional in contrast to what has been traditionally viewed as the substance of administration. Obviously, other choices were possible and perhaps preferable.

All of the contributions were written particularly for this book. The authors were selected both for their expertise in the generic aspects of administration and in their application to the field of mental health. In fact, a major objective of the book is the adaptation of general administration to the mental health scene.

It is my hope that this volume will help stimulate other publications in this important area. For the volume and quality of the literature in a particular field is often indicative of its ethos.

Saul Feldman

INTRODUCTION

D URING THE PAST DECADE, mental health services have changed dramatically and the administration of these services has grown far more difficult. Mental health programs are spending more money, employing more people, serving more clients in more varied ways and providing services of greater scope than ever before. In marked contrast to its predecessors, the prototype mental health organization of the 1970's is a complex, frequently decentralized service system with various levels of accountability and close ties with other human services.

While this increased complexity is likely to characterize the delivery of mental health services for a long time to come, it has not been accompanied by the necessary administrative expertise. As a result, the potential of greater resources and advanced clinical knowledge is hampered by administration that was barely adequate even in the *horse and buggy* days of mental health. At the same time, the need to increase the effectiveness of administration in mental health is widely acknowledged; in fact, it may be one of the few issues in the mental health field on which everyone can agree. But very little progress has been made. The ability gap is growing wider as mental health services continue to expand in size and complexity.

Unfortunately, an adequate solution to the problem is difficult for several reasons. First, mental health services are generally administered by mental health professionals with little knowledge or experience in administration. They are often promoted to executive positions by virtue of their seniority or clinical ability and are attracted to administration by the salary, status and the power *to get things done.* On the other hand, when trained administrators are employed, they may have little knowledge of or identification with the field of mental health. With both a mental health professional and business manager working together, each may be expert in his own area but there is often no common frame of reference to permit a unified approach.

Second, there is little useful literature on administration in mental health. Up-to-date, relevant information is very hard to find. The writing is so sparse that any new training programs developed would have almost no pertinent teaching material available. While the literature in other fields does have some relevance for mental health, it is not directly transferrable to the mental health setting. The necessary adaptation has not taken place and as a result, administration in mental health has benefited only slightly from the work in other related areas.

Without a literature, improvements in mental health administration come very slowly, if at all. Progress in any field is dependent upon the stimuli ordinarily provided by published research, descriptive articles and case studies.

A third reason for the slow development of good administration in mental health is the shape and substance of the field itself. Administration in general and mental health administration in particular have not been well defined or conceptualized due to the broad and varied nature of the subject matter. While the substance of administration has a strong generic base, it is modified by the characteristics of the field in which it is applied. The generic administrative processes (planning, budgeting, decision making, etc.) are shaped by the environments in which they take place. As a result, administration in mental health is different from administration in other fields while sharing a common base. The nature and effects of these differences are little understood and require careful research.

The problem is compounded by the many conflicting definitions and usages of the term administration. It is defined on the one hand as a mechanistic process divorced from program and policy and on the other, as organizational leadership inseparable from policy and central to program effectiveness. As used in this volume, administration is a leadership process, interwoven with the achievement of program goals and central to organizational effectiveness. In effect, administration *is* program and program *is* administration.

Fourth, administration is shaped by the needs and values of the parties to the process as well as by the particular field in which it is applied. It is normative and defies neat, precise measures, despite the advances in quantitative analysis and new technology. While its mercurial qualities together with the universal yearning for order and certainty have stimulated a dependence upon so called administrative *principles,* administration is actually situational and there are few, if any principles in the sense of immutable truths. One *principle* conflicts with another and they are better used to justify actions already taken than to help with decisions still to be made. In fact, uncertainty is omnipresent in the administrative task and the capacity to tolerate ambiguity is essential to success in administration.

A fifth obstacle to improving the administrative state of the art in mental health is the paucity of training programs. Due at least in part to the difficulties in defining the field and the lack of a literature, few training programs in administration have developed. Indeed, the essential question—*training for what?*—still remains unanswered.

What mental health administrators should know (or at least be taught) must be a function of what they do. The content of training programs in mental health administration must be determined by the nature of the administrative task. Knowledge of the way mental health administrators spend their time, the major decisions they make, the structures within which they work and the primary people with whom they interact is not yet available, at least in any comprehensive sense. Given the tendency of teaching programs to become entrenched once established, new training programs must be related to the *real world* of mental health services in which the administrator functions. It is a world very different from its counterpart earlier in the century.

In this *real world,* contemporary mental health services seem to be moving (some less rapidly than others) in the following directions:

1) Increased scope and resources;
2) Larger and more diverse staffs;
3) Complex organizational patterns;
4) Multiple funding sources;

5) Multi-unit systems coordinated with other services;
6) Sophisticated management information and evaluation;
7) Close involvement with government at all levels;
8) Greater community involvement; and
9) Increased sensitivity to change.

While several of these characteristics have been most prominent in the federally funded community mental health center, they are beginning to prevail in other mental health services and may well dominate the entire human services field in the near future.

Increased Scope and Resources

The scope of mental health services has broadened considerably, both in the range of services provided and in the people served. Community mental health centers, mental hospitals and outpatient clinics are increasingly offering a wide spectrum of services far beyond their traditional borders. As a result, they are serving greater numbers and a more varied clientele than ever before.

Increased resources have become available to actualize these programs of greater scope and size. The average community mental health center, for example, has an annual budget of nearly $1 million, substantially more than the traditional outpatient clinic. While large budgets are not unusual for mental health facilities (as the budgets of many state mental hospitals attest), the expenditures of community programs are related more heavily to services than to the maintenance of large physical plants.

With this increase in available resources and a wider range of programs on which they can be expended, planning and budgeting in mental health become much more important. In his chapter on planning, Ralph Littlestone defines the task as: "The fundamental planning objective is meeting client needs." He describes planning as dealing with the future; decisions made today will determine the shape of things to come. As Littlestone puts it, "Planning is reasoning about how an organization gets where it wants to go."

Planning and budgeting are closely related, particularly in the program budget model advocated by Feldman. Properly used, the budget process can be a key instrument in the attainment of program goals. The program budget can "result in a more adequate utilization of resources" and. . ."can stimulate mental health executives to problem solve in a more meaningful and productive fashion."

Larger and More Diverse Staffs

In accord with larger budgets and more expensive programs, staff size has grown apace. For example, the average community mental health center employs 108 people and staffs of over 150 are not unusual. Further, these staffs are far more ecumenical than in the past. Working along with the traditional mental health professionals are people from a wide variety of occupations and professional disciplines. According to H. G. Whittington, the success of the mental health executive ultimately depends on the performance of this staff.

But the mental health executive has an unusually difficult job in managing staff. In mental health, as in all human services, staff members are accustomed to autonomy and defy imposed stereo-typed requirements. Too often, they regard the organization—and the executive—as the enemy. Each staff member has the power to facilitate or frustrate the policies of the agency. Dr. Whittington makes it clear that the mental health executive, though he considers himself an expert in human behavior, has his job cut out for him.

Dr. Whittington outlines some of the qualities necessary for successful personnel management. The mental health executive should have won his spurs as a competent practitioner. He should be able to convince his staff of his own involvement, concern and availability. He should be a good communicator and should be able to clearly define the organization's superordinate goals for the staff. He should encourage diversity and innovation, maintain a system of rewards and (if needed) penalties, and he should keep his staff informed. Finally, he should always attempt to move decision-making as far down the hierarchical ladder as can be managed. While on the one hand the leader must make decisions and demonstrate to the staff that he is capable of doing so, the authoritarian model does not work with mental health professionals. They will accept consultation and collaboration, but supervision in the routine sense simply does not work.

Complex Organizational Patterns

Increased organizational size if not properly managed can be dysfunctional to services intended to be accessible and responsive to community needs. Mental health programs are increasingly modifying their organizational structures to help cope with the problems often associated with size. Decentralization is one method they are turning to increasingly. This decentralization takes several forms but two seem most common; the development of satellites or *storefronts* in the community and the deployment of staff into teams assigned to a specific territory but operating from a central base.

David Mechanic addresses himself to the organizational problems associated with an expanding program that can threaten its effective operation. Basically, he views an organization as a social grouping developed around the pursuit of specific goals. While it is more independent and less tied to specific people than a family or tribe, for example, people are what it is all about. Despite Max Weber's theoretical constructs about the nature of bureaucracy, an organization depends largely on the strengths and weaknesses of the people in it, and how well they are managed.

Along with Whittington, Mechanic feels that this is particularly true of human service agencies, employing professionals with their own standards and convictions about how their skills should be used and determined to make their own decisions. The wise mental health executive will not attempt to control them, for this attempt is bound to fail, but rather will seek to win their loyalty and commitment to the organization and its goals. Decentralization can make this more difficult. Staff members working out in the community, away from the central organization may begin to identify less with its goals and more with those of the milieu in which they are closely involved.

According to Mechanic, the ambiguous nature of mental health services and the strong professional orientation of the staff require that organizational rules be handled with extreme care.

Unless the rules are very broad and flexible, sooner or later a staff member is bound to break them. It would be fatal for the executive to insist on literal adherence to rules. The enthusiasm of the staff is vital to the maintenance of a positive organizational atmosphere because, as Mechanic puts it, the communication of hope to the patient is essential.

Under the circumstances, the wise executive will have a minimum framework of broad rules and will exercise flexibility in enforcing them. In addition, in order to ensure a continuing sense of mission, he will seek to maintain that attitude by giving his staff a feeling of participation in the organization's major decisions.

Multiple Funding Sources

The contemporary mental health service agency is dependent upon a wide variety of funding sources for its survival. In contrast to earlier patterns, funding has become highly pluralistic. Many community mental health centers for example, obtain funds from ten or more different sources, with different fiscal years, reporting requirements and special needs.

In the chapter on financing, Ernest Harvey describes this growing multiplicity of funding sources for mental health services and its impact on administration. He points out that increased Federal participation has been the most significant change in recent years, a result of the community mental health centers legislation in the 1960's. However, Federal funds are *seed money,* that decline on a gradual basis. This requires community mental health centers to develop alternate sources of support to ensure their survival. Fund raising and grantsmanship thus become important aspects of the administrative task, together with the management capability necessary to account for a wide variety of funds.

According to Harvey, the prospects for community mental health centers to survive without substantial federal support are far from bright. A study of sixteen early centers reveals some of the difficulties they face in their quest for alternate sources of funds. State funding, traditionally the most substantial contributor to mental health services, appears to have reached a plateau. Local government funding has been growing perceptibly in some states as the result of enabling legislation, but suffers from too narrow a tax base. Private philanthropy has made substantial contributions in the past but cannot be expected to fill the gap. Fees, insurance payments, Medicare and Medicaid have had only a minor impact. However, the advent of revenue sharing and some form of national health insurance (if it includes coverage for mental health) can help substantially.

Multi-Unit Systems Coordinated with Other Services

Perhaps the most striking feature of the new look in mental health services is the development of existing programs into co-ordinated systems of care. At least in some parts of the country, the major problem has not been so much the paucity of mental health services as the insulation of those already in existence. Mental health agencies are now working together and integrating their services more closely than ever before. While eminently desirable however, the barriers against this coordination are formidable.

These developing mental health systems are also working more in concert with other programs as well, in the recognition that mental health must be a partner in a coordinated system of human services. Gregory O'Brien describes the new importance of these interorganizational relationships and the qualities that program directors and key staff must possess to bring them about.

Since virtually no caregiving organization today is fully autonomous and self-sufficient, its relations with other programs are crucial. To that end, the mental health executive must develop a climate of trust and mutual benefit with other organizations. To help with this, he must be aware of all the criss-crossing interorganizational linkages maintained by staff members in his organization.

O'Brien feels that the interorganizational environment and the nature of the focal agency's interactions with it may influence its own internal program goals. Schematically, he describes the focal organization as an *open system* with *system boundaries*. And interaction consists of resources (patients, information, clinical skills, etc.) taken across these boundaries, modified and then returned. The *organizational set* is made up of the individuals and organizations in the environment with whom the focal agency is most concerned. And the relationships of interdependence and independence between organizations are fluid and ever shifting.

With its growing financial contribution to all human service agencies, government has assumed a sharply increased role in determining the nature of interorganizational exchanges. With increasing frequency, agencies are no longer free to choose whether they will or will not have relations with other entities. The federal government mandates such relationships as a requirement for funding in order to ensure a comprehensive and full range of services.

O'Brien distinguishes four general models of interorganizational relationships. They are (1) voluntary exchanges of resources and information at random; (2) voluntary exchanges with efforts to standardize mechanisms of exchange; (3) forced (mandated) exchanges where the participation is required but there are no means for the resolution of conflict; and (4) hierarchical coordination, the most formal and rigid type where both the relationship and the mechanisms for conflict resolution are mandated.

Since almost all organizations relate to each other on a variety of levels, most of them experience all four types of interorganizational relationships. O'Brien suggests that the type 2 and 3 models offer the greatest opportunity for the mental health executive to build relationships of mutual benefit.

Sophisticated Management Information and Evaluation

Another feature of the modern mental health organization is its increasing use of computers and sophisticated technology to obtain a wide range of information about its operation. Wilder and Miller discuss this growing need for effective, purposeful management information. They feel that mental health organizations too frequently accumulate vast amounts of data but still do not have enough management information; most of the data are not relevant to the objectives of the organization.

To develop a management information system, the agency executive and the senior staff must survey their program purposes, their goals and priorities, and their allocation of resources. They must then determine just what information is required to help them in the planning process, not only for the whole organization but for each of its major functions. The information requirements should be formalized and incorporated into the job descriptions of the responsible staff members.

In building a management information system, it is just as important to determine what data are not needed as it is to identify the important information. The basic questions that should be asked include: What are the objectives of the organization? Does it have the human and physical resources to do the job? Will the methods employed produce the desired results? Is the time right to introduce and carry out the program? After a reasonable time, will it be possible to determine if anything was achieved? The information pertinent to these questions must be simple, accurate and timely.

From the beginning, the administrator must determine who is to participate in the information system, and who is to collect the data. More often than not, the research unit is not the place for data gathering. Since the research staff does not have the responsibility for carrying out the program, they find it difficult to resist the temptation of collecting more and more data that may be of value *some day*. The responsibility for collecting management information should lie with those who implement the program, and the system should be flexible, economic and confidential. Again, it is the responsibility of the agency executive to see that the system is properly designed and implemented, that the staff understands its importance and that the cooperation of all appropriate staff members is won.

Management information is also essential for program evaluation, an activity that Paul Binner feels has been given far too little attention by mental health programs. Binner points out that in community mental health centers, only 2 percent of staff time is spent on evaluation. This is true despite the benefits of evaluation that Binner feels are substantial.

Among these benefits is the greater familiarity with the agency gained by the executive in the process of designing the evaluation framework. Evaluation may also help gain outside support for the program, it may help diagnose organizational problems and uncover useful procedures. It may also help change inappropriate programs and goals before valuable resources are wasted.

At the same time, the executive should be under no illusion that evaluation is neutral and objective. According to Binner, it is an adversary proceeding, and those responsible for evaluation have their own agendas and biases. However, this too is helpful because it elicits a variety of staff expressions and points of view that can be of value in the decision process.

The first and fundamental step in evaluation is the establishment of a contract, i.e., an understanding of what is to be accomplished with the resources provided. The contract is concluded between the organization and the parties to whom it is accountable. It should include agreement on the people to be served, the amounts and kinds of service to be provided, the objectives of the program and the criteria by which the organization will be judged.

Binner acknowledges that some evaluation procedures are too complex for the tools at hand, that the resources are few and that there are no universally accepted guidelines. Despite these shortcomings, he believes that good evaluation can and must be done and that it is central to successful management.

Littlestone also emphasizes the importance of information and evaluation but within the framework of planning. He sees the basic planning model as defining the problem, collecting the pertinent data and choosing the best solution. Evaluation has improved the effectiveness of planning by making results verifiable —it provides a yardstick by which to measure them.

Close Involvement with Government at All Levels

The real world of mental health services in which the administrator now functions is also featured by a close and intensive involvement with government at all levels. Today, mental health along with other human services has become politicized to a greater degree than ever before. As human problems impact with ever greater insistence on the public mind, and as the public expenditures and public visibility of human services have expanded, they have moved into the center of the political stage.

Morgan and Connery describe the evolution of mental health programs from a preoccupation with state government only to a concern with other levels as well. No longer does the fate of the mental health budget depend solely upon the funds appropriated by state legislatures. Federal financing, on the one hand, and support by local government, be it the county board of supervisors or the city council, on the other hand, have assumed a position of growing importance. Thus, the involvement of mental health agencies has expanded to all levels of government, as well as to the interaction between them.

Morgan and Connery provide a view of this governmental system upon which mental health programs have become so dependent. With emphasis upon the decision making processes, they review the operations of government at all three levels. In order to compete for funds with other programs, the mental health executive must understand how the system works and where his participation can have the greatest impact. But this is no simple task. The pluralistic nature of the governmental system, the overlapping, fragmented political jurisdictions at the local level and the inexorable tendency toward legislative inertia all make positive action extremely difficult.

Greater Community Involvement

The advent of *consumerism* is profoundly affecting mental health services. Terms such as *citizen participation, community control* and *relevance* have become a regular part of the mental health scene. The objective is the delivery of mental health services responsive to the needs of the people served.

The term *community* however, is sufficiently broad and vague to hold out the promise of something for everyone. At the *conservative* end of the scale it means mental health care in the community for people who would otherwise go to the state hospital.

At the other end, it means community control of the delivery system and there seems to be a wide range of definitions in between. Whatever the definition, some form of community involvement in mental health services has become widely accepted, at least in theory. However, seemingly, *simple* questions have not yet been answered. These include: What is a community? Who are its legitimate representatives and how can you tell? Under what conditions and in what ways do you involve the community in the decision making process? What kind of involvement works best and where?

Seymour Kaplan feels that there are many more questions than answers about community participation, including the definition of *community* and *participation*. However, it is his conviction that a greater involvement of consumers and the public at large in the delivery of human services is bound to result in better services. Kaplan points out that if a community is to be defined as a Gemeinschaft, i.e., a body of people with social cohesion and a common psychological identification, it is rarely to be found in contemporary America. For practical purposes, this organic entity has been replaced by substitutes such as geographic catchment or service areas and target populations. In this setting, community participation may take the form of participation as a consumer, as a volunteer, as an indigenous non-professional, as a board member, or as an organizational member.

Kaplan traces the genesis of the community participation concept to the "Health New Deal" of the 1960's, i.e., the Community Mental Health Centers Act in 1963, the Equal Opportunity Act in 1964 and the Medicare and Medicaid legislation in 1965. He feels that the demand for community participation may be primarily to improve services or it may be to gain political power. In either case, the civil rights movement and the militancy of the 1960's have had a profound influence on human service agencies. While there have been upheavals and problems, there have also been major attitudinal changes that have made services far more responsive.

In the use of community participation for political ends, the services are secondary. The real objective of the community group is to gain political power with control of the organization as merely a tool. Thus far, mental health organizations have not become the focus of such a contest. But Kaplan cites the situation in the New York City school system in the 1960's as one example of this political conflict.

Increased Sensitivity to Change

The capacity of a mental health program to change with the society around it may be the most critical determinant of its growth and viability. In the chapter on Innovation and Change, Howard Davis considers some of the ways in which the administrator can manage change and turn it to the advantage of his organization. While it may be impossible to predict specific changes, organizational change is not a random set of developments continually facing the executive with totally new demands. Change can be managed effectively and indeed, the key to successful management is whether the administrator manages change or change manages him.

The management of change is not an esoteric, haphazard process where results depend solely upon chance. There is evidence that the employment of planned change is effective. But there are no quick tricks; the field of change is evolving into a technology with its own techniques and processes. Among the techniques discussed by Dr. Davis are manipulation, power equalization approaches such as participative management, sensitivity training, organizational development and the experimental social innovation model. He presents a guideline for the management of change that is primarily a *people* approach, recognizing organizations not only as charts and policy manuals but as groups of individuals.

In the final analysis, change may be what mental health services are really all about; for constructive change through greater understanding is the essence of the profession. Alfred North Whitehead once said, "The art of progress is to preserve order amid change and change amid order." This above all is the challenge for the mental health executive in the 1970's.

SAUL FELDMAN

ACKNOWLEDGMENTS

I AM INDEBTED to the contributors in this volume, all of whom so clearly recognized the need for such a work and so willingly committed themselves to it despite their other considerable burdens. I particularly appreciate their tolerance for so finicky an editor.

Isabel Davidoff has been a great help with her editorial suggestions and general assistance.

I am grateful to Judy Kligman for overcoming so well the obstacles inherent in typing a multi-authored, many referenced manuscript.

CONTENTS

THE ADMINISTRATION OF
MENTAL HEALTH SERVICES

CHAPTER 1

PLANNING IN MENTAL HEALTH

RALPH LITTLESTONE

PLANNING IS CONCERNED with the future and with the impact of the present on the future. Since the primary responsibility of an administrator is the continuing viability of his organization, he must of necessity include planning as one of his most important functions.

The decision an administrator makes today determines the organization's substance tomorrow. Some decisions irrevocably affect the future for many years. The decision to construct a hospital is one example. The hospital may take five years to finance, plan, build, and occupy. Its useful life will extend at least another twenty years. It is a major investment not easily abandoned. By its nature, it will influence the essentials of the organization's program.

A decision to close a facility will likewise have major long-term consequences. The economic and political impact caused by terminating the payroll for a substantial population invokes powerful forces when such change is attempted.

While less dramatic, other administrative decisions also have significant long-term consequences. The kinds and numbers of staff selected to operate a program will have a fundamental impact on the nature of that program. The relation of a facility to its clientele and the role of citizens and professional organizations in program planning, evaluation and administration are also of far reaching import. A decision to operate in a certain way with respect to these procedures will have enduring consequences. A decision to change the relationship may either strengthen or disrupt

3

an organization for a long time. Procedures and expectations, once established, are not easily changed. Decisions made today that affect an organization's existence tomorrow is the substance of planning. The ability of an administrator to make sound decisions will depend upon his knowing what decisions are possible, the consequences of each, their impact on his organization, and which decisions, taking everything into account, are likely to move the organization most quickly and effectively in the direction it wishes to go to meet its objectives.

Traditionally, planning is described as a process of identifying alternatives, specifying the advantages and disadvantages of each, and then, based on this information, a decision is made. For each alternative there is a variety of legal, political and economic considerations to be assessed. These may include the quality and quantity of the service or product produced by the organization, the impact on those who produce it and the impact on consumers. Even in classical profit making organizations, the latter factor has assumed a scope not considered in early planning models. At least in theory, it has now gone far beyond concern with the direct consumer of the product and includes ecological or environmental considerations as well. The recognition that there is a host of forces that must be taken into account in an organization's planning in addition to those objective factors ordinarily included in the traditional planning model has led to a proliferation of planning models—some new and others with new names for old processes.

The major distinction between the newer and more traditional schools of planning can be considered as the difference between planning as a unilateral intellectual activity relatively isolated from its environment and planning carried out with or by those affected. Whether planning as an isolated activity has ever been successful is dubious. For planning to be effective, it must include data on all of the key factors that will determine the organization's future viability. When such factors as employee and client attitudes and the organization's impact on its environment are ignored in the planning process, then the result may be nothing more than an intellectual exercise. The difficulty, of course, is assigning values in the planning process to the organization's impact on employees, consumers and third parties affected by its activities.

Since there is no way to assign an exact value to this impact, the give and take participatory process serves as a substitute. Elaborate theories have been advanced calling for the involvement in its planning of those affected by the organization. This results in an investment in the outcome by those participating, a shared investment toward a common goal. This is the process of cooptation, a process which is not one sided. Management is coopted as well as the other participants since it makes, directly or implicitly, a commitment to abide by the consequences of the sharing process.

The Nature of Planning*

One of the most comprehensive books on corporate planning is George A. Steiner's (1969) *Top Management Planning.* In discussing the generic nature of planning, Steiner observes that all planning is concerned with the future, the futurity of present decisions. Planning examines future alternative courses of action open to an organization. In choosing from among these, a frame of reference is established for *current* decisions. Also, planning examines evolving chains of cause and effect likely to result from current decisions. Planning is reasoning about how an organization will get where it wants to go. The basic task of comprehensive planning is to visualize the organization as the managers wish it to be in the future. Planning inherently involves assessing the future and making provision for it. The essence of planning is to see opportunities and threats in the future and respectively exploit or combat them as appropriate.

Planning is a process that begins with setting objectives; then defining strategies, policies and detailed plans to achieve them; establishing an organization to implement decisions, and reviewing performance and feedback to introduce a new planning cycle. Planning may be defined as deciding in advance what is to be

---

*The discussion in the section on The Nature of Planning is largely an adaptation from Steiner (1969).

done, when it is to be done, how it is to be done and who is to do it. It is continuous because changes in the environment are continuous.

Planning is a philosophy, an attitude, a way of life. It necessitates dedication to acting on the basis of a contemplation of the future and a determination to plan constantly and systematically as an integral part of management. The first step toward adequate planning is the establishment of a planning climate (Besse in Steiner, 1969).

Plans can be divided into three structural blocks—strategic plans, medium range programs and short range detailed plans and budgets. All are interrelated. A cardinal purpose is to discover future opportunities and make plans to exploit them. Correspondingly, basic long range planning is the detection of obstructions that must be removed from the road ahead. Strategic planning is the process of determining major objectives of the organization and the policies and strategies that will govern the acquisition, use and disposition of resources to achieve those objectives.

There is a difference between planning and plans. Planning is a process. Plans are a commitment to specific courses of action growing out of the process. Inherent in the planning process is the rigorous obligation to come to a specific action to be taken *today*. Planning without plans is a waste of time. But the planning process itself is the cardinal emphasis and plans are ancillary to it (Breech in Steiner, 1969). Although planning should lead to action, a large part of planning does not result in *written* plans.

Steiner makes the interesting point that two restraints on comprehensive planning were removed after World War II that helped make such planning possible. The first was the idea that business no longer stood helpless in the face of market forces. A company could, according to Ernest Breech, *"make* trends, not . . . follow them. With a well-staffed management team in which an aggressive risk-taking spirit is backed up by cool-headed analytical planning, there will be no problem too tough to be solved" (Breech in Steiner, 1969). This is the philosophy that business can, to a great degree, determine where it wants to go in the future and do things to assure that it gets there.

The second restraint was the economic booms and busts that have been replaced in the last twenty-five years with remarkable economic stability. A major historical barrier to long range business planning was thereby removed.

Along with this change in economic conditions and attitudes toward influencing the future, Steiner cites the effect of rapid technological change which is accompanied by overnight obsolescence and the birth of new industries. As a result, the impact of decisions is so rapid, so far reaching, and so costly, that pressure on management to be right is very great. Other factors such as the mounting complexity of business management, growing competition, population changes, increasingly complex government regulations and labor union activities all act together to compel greater attention to planning.

Planning is not making future decisions—planning is concerned with making current decisions in the light of their futurity. The basic problem of planning is not what should be done in the future, but rather what should be done now to make desired things happen in the uncertain future. Decisions cannot be made only for the present—once made the decisions may have long term irrevocable consequences. Planning is not an attempt to eliminate risk. Alternatives should be selected which will maximize the objective with minimal risk. Planning is not a blueprint for the future. It should be dominated by flexibility to alter current decisions over time so as to take advantage of changes in the organization and its environment.

Time is a key dimension in planning. Weyerhaueser is planning for tree growth 75 years in the future while U.S. Steel has estimated iron ore needs in the year 2000 to make current commitments. Steiner differentiates this type of planning, long range projections which become premises in the planning process, from actual plans for specific periods. Long range projections are made of the economic environment, customer demand or new technology extending ten to twenty years. Long range objectives for ten years are common. It is unusual, though to find detailed plans beyond five years. Lockheed asks each of its divisions to develop annually a ten year plan. Its plans for a supersonic transport covered twenty-five years.

Although the line between planning and forecasting is sometimes hard to draw, planning is not forecasting. The one thing that is certain about forecasts is that they will be wrong. In planning, the effort must be to find the most probable future course of events bearing upon planning and to use that guidance in developing plans. Planners must realize that the future does not lie somewhere along a straight line projection. Forecasting attempts to see probable events in the future, but the entrepreneurial problem is to innovate and find the unique event that will change the probabilities (Drucker in Steiner, 1969).

Two Branches of Planning

Planning today might be conceptualized as the merger of two branches of planning experience and thinking—business or corporate planning on the one hand and community organization planning on the other. These branches developed in settings that produced fundamentally different planning approaches. Corporate planning, with its roots in industry, emphasizes the manufacture and marketing of tangible products. Planning in this setting is viewed as a logical process of setting objectives (production and marketing goals), assessing resources (men, materials, money), considering different ways to combine these resources most effectively and economically to meet the objectives, choosing the best way, proceeding with the plan, assessing the outcome, then making necessary changes or adopting a different alternative if the first choice is not effective.

Planning as a community organization process developed as part of society's response to such human problems as poverty, illness, unemployment and poor housing. The nature and quality of the response is a reflection of the moral values of the time. The techniques used have ranged from appeals to the public conscience and enlisting support from civic and business leaders to organizing those affected by the problems into power groups.

Too frequently, the planning literature treats these two aspects of planning as opposites. In his comprehensive book on corporate planning, Steiner adheres to the traditional planning process. While he does comment on the relationship of corporations to the public, he does not bring into his extensive discussion the concepts of community organization which make up so much of the current body of planning literature. On the other hand, Roland Warren (1971), impatient with this distinction, merges them into what he calls the *concrete-processual* model. In his classic work on community organization, Murray Ross (1967) describes the planning process as including the logical steps of the corporate model but, as his major theme, stresses the involvement in the process of those affected. Through this involvement, consumer groups would gain cohesiveness and strength, their bargaining position would be improved and their demands sharpened.

Recent years have seen the growth of *ecological* issues raised by the public, protests by or on behalf of impoverished residents displaced by slum clearance, proxy fights to influence corporate policy for the *public good,* and active consumer advocacy by Ralph Nader and others. How this will be reflected in the corporate planning texts of the future remains to be seen. Whether these forces will be powerful enough to affect future corporate policy is also undetermined.

Steps in the Planning Process

Approaches to planning are often divided into the two models discussed: *rational planning,* stressing the development of facts and their analysis, and *participatory planning,* emphasizing the planning process. Comments on the distinction between these two approaches were made earlier where it was suggested that these models are derived from two distinct trends which may be merging under the heading of *social policy planning.* As far back as 1955, Ross combined these two models while stressing the importance of process.

Ross, (1967), defined planning as the process of locating and defining a problem or set of problems, exploring its nature and scope, considering various solutions, selecting what appears to be a feasible solution, and taking action with respect to the solution chosen. He then defined *community organization* in such a way that planning became part of the community organization process. He said "there are essentially two aspects to the community organization process: one having to do with planning, and the second with *community integration.* In our view these two essential aspects of community organization . . . are inseparable parts of the one process—in fact, one can state that only when these two aspects are interlocked and merged into one process is community organization . . . present."

"Community organization . . . is . . . a process by which a community identifies its needs or objectives, orders (or ranks) these needs or objectives, develops the confidence and will to work at these needs or objectives, finds the resources (internal and/or external) to deal with these needs or objectives, takes action with respect to them, and in so doing extends and develops cooperative and collaborative attitudes and practices in the community."

Community integration is defined by Ross as ". . . the achievement of such insights and skills by members of the community as will permit a creative use of tension and conflict in the community. . . . Development in the community of the capacity to function as a unit with respect to its needs, problems, and common objectives."

The role of citizens and consumers is the object of much discussion. It is a topic that provokes a wide range of opinions. Peter Rossi (1965) wrote that "Citizen participation is a good way for a professional to operate to get things done, but there is no superior wisdom in the local masses, merely superior strength." Saul Alinsky (Sanders, 1970), too, said "I do not . . . glorify the poor." But, he said, "You have to have power . . . you'll only get it through organization." Organization is done around issues, discontents. Without such organization, planning through participation is ineffective because the participants are unequal in power. Even with organization, minorities will still be minorities. They "need allies from the middle class."

In their work on *Goals and Means for Social Change,* Blum, Miranda, and Meyer (1970), discuss self help organizations. They indicate that these have two major goals—increasing the socio-economic mobility and the status of (1) defined *groups* in society, and (2) individuals. They assert there are three means to do this—(1) concurrence, (2) negotiations, and (3) contest. Pursuit of *group* mobility goals, they say, poses a major threat to the ideology of the larger society because these goals are alien to basic ideology and economic interests. It is likely that successful efforts must involve contest. Contest is designed to bring about *negotiation* which occurs when the power situation cannot be resolved unilaterally or resolution is too costly. Confrontation is designed to lead to negotiation or concurrence, not to achieve the goal directly, otherwise it is dysfunctional. *Individual* mobility is not as threatening. Coalitions of self help groups are necessary to achieve group mobility. They must band together to negotiate and contest.

Roland Warren (Scobie, 1971) analyzing this area of planning strategy, presents three types of planning situations based on the degree of consensus.

1. Value consensus—agreement on objectives, methods and importance of the issue.
2. Value differences—agreement on objectives but not on methods or importance or saliency of the issue.
3. Value dissensus—disagreement on these.

Warren indicates that collaborative methods might work in (1), not in (3), and partially in (2). (2) calls for *campaign* strategy to convince and pressure the adversary without alienating him if possible. (3) calls for *contest* strategies. To employ collaborative or campaign strategies in face of basic value differences would be ineffectual and a waste of resources.

Scobie (1971), points out that not all strategies are available or appropriate for use by all types of organizations. A comprehensive health planning agency, for example, is unlikely to employ a social action model although groups supported by it might. "Regardless of one's goals, it is unlikely that change will occur unless sufficient resources are available to overcome resistance." *This is the measurement of feasibility,* the heart of the analysis of alternatives.

In the rational planning process, the steps are viewed much the same by different authors. The variations are in choice of language and in the fineness with which the steps are broken down. Steiner (1969) presents what he calls the simplest model with three steps: (1) determine and define the problem, (2) collect all pertinent factors available to solve the problem, and (3) decide which actions to take to solve the problem. One of the more interesting versions is the Defense Department's "Commanders' Estimate of the Situation."

Estimate of the Situation

Reference: Map, chart, or document. (As necessary for understanding of the estimate.)

1. MISSION

A statement of the task and its purpose. If the mission is general in nature, determine by analysis what tasks must be performed to insure that the mission is accomplished. State multiple tasks in the sequence in which they are to be accomplished.

2. THE SITUATION AND COURSES OF ACTION

   a. Determine all facts or in the absence of facts logical assumptions which have a bearing on the situation and which contribute to or influence the ultimate choice or a course of action. Analyze available facts and/or assumptions and arrive at deductions from these as to their favorable or adverse influence or effect on the accomplishment of the mission.

   b. Determine and list significant difficulties or difficulty patterns which are anticipated and which could adversely affect the accomplishment of the mission.

   c. Determine and list all feasible courses of action which will accomplish the mission if successful.

3. ANALYSIS OF OPPOSING COURSES OF ACTION

Determine through analysis the probable outcome of each course of action listed in paragraph 2c when opposed by each significant difficulty enumerated in paragraph 2b. This may be done in two steps—

   a. Determine and state those anticipated difficulties or difficulty patterns which have an approximately equal on all courses of action.

   b. Analyze each course of action against each significant difficulty or difficulty pattern (except those stated in paragraph 3a above) to determine strength and weaknesses inherent in each course of action.

4. COMPARISON OF OWN COURSES OF ACTION

Compare courses of action in terms of significant advantages and disadvantages which emerged during analysis (par. 3 above). Decide which course of action promises to be most successful in accomplishing the mission.

5. DECISION
   Translate the course of action selected into a complete statement, showing *who, what, when, where, how,* and *why* as appropriate.

Source: War Department, Staff Officers' Field Manual, FM 101-5, U.S. Department of Defense, Washington, U.S. Government Printing Office (1960 edition), page 142.

Planning and Evaluation

Evaluation is ordinarily presented as the last step in the planning process, if it appears at all. This is true both in the literature and in practice where evaluation is commonly undertaken at the time pressures arise to demonstrate results. According to Orville F. Poland (1971), "An examination of four widely used textbooks in public administration indicated that none includes a chapter on evaluation." He asked, "Why does public administration ignore evaluation?"

Both evaluation and the standard setting process can serve an important function beginning with the first step in the planning cycle. If, from the outset, evaluation is considered concurrently with other planning steps, a rigor is introduced that will aid in testing the feasibility of each step in the planning process. The planning cycle, revised to include evaluation, would appear as follows:

Planning Cycle

Planning Step	*Concurrent Evaluation Action*
1. Identify the problem	1. Quantify in order to measure change
2. Specify goals	2. Quantify and develop criteria
3. Devise alternate solutions	3. Quantify and specify criteria Specify data requirements
4. Select preferred solution	4. Specify Criteria Data requirements Devise data collection system

5. Implement	5. Collect data
6. Evaluate	6. Analyze data and assess against criteria
7. Revise plan	7. See 4
8. Implement	8. Collect data

If a program is to be evaluated, its performance must be quantifiable and measurable. If this cannot be done, serious questions should be raised about its feasibility. If measurable criteria cannot be established at the outset, it is not likely this can be done later when results are demanded to justify continued support.

In order to evaluate a program, the following must be specified.

—The problems or questions the program is addressing,
—The goals of the program,
—The criteria for judging success or failure,
—The data needed for this purpose.

To illustrate the implications of this approach to planning a community mental health center, the following simplified example is given of what might be specified under each of these four headings before beginning other steps in the planning cycle.

1. The Problem

There is high prevalence of mental illness in the neighborhood.
Treatment is delayed until illness is acute.
The mentally ill are being sent to a distant state hospital.
Children with learning and behavior problems are dropping out or being expelled from school.

2. The Goal

a. To make a full range of mental health services easily available to residents of the neighborhood.
b. To reduce admissions to state hospitals from the neighborhood.
c. To reduce admissions to all mental health facilities.
d. To minimize disruption of normal living patterns at home, on the job, and at school.

3. Criteria

a. Admissions to state hospitals from the area. (These should be reduced to a specified level.)

b. Admissions for serious mental illness. (These should be reduced to the state hospitals but increased, in the short run, to local services.)
c. Admissions to all mental health programs. (These should go down in the long run.)
d. Days in school, at work, at home. (These should go up.)
e. Functioning at grade level in school. (This should improve.)

4. Data Needs

Rates by
—Census tract
—School districts
—Catchment area
for

1. Admissions to State Hospitals (by diagnosis, age, sex, ethnic group)
2. Admissions to all mental health services (by diagnosis, age, sex, ethnic group)
3. School attendance, learning and behavior problems in school, below grade rates
4. Time lost from work and homemaking for reasons associated with emotional disturbance

STANDARDS—PROGRAM AND COST

Hand-in-hand with evaluation, standard setting is an essential but neglected step in the planning process. A recent controversy in Washington, D. C., over child care centers illustrates a problem common to planning and administration of human service programs in all fields. A contract was negotiated with a private firm to operate a child care program for delinquent and dependent children. The program is being carried out in several group homes which offer room, board and supervision by counsellors. The counsellors have complained that the firm is using contract money to increase its profit while food, clothing, recreation and housing allowances for the children are inadequate and the counsellors are underpaid. The corporation claims it is losing money (Washington Post, 1972).

This event was predictable. It has happened before. It is inevitable in the absence of standards and the cost estimates that standards make possible. Other human services have the same problem. For example, the rates charged by nursing homes vary extensively. The relation between the rate charged and the services given is an unknown. Within the same nursing home, a private patient may pay more than a patient supported by Medicaid or Medicare. Reimbursement rates under these public programs are set by public agencies, largely on a subjective basis. Nursing home operators have claimed they are allowed too little to offer a first rate program and stay in business. They may be right but no one really knows.

Local mental health programs supported by state matching funds vary substantially in cost per unit of population served. These variations are not reflected in objective measures of benefits or results such as their impact on admissions to state mental hospitals. A county receiving the most state money per capita may have one of the highest state hospital admission rates. The same may be true in the community mental health program. The median amount of Federal support of individual community mental health centers in 1971 was $647,000. The range, though, from one to the other, was tenfold. There is no known relationship between these amounts and the benefits to those served. What is lacking are standards on which to make useful judgments. What is a quality program? What are the elements essential to such a program? What should such a program cost? What manpower is needed? What facilities and equipment are required? What does it take to make a decent program go?

There are enough mental health and other human service programs in existence so that it should be possible to describe their operations, compare them with standards for desirable programs, and support a number of demonstrations to find out how *decent* programs would operate and what they would cost. Such findings would then become the basis for program, manpower, facility and fiscal plans and projections. They would be the basis for grants and for contracts, for negotiations and re-negotiations if the amounts should prove too low or too high.

Twenty years ago, Bradley Buell (1952), wrote "There are as yet no standard criteria for measuring rehabilitation results. In all these areas, methods must be developed and tested objectively, but in none of them do we anticipate insuperable difficulties."

Yet the state of the art of output evaluation of human service programs is still so embryonic that input and process measures must, for the most part, be the criteria of choice today. If the output measures were effective, then it should make no difference to a funding agency what processes are used so long as the product is competitive. At this time it is both desirable and possible to set standards for child care homes, e.g., that would specify the amount and quality of food, clothing and housing and the amount and kind of activity programs and counselling such homes should offer. These are input and process measures. Their costs can be determined and the resources required now and in the future can be estimated.

Standards, for this purpose, are defined as those elements considered essential to successful program operations. The elements consist of physical items, such as supplies and space, and *activities.* Most attention has been paid in the past to physical conditions, largely safety features, especially related to fire danger and sanitation. The question of what takes place during the waking hours of the inmates of facilities has not been the focus of concern of licensing, accrediting and other standard setting bodies. In 1952, Buell wrote of the "evils of low grade commercial nursing homes." "The 1950 amendments to the Social Security Act" he said, "stipulated that a state authority must be responsible for establishing and meeting standards in all public and private institutes housing recipients of such (assistance) payments." He predicted optimistically that "an improvement . . . may, therefore, be expected." Recent exposures of nursing home conditions by Ralph Nader's investigators and the attention brought to them by President Nixon show that twenty years later the problem is still present.

There are compelling reasons beyond those discussed above for attention to program standards by mental health and other human service organizations. The mentally ill, the retarded, the physically handicapped, delinquent and dependent children, law offenders, and very large numbers of aged are literally at the mercy of society. They are too often isolated, out of public view and dependent on standards and their enforcement by public agencies for their lives and their future in the most profound sense. Standards are far from academic.

Context for Mental Health Planning

Mental health programs are administered at levels ranging from national to neighborhood. The kinds of programs and the nature of decisions, the factors that affect decisions and the participants in decision-making are necessarily influenced by the program's location and its scope.

The one factor that all mental health planning has in common is the program's ultimate target. The reason mental health programs and facilities exist at all, at any level, is because there are people who need help. It is easy to lose sight of this in program planning, and in other aspects of administration. Administrators and planners, particularly at higher levels, are not ordinarily in direct and daily contact with those whom the program serves.

In planning, the essential question always is, What effect will this decision have on the people to be served—patients, families, those at high risk? If the action considered does not provide this clientele more service or better service, then the essential test of relevance is not met. This is true for training and other indirect services as well. The criterion as to whether the service is worthwhile must be tested against the standard of improvements in the mental health of the recipient. If a decision is made to carry out a certain activity and if it is claimed that this will improve service for those in need of help, then it should be possible to test the results. Do the people who need the help get it and does it make a difference? Program plans should be so designed that these questions can be asked and answered.

In this connection, there is a problem in mental health and all human services. There is a limited number of facts on which sound program plans can be based. There are few evaluation findings in mental health that provide a basis for extending past programs and practices into the future. One is faced, therefore, with the alternatives of doing nothing, doing more of the same, or trying new approaches and hoping they will be successful.

A Framework for Mental Health Program Planning

One common framework for planning mental health programs is based on a medical model. The steps in this model are: (1) Case finding; (2) Treatment; and (3) Aftercare. This formulation, particularly associated with the mental health field, has several defects. *Aftercare* is essentially equivalent to post-state hospital care. This places the hospital at the center of the mental health universe. The model tends to ignore the importance of essential non-medical services and it omits *prevention* as an ingredient in the range of mental health services.

Correcting for these defects, a revised framework includes: (1) Prevention; (2) Case finding; (3) Treatment and Non-Medical service. In this model, *Aftercare* is omitted both because of the distortion its use introduces and because differentiating between treatment and aftercare is not useful.

The two major changes in the model are the addition of *Prevention* as the first step and the recognition that services in addition to treatment are required by the mental health clientele and they should be provided concurrently. Presenting the steps as sequential is, in itself, a faulty concept. All, in fact, go on at the same time.

This model, even though it introduces prevention, still emphasizes pathology. Buell (1952), from the social welfare field, made an instructive comment about a similar focus in his own work.

> Our own use of pathological terminology is deliberate, however, because we believe it is conducive to more precise thinking. Pathological conditions exist, it is possible to get data about them, study their causation, observe and test efforts to correct them and prevent their occurrence. The practical danger of using more optimistic sounding phrases lies not only in the fact that the concepts may be more vague, but also, and more importantly, in the fact that a program which does not accept ultimate responsibility for the prevention or protection against pathology conditions is removed from the compulsion to measure specific results.

Another matrix for planning is the breakdown into service,

training, and research. In response to a variety of forces, this model has been elaborated further by identifying special problem or priority areas such as alcohol, drugs, children, aged, and minorities.

Still another reference point for mental health planning is the *client needs system.* For those with mental health problems, what are their requirements? There are the basics everyone needs such as food, shelter, clothing, love, recreation and good health. And there are the services specifically planned to alleviate stresses associated with mental disability. These two sets are closely related assuming that stress is a function of the extent to which basic human needs are not satisfied. Building in a consumer point of view changes the question from "What does the staff have to offer that the client can be given?" to "What help does the client need, when and where, and what must be done to provide the service?" A simple example is clinic office hours. Many needy patients are excluded by the 9:00 to 5:00 weekday pattern. If the needs of a workingman or school child are examined, evening or weekend hours might be found more suitable.

All of the frameworks discussed so far except the client needs system represent a provider point of view. Mental health programs, though, have as their *raison d'etre,* the meeting of client needs. This is the fundamental program planning objective. To plan to this end, client needs must be understood and a response system devised which will force continuing focus on the client and his needs. The concept of *population* coupled with *accountability* is one such approach.

The Population Base

It is in this sense that the catchment area idea is important. Catchment area, as used in the Community Mental Health Centers Program, is a geographic area with a population of 75,000 to 200,000. The same concept was adopted by the Office of Economic Opportunity for Neighborhood Health Centers (NHCs) but with smaller areas and populations. The Mile Square Neighborhood Health Center in Chicago, for example, serves one square mile with 25,000 residents. Catchment areas should be small enough so that services are physically accessible and the population discrete. Limiting the boundaries and the size of the population makes it easier to assess needs and to measure the impact of the program on individuals and families as well as on the neighborhoods. Where individual problems have their origin in area wide conditions, plans for corrective action can be addressed to the broader base.

Using the population as the basis for planning permits another type of analysis—the assessment of alternative ways to provide services. This can be illustrated with examples from some current efforts at health planning.

Assume that an area bounded by a square includes 100,000 residents who are a cross section of the U.S. population. The object is to provide adequate health services to this population. For this purpose, only two dimensions will be considered, service delivery mechanisms and financing. These are illustrated below.

Delivery	*Financing*
Individual Private Practice	Personal Resources
Group Practice	Prepaid Plans
General Hospitals	Medicare (a prepaid plan)
Neighborhood Health Centers	Medicaid (government support)
	Other Government Support

If these are applied to the hypothetical population of 100,000, a picture such as the following emerges. The blank spaces show uncovered people or gaps in service.

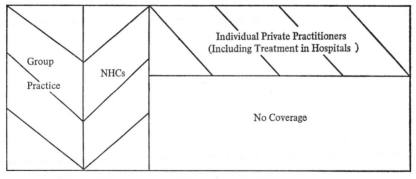

Figure 1-1. Population Covered by Health Service Systems.

To understand the diagram above, financial coverage must be examined at the same time.

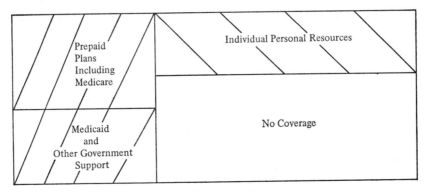

Figure 1-2. Financial Coverage.

The population not covered is the same in both diagrams because lack of coverage in this case is due to inadequate financing. If the object of the plan is to cover 100 percent of the population, then provision must be made for the uncovered portion. In this instance, it is assumed that those without coverage consist primarily of the *in between* people; earning too little to afford private care and too much to be eligible for Medicaid and Neighborhood Health Centers. (Because of their essentially emergency nature and chance location, county hospitals are not included here as part of a planned system for delivering health care to the total population.)

To fill the gap, one alternative is to provide sufficient income to the uncovered population so it can purchase its care directly or by prepayment. Another alternative is to raise the eligibility ceiling so the uncovered population can be served by Neighborhood Health Centers or through Medicaid. There are, of course, other possibilities. Such a method of analysis must be pursued in some form to be sure that the plans will indeed meet the objective of making care available to the entire population.

Another alternative open to health planners is the community mental health center model of a financing and delivery system. In concept, it is designed to serve the total population of its catchment area not otherwise provided for. It has no income eligibility limits such as Neighborhood Health Centers have, it has a sliding fee scale for those who can pay, it collects from third parties, it makes no charge for those who cannot pay. Its delivery program is designed to provide for all of the mental health service needs of its clientele. The existence of such a model, in theory, would fill all gaps.

In fact, service needs of clients are such that they cannot be met by any one system as human services are presently structured. To illustrate this, some findings from a study of multi-problem families are presented below.

Ninety-six families living in a large Eastern city and the agencies working with them were interviewed by the National Study Service in 1970. The families had in common some manifestation of mental illness or emotional distubance. It was not intended to be a representative sample but the findings are compatible with Bradley Buell's studies of multi-problem families twenty-three years ago and others done since. Seventy-one of the ninety-six families had 6 or more major problems; employment, housing, physical health, school difficulties, family relationships, mental health, legal, delinquency, insufficient income, family deficits, addiction, poor housekeeping, and other. Each of these problems is responded to by different major delivery systems that together make up the community social agency structure. The lack of coordination among these systems was documented in a case study of young children in a large West Coast city (Stewart and Baker, 1965). In one instance, the father was in a state prison, the mother in a state hospital and the child in the children's unit of the same state hospital. Placement plans were being made at the same time for all three without any joint planning among the professional staffs. There is no reason to expect that in 1972 things are substantially different.

If these represent the facts about the service needs of the mental health clientele, then this is the starting point for planning. Although the National Study Service sample probably has a higher proportion of low income families than would be found in a cross-section of the general population, at the same time, these are the families that claim the attention of public agencies. Six percent of the families in several communities were found by Buell (1958) to make up more than 50 percent of the social agency caseload. Those of higher income often have other things going for them—jobs, employers, and intact families who worry about them (Littlestone, 1965).

The multiple nature of client problems and the difficulty clients have in obtaining service have, over the years, inevitably pointed to a multi-service structure, the one-stop-shop, as a possible answer. The Research Division of the Social and Rehabilitation Service (SRS) has identified 3000 agencies that offer two or more different services. In 1966, President Johnson initiated a national program to establish fourteen multi-service centers across the country with the combined effort and funds of five Federal agencies. Before that, the Office of Equal Opportunity supported neighborhood service centers on a smaller scale in communities throughout the nation. When Elliott Richardson was appointed Department of Health, Education, and Welfare Secretary, he made integration of human services a major objective of his administration.

Despite extensive experience with multi-service centers, there has been no adequate evaluation of such programs.

Studies undertaken for SRS (O'Donnell, 1971; O'Donnell and Sullivan, 1969) are an important step in this direction. The National Institute of Mental Health is now collaborating with SRS, building on the work already done and carrying it another step, to evaluate the viability of the multi-service center concept and to investigate its application to mental health programming.

Because mental health clients present the range of problems described in the National Study Service study, it is not surprising to find that community mental health centers have many of the characteristics of a multi-service center. A tradition in the mental health field, at least in public and voluntary agencies, has been the combination of psychiatry and psychiatric social work. Providing psychiatric treatment to a family facing the stress of unemployment, overcrowded and substandard housing, delinquency, or expulsion of children from school without helping with these problems would be unrealistic. In planning for community mental health programs, the social case work function has automatically been included. In fact, it may be the most essential function. Many community mental health centers have extended this function to include the process of community organization as well as the case work function. Some problems must be solved, not at the case level but at the community, state or national level. The latest forms that planning has taken, such as advocacy and consumer participation, are found in most community mental health centers while they work on individual problems as well.

Just as *integration of human services* has become a watchword, and for good reason, its opposite, the *categorical* approach has become the pejorative. Integration is good. Fragmentation is bad. Singling out a problem is categorical, it is fragmentation. Problems single themselves out when they affect enough people. When they are not resolved, pressure to concentrate on them is inevitable. This is why such problems as cancer, heart disease, smoking, and mental illness have already been singled out for special financial and organizational attention. This process is just as true for categories within categories. The National Institute of Mental Health is what is known as a mission oriented agency. It was established twenty-five years ago in response to then existing forces. Because pressures have mounted on categorical problems inside the mental health field, there is now a National Institute on Alcohol Abuse and Alcoholism, there will be a new drug institute, there is special funding for poverty area and children's programs in community mental health centers, a bill has been introduced to do the same for aging, and the responsibility for mental retardation was removed from the National Institute of Mental Health.

Forces are at work at all levels, in communities and in the nation, which, at any one time are in uneasy equilibrium. There are the problems and those affected. There are the responses, the resources and those who pay. Despite the attractiveness, the rationality of integrated, noncategorical programs, there is little evidence that the political force needed to fund a concept at an adequate level can effectively match the force that can be mobilized to support the concrete categorical needs as perceived by individuals, families and their political representatives.

SUMMARY AND CONCLUSION

Planning is concerned with the impact of present decisions on the future. It addresses both desirable directions and contingencies. It is likely that if a plan is available when demand arises, and it is at all responsive to the issues, it will be used.

A comprehensive theory of planning will take into account the process of planning, the facts that bear on decisions and the forces that determine decisions. Planning at any level takes place in a matrix that has both horizontal and vertical dimensions. Interdependency is evident in both directions.

A number of planning theories have evolved which differ because they were developed for different settings by individuals with varying backgrounds of experience and training.

Rational planning assumes that it is possible to make decisions based on marshalling the relevant facts that bear on a problem and choosing the best way to advance toward a specified goal. This approach has been most highly refined in the field of business where the setting is conducive to its application. In government, a similar approach has been applied to military planning. In both settings, the emphasis is on logistics. Another field identified with planning theory is city planning; however, the design and adoption of functional and aesthetically planned environments has rarely been applied successfully.

Another body of planning theory has developed under the heading of *community organization.* Community organization theory developed in a setting vastly different from business and the military. It arose in a field where the subject matter was the resolution of human problems rather than the production and distribution of things. The theory was developed by those with backgrounds in the human services, primarily social welfare. Community organization emphasizes the planning *process* and its use to build relationships and strengths in and among groups affected by social policy decisions.

A recent development is *advocacy planning.* It consists of

making the skills and experience of planning technicians available to groups affected by social policy decisions, groups that do not themselves have the sophistication to play the bureaucratic planning game.

Social policy planning is another recent development. It is an attempt to apply planning theory to the formulation and adoption of policies affecting humans at levels ranging from community to national. It combines the concepts of rational planning and community organization.

Systems analysis and the related field of operations research have contributed concepts and techniques which are being applied to planning. The application of systems analysis to the behavioral field is still so imprecise, though, that at this time it must be looked at as another framework to add to the list as an aid to planning.

Two important elements of the planning cycle, *evaluation* and *standards,* have been neglected in the literature and in practice. Their relationship to the other steps in the planning process is discussed and illustrated. While a rational approach to a comprehensive theory of planning is not difficult to conceive, its successful application is. Its breakdown in practice has led to a fall back position, *pluralism,* as an alternate approach to planning. The role of the planner here is to help ensure that those forces necessary to achieve a balance are in operation and have the appropriate weight. The planner also provides technical and factual input for decisions.

All of the terms and concepts presented here are arbitrarily selected. Others are used and defined differently by writers in the planning field. Applying them to mental health requires a further body of selected definitions, concepts and assumptions. Various frameworks to serve as a checklist for mental health planning are presented as well as a point of view about the importance of the client population as the center of the planning universe.

REFERENCES

Buell, Bradley: *Community Planning for Human Services.* New York, Columbia University Press, 1952.

Buell, Bradley: Reorganizing to prevent and control behavior. *Ment Hyg*, *42*, 1958.

Blum, Arthur; Miranda, Magdalena and Meyer, Maurice: Goals and means for social change. In Cox, Fred *et al.* (Eds.): *Strategies of Community Organization*. Itasca, Peacock, 1970.

Littlestone, Ralph: Sensitive Aspects of Planning Emergency Services. Sacramento, California Department of Mental Hygiene, 1965.

Littlestone, Ralph: Mental Health Center Funding and Evaluation. Unpublished manuscript, National Institute of Mental Health, Bethesda, 1970.

National Study Service, Inc.: *The Troubled Family in River City*, Forthcoming.

News Item: Washington Post. Washington, D. C., 1972.

O'Donnell, Edward: Service integration: The public welfare agency and the neighborhood center. *Welfare In Review, 9,* 1971.

O'Donnell, Edward and Sullivan, Marilyn: Service delivery and social action through the neighborhood center: A review of research. *Welfare In Review,* 7:1-12, 1969.

Poland, Orville F.: Why does public administration ignore evaluation? *Public Administration Review,* March/April, 1971.

Ross, Murray G.: *Community Organization*, 2nd ed. New York, Harper and Row, 1967.

Rossi, Peter H.: What makes communities tick? In Katz, Alfred H., and Felton, Jean S.: *Health and the Community*. New York, Free Press, 1965.

Sanders, Marion K.: *The Professional Radical*. New York, Harper and Row, 1970.

Stewart, Elizabeth and Baker, Paul: Coordination of Local Mental Health and Mental Health-Related Services. Sacramento, California Department of Mental Hygiene, 1965.

Scobie, Richard S.: Social Planning in the Community Context—Six Principles for Mental Health Planners. Paper presented to the Mental Health Planning Conference, National Institute of Mental Health, Bethesda, Maryland, September 9 and 10, 1971.

Steiner, George A.: *Top Management Planning*. London, Collier-MacMillan, 1969.

Warren, Roland L.: *Truth, Love, and Social Change*. New York, Rand, McNally, 1971.

CHAPTER 2

BUDGETING AND BEHAVIOR

SAUL FELDMAN

MENTAL HEALTH ADMINISTRATION has failed to keep pace with the growth and progress so characteristic of the mental health field as a whole. Poor management, inadequate organization and the inefficient use of resources too frequently retard the effectiveness of well conceived clinical and community programs. Mental health agencies, larger and more complex than ever before, are still administered by staff with no training and little relevant experience in administration.

Nowhere is this more evident than in the area of budgeting, an activity so important to the success of any organization. Budgeting practices in mental health agencies have a prosaic uniformity that transcends other major differences between them in program, geography, size, auspice and funding. This immutability of the budget process is primarily a function of the widespread use of the object or line item budget. The object budget is viewed primarily as an instrument of expenditure control. It establishes a financial frame of reference that fixes the limits of expenditure and establishes behavioral guidelines. As one mental health executive explains it, "I couldn't imagine doing my job without a budget. It sets expenditure limits and we see how we are operating by comparing what we actually spend with what is budgeted. It enables me to know what is going on financially."

The Object Budget

The object budget first appeared in the early 1900's and has remained relatively unchanged since. Essentially negative in its effect upon operations, it rigidly controls expenditures, limits the discretion of the executive and imposes a stereotyped, mechanical framework upon administrative behavior. The object approach emphasizes control and accountability with the objects of expenditure serving as ends unto themselves. Salaries are paid, supplies are purchased and other expenses are incurred, all unrelated to programs and services. The budget is insulated from organizational objectives and there is a sharp dichotomy between program on the one hand and costs on the other.

The emphasis is on the budget as a determinant as well as an enforcer of administrative accountability. This orientation is a derivative of the early twentieth century when, in an era of reform, the dominant budget philosophy stressed reduced opportunities for administrative misconduct. As Burkhead (1962) has pointed out in his discussion of the object budget:

> It served admirably to establish a tight control over expenditures and limited sharply the discretion of government officials. The object classification was a direct product of an era when both legislators and the citizenry at large were filled with distrust for administrators. It was a great technical step forward in budgeting since it permitted the installation of . . . accounting systems which could be linked with budget accounts and thus limit defalcations.

In the object budget, expenses are grouped according to objects of expenditure and include such categories as personal services, equipment, supplies and materials, and other expenses. These major groupings may be further subdivided into more specific items. For example, the category of *other expenses* may include rent, postage, repairs, insurance and a variety of others. The personal services section may be divided according to the various categories of personnel employed. In larger organizations, the budget items may be classified according to organizational units such as departments or offices.

Budget definitions which reflect this object approach view the budget as an "instrument of administrative control," (Public Administration Service, 1962) and "a bound estimate of expenditures and receipts for a given period" (Dimock, Dimock, and Koenig, 1958).

BUDGETING IN MENTAL HEALTH ORGANIZATIONS

Budget Preparation

In most mental health agencies, the budget process generally begins with a notification from the State, city or other funding source indicating the date by which the budget request for the coming year is due and the forms on which the request must be submitted. Generally, the budget request is due within one to three months from the date of the initial notice, and this is usually about five to seven months before the beginning of the next fiscal year.

The basic information used in preparing the budget request includes the approved budget for the current year, the actual expenditures incurred by the agency to date and an estimate of expenditures for the rest of the year. Using these data, a tentative budget is prepared. The expenses are listed in the required order and estimates are made of these expenses for the following year. Staff salaries, the most significant part of the budget, are calculated by adding a predetermined increment to the salaries for the current year and the other expenses are calculated in much the same fashion. Thus emerges what one mental health administrator has characterized as the *survival budget*. It is the minimum amount of money required to fund the program *as is* during the forthcoming year.

Often the next step will be a review by department heads and administrative staff to evaluate the possibility of additions to this survival budget. Only rarely will other staff members be involved in these discussions. The department heads are asked to identify new programs they would like to begin during the next year and their projected costs. It then remains for the agency director and his staff to decide which of the new programs proposed will be included in the budget request. These new programs are generally referred to as expansion items in contrast to budget increases which come about through routine salary increments. Most frequently, mental health agencies are not provided in advance with any guidelines from the funding bodies as to the availability of such expansion funds.

In the final analysis, the decision on how much to ask for and for what purpose represents an amalgam of several factors—the anticipated availability of funds, staff interests, community needs and *what will go*. Guesses are made as to whether additional funds will be available and if so, the type of program most likely to attract them. If a budget item can meet these twin criteria—if it is *sexy* enough and funding is at least within the realm of feasibility —then it may be included in the budget request. If it does not satisfy at least both these criteria, then it will almost certainly be eliminated.

In essence, it is the perception of what is *reasonable* that is often the single, most important determinant of the budget request. The agency director's behavior is strongly motivated by what he perceives will be the effect of his budget request on his board of directors and the funding sources and in turn their opinion of him. He is concerned that if he appears *unreasonable* and asks for *too much,* he may incur their displeasure. Since they frequently exercise control over his salary, his personnel benefits and even his job, his sensitivity to their feelings is quite understandable. His goal, therefore, seems to be a budget request reflecting a fractional response to need while of a magnitude that is non-threatening, or *reasonable*.

This factor of reasonableness is in turn dependent upon the agency director's perception of the financial reality. He estimates the amount of money likely to be available and then tailors his budget request to it, perhaps adding a *reasonable* bit more. Through this precensorship, he, in effect, seems to abrogate at least a portion of that which would ordinarily be the responsibility of a board of directors or other authorizing body. As a result, boards are frequently presented with a very limited range of budget alternatives from which to choose. Their discretion has already been severely limited by the budget preparation process. As the director of one mental health agency remarked, "Perhaps I act too much like a board member myself. Maybe I should present what is really needed and let them make the cuts."

Emphasis on the Current Budget

In preparing the budget request, the current year's budget is used as the primary frame of reference. Budgeting almost never starts from scratch, where the entire budget would be reformulated each year. This utilization of a safe base upon which to build a new budget is a generally accepted practice. Thus, new budget requests are incremental—the new budget is actually the old budget plus an increment. What is at issue from year to year then, is not the total budget request but rather that portion of it which exceeds the last budget. The concern is not "how much should we ask for" but rather "how much more than this year can we get."

Budget Authorization

After the budget is prepared, it is generally submitted to a board of directors or other governing body for approval. In some mental health agencies, the board is actually involved in the preparation of the budget. In effect, it is a shared responsibility with no real separation of function between the executive and the board. In other organizations, board members have no involvement with the budget at all until it is actually presented to them. In general, the involvement of the board of directors in budget preparation varies from place to place but once the budget is submitted to the board, the approval process is quite uniform.

The budget request is either submitted to a subcommittee of the board or to the entire board itself. Where a subcommittee is used, the agency director meets with the group to present and discuss the budget. Subcommittee members often do not receive copies of the budget in advance but nonetheless, only in rare instances do their deliberations require more than one meeting. Where a subcommittee is not used, the budget request is submitted directly to the entire board, generally at a regularly scheduled meeting. For many of the board members, this meeting represents their first and only contact with the budget.

It is not surprising then that the role played by boards of directors in the budget approval process has no significant impact either on the size or substance of the final budget. Boards spend very little time and seem to be only minimally involved in budget considerations. Whatever involvement does take place frequently relates to budget questions of very minor importance and to budgetary details. There may be a great deal of interest displayed by board members in clerical and secretarial salaries, for example. This type of discussion focuses on whether proposed increments for the clerical staff are excessive and can become quite heated despite the insignificant portion of the budget it actually represents. Other issues of a similar nature occupy the major portion of what little time is spent by boards in the budget process.

Budget Execution

It is the agency director who is ultimately responsible for the proper spending of the budget. He is generally assisted in this task by either a bookkeeper, business manager or perhaps an accounting department. In the total budget process, it is budget execution that commands the greatest time and attention. Staying within the various expenditure limits, properly allocating disbursements over a particular time period and making appropriate expenditure decisions is a continuous activity.

Mental health executives feel that the orderly expenditure of their funds in a systematic way over the fiscal year is an important criterion by which their administrative performance will be judged (Feldman, 1967). Further, should overspending take place, supplemental funds are quite difficult to obtain. Agency directors who request such funds are concerned that they will be viewed as inefficient and the request itself may be seen as an admission of poor administrative functioning.

Discretion in Executing the Budget

In good measure, the degree of discretion available to a mental health agency in making expenditures is very much affected by its dependence upon government funds. Budgetary discretion seems to decrease as fiscal involvement with government increases. A mental health agency funded even in part by government may have little flexibility in spending its budget. Permission for even the slightest change may be required—a shift of as little as $50 may not be possible without a letter in triplicate justifying the change.

Restrictions are at least equally severe on changes in the personal services section of the budget. If the budget prescribes that a staff position be filled by a psychiatric social worker, a psychologist may not be hired without permission even though he may be eminently qualified. In some jurisdictions, the qualifications of every prospective staff member must be approved by the appropriate government agency prior to employment. Salaries, increments and personnel benefits are carefully delineated for each staff member and must be rigidly adhered to.

As a result, the agency director does not truly carry the executive responsibility either for hiring peronnel or for the conditions of their employment. Mental health executives feel these restrictions on their behavior are unreasonable and limit their effectiveness. As one administrator indicated, "The word *director* in my title is really a misnomer. I must ask permission for practically everything I do. I feel frequently as if I am in an administrative strait jacket."

Where mental health organizations do not receive government funds, the restrictions upon their administrative flexibility are far less severe. In these agencies, the extent of the director's discretion in executing the budget is primarily a function of his relationship with the board of directors. Where the relationship is a positive one, he will enjoy a great deal of discretion. While government may still exercise some control through a licensing function, this type of control is far less restrictive. Staff members may be required to meet certain standards, but the conditions of their employment are generally at the discretion of the agency acting within preexisting guidelines. Shifts between expenditure lines may be made without board approval. In general, major expenditures and those connoting some change in policy will be discussed and clarified with the board.

The Parties to the Budget Process

In essence, budgeting in mental health agencies is a routine task with numbers in which the participants have little difficulty assuming their accustomed roles. It is done because it is required and as with all such tasks, the wish is to be finished as rapidly as possible and to proceed with more pleasurable activities. The budget is understood primarily as a means of obtaining the resources required to fund the program and to control expenditures.

It plays no significant role either as a management tool or an instrument of policy. While the budget is used to control expenditures, it does not relate them in any way to program. In essence, the budget process has a prosaic uniformity that insulates it from its environment and perpetuates a budget system that is ineffective and devoid of operational significance. Some of the reasons for this state of affairs emerge as we examine the roles of the primary parties to the budget process.

The Executive's Role

The term executive is used to describe the individual who is accountable for the financial and administrative functioning of the agency. In many mental health organizations, this is the same person who carries the ultimate programmatic responsibility as well. For the most part, mental health executives are psychiatric social workers, psychiatrists or psychologists with no training in budgeting or administration. They are primarily interested in and stimulated by the development of clinical programs and activities. Their lack of sophistication and interest in administration militates against more than a peripheral involvement in budgeting and promotes an acceptance of the budgetary status quo. A non-demanding, routine budget process leaves more time available for them to engage in activities of greater interest and importance to them.

When the mental health agency has a business manager, he may be delegated the entire responsibility for budgeting. While this is convenient, it ignores the major importance of the budget as an instrument of policy. Business managers may be comfortable with the technical aspects of budgeting, but they do not typically have either the program knowledge nor the frame of reference to use the budget as a positive influence on the nature and effectiveness of the program.

While mental health executives express a desire for greater discretion in executing their budgets, there is some question as to whether this would be desirable. Their general lack of training and interest in budgetary matters and their insensitivity to the impact of the budget on policies and programs may, if anything, argue for less discretion if only to reduce the margin for administrative error.

The Board of Directors' Role

In common with the agency director, boards also contribute to the maintenance of the budgetary status quo. They play a relatively inconsequential role in the budget process; the budget they ultimately approve is generally a facsimile of the one submitted to them. They go through the motions of budget approval, focusing their interest on items of relative unimportance.

There seem to be several factors involved in this budgetary apathy by boards. For one, the agency director sharply limits the board's function in his preparation of the budget. His emphasis upon *reasonableness* and *what will go,* generally results in a budget request of very limited proportions that discourages meaningful board action.

Secondly, board members are generally not responsible for financing the operations of the mental health organizations with which they are involved. For example, just 2 percent of all the funds expended by community mental health centers comes from charitable contributions. Since it is reasonable to assume a close relationship between fiscal responsibility and budgetary involvement, the less money a board raises, the less its expected degree of significant involvement in the affairs of the organization.

A major communication problem between agency directors and their boards may be the most important factor contributing to the lack of meaningful involvement by boards in the budget process. These two primary parties to the budget have not found a mutually intelligible language with which to communicate. It is generally considered desirable to recruit people successful in business and industry to serve on the boards of mental health organizations in the hope that they may contribute their prestige, their connections and perhaps their funds. These board members come from a profit oriented environment where there is an emphasis on the relationship between costs and production, between means and ends. As board members of a mental health organization, they are asked to review budgets presented in a manner alien to their own business understanding; budgets presented with objects of expenditure as ends and no connection between costs and programs. As a result, they are not able to evaluate the relative costs and desirability of the agency's various programs and services. The budgets they review do not contain the data that would make such an analysis possible. They can clearly identify expenditures such as salaries and rent, but cannot relate these to anything else. As one board member has written:

> I wonder how many trustees have shared my experience of masking feelings of impotence and ignorance as I solemnly reviewed the lists of figures. From time to time I would ask why a figure differed from the corresponding one a year earlier. If the income did not equal the outgo, I refused to approve the budget. But as soon as the budget was in balance, I approved it, without any real reason for knowing that the year could or should come out that way (MacLeod, 1971).

A frame of reference so vital to the success of his own business is not applicable by the board member to the mental health agency. The tools with which he ordinarily evaluates alternatives and makes decisions in his own enterprise are inoperable when applied to the mental health setting. In his business, he can decide to increase the production of product *A* and not product *B*, but cannot evaluate the relative desirability of various mental health programs. Similar communication problems exist for other board members as well. Clergymen, physicians, community representatives, and others who serve on boards are not able to relate costs to programs and to intelligently set priorities.

They accept these limitations on their behavior because they become convinced, frequently with the aid of the agency director, that mental health organizations are different from other enterprises. These differences it is implied, are so great as to render relatively useless their normal tools of inquiry and understanding. They come to feel that there is a *delicacy*, a *mystique* about mental health programs that defies the understanding of everyone but a mental health professional. They are *outsiders, ordinary laymen,* whose experience and sensitivity is simply not transferable to an understanding of this *unique* environment.

No wonder board members so frequently confine their participation in the budget process to those issues with which they feel comfortable, such as salaries for secretaries and clerks. This is the major role left open to them. At least in this sense, it may be that the agency board has become an anachronism. The barren, routine budget process, the mystique that still surrounds mental health services and the ascendance of government financing have so truncated the board function as to make it almost meaningless.

The Role of Government

Government is the third major party to the budget process and a primary contributor to the rigidity and ineffectiveness of budgeting in mental health organizations. Public support for mental health services has increased rapidly in the past decade; almost 80 percent of all the funds available to community mental health centers comes from Federal, State and local government. Other mental health facilities are also very dependent upon public funds. Through this funding responsibility as well as its approval and licensing functions, government exerts a major influence upon the operation of mental health programs.

Little wonder then, that the object budget required by government funding agencies at all levels, is the dominant factor in budgeting and prescribes the manner in which the budget process is conducted. Since the budget request must be structured by objects of expenditure, the behavior of the parties to the budget process is compatible with this requirement. They think in terms of salaries, rent and other costs but not how these relate to the agency's programs. This inability to identify costs with programs and inevitably, the failure to comparatively evaluate programs are engendered by the object budget and reinforced by the lack of budgetary sophistication. The absence of any government requirements for meaningful program cost data or performance reports adds to the dismal process.

In essence, government's need for operational accountability and control results in the use of the object budget which fosters a routine, mechanistic view of budgeting. This perception of the budget process as routine reinforces the view that mental health executives need no competence or interest in budgetary matters. As a consequence, the mental health professionals who become administrators readily accept a system compatible with their needs to be only minimally involved in budgeting. This lack of involvement and interest in budgeting results, in turn, in a skeletal budget request that has little meaning to the board of directors. The board, a voluntary group serving in an *after-hours* capacity, becomes apathetic and relatively uninvolved in the operations of the mental health agency. This apathy by both the board and the mental health executive serves to reduce the demands made upon government for greater discretion in the management of budgetary affairs. Government, not subject to pressure for change, perpetuates and reinforces the object budget as a means of control.

In this fashion, a circular, self-reinforcing system of interlocking needs is maintained that effectively binds the participants to relatively fixed patterns of behavior. Resistant to change and insulated from its environment, the system perpetuates a chain of events resulting in the use of budget practices inimical to the growth and progress of mental health programs.

THE PROGRAM BUDGET

In marked contrast to the object budget's focus on expenditure control, program budgeting can be a visible, dynamic process intrinsic to effective organizational functioning. The program approach emphasizes the budget as an instrument of policy and is concerned with the identification of costs with programs. The program budget is most effective in those very areas where the object budget is most deficient. It strongly emphasizes the relationship between means and ends, things purchased and services provided. This concept is expressed in a variety of ways: the allocation of costs to benefits, inputs to outputs, expenditures to achievements and resource utilization to accomplishments. The program budget "shifts the emphasis from the means of accomplishment to the accomplishment itself" (Burkhead, 1962) .

In essence, program budgeting emphasizes:

1. The budget as a management tool not merely a control device;
2. The budget as a statement of organizational goals and activities;

3. Budgeting as a continuous function rather than only once each year;
4. The budget as a major instrument of policy;
5. The budget as an integral part of the political process, and;
6. The use of the budget as a measure of organizational functioning.

In this sense, a budget is defined as a financial plan reflecting organizational goals and policies for a forthcoming period and providing a basis for the analysis of costs and activities.

Decision Making

Program budgeting provides quantitative data helpful in making decisions about which programs to implement and to what extent. While the availability of such data alone does not permit a definitive choice among alternatives, it can facilitate the making of difficult decisions. At the very least, program budgeting identifies the cost of each program so that useful comparisons can be made. As MacLeod (1971) has indicated,

> Program budgeting permits disciplined organization of the economic data relative to a decision involving the allocation of resources. Using it, one can gather costs by program, evaluate the impact of the program's expansion or contraction . . ., and estimate with some degree of confidence the program's future economic demands.

In much the same vein, Smithies (1965) has described program budgeting as involving "the use of budgeting techniques that facilitate explicit consideration of the pursuit of policy objectives in terms of the economic costs both at the present time and in the future." By emphasizing the things a mental health agency does rather than the things it buys, program budgeting helps mental health executives use systematic common sense in directing their agencies.

Current Importance of the Program Budget Concept

While program budgeting as an idea appeared in the early 1900's, it was not until the 1960's that it began to dominate the budgeting literature in business and public administration. With relatively few exceptions, budget theorists now subscribe to its concepts, endorse its philosophy and urge its adoption. Program budgeting has become the prototype of modern, sophisticated budget theory with emphasis upon its utility as an instrument of rational decision making.

According to the Committee for Economic Development (1966), the program budget should be,

> . . . a focus for rational policy decisions and . . . a tool for effective management. In its broad sense, the budgetary process is intimately associated with every phase of planning, from the identification of major . . . goals to the selection of immediate priorities. It is involved in the conduct of current operations; without it results cannot be appraised. It determines the way in which scarce resources are allocated among competing needs and how effectively these resources are subsequently used. In these terms, it is an essential instrument—in many respects the primary one for defining . . . purposes and achieving . . . objectives.

In business, the concepts of program budgeting are widely accepted. The budget is viewed as a management tool useful in the maximization of profits and the improvement of managerial performance. This program approach is illustrated by Sord and Welsch (1958) who wrote, "Management . . . is definitely commited to budgeting as an instrument of managerial planning and control. The budget is a device that is primarily used . . . for securing a coordinated, balanced and unified plan of operation." Chamberlain (1962) describes the three important functions of a budget as: " (1) The posing of specific goals; (2) The planning of specific paths to these goals; and (3) Continuing attention to the changes in the underlying assumptions. . . ."

Thus, program budgeting is an integral part of the literature in both public and business administration. Program concepts are as mature as budget theory itself and have been prominent in the literature for the past fifty years. Despite this longevity and theoretical importance, the program budget approach has had relatively little impact on budget practices in the mental health field. Budgeting within mental health organizations is committed to the old object budget with all of its frailties. Of the planning, management, evaluation and control functions of the budget, in mental health organizations it is very clear that the control function predominates.

Form and Behavior

The object budget exercises a pervasive influence upon budgeting practices in mental health organizations. It results in a mechanical stereotyped budget process removed from the mainstream of organizational functioning and concerned with means rather than ends. When the mental health executive begins to prepare his budget request, the form of the document he must submit has a major impact on his behavior. He will list the projected expenditures in the order called for by the budget form and then estimate the amount each item will cost. Since the budget request form is stated in object terms requiring the submission of data organized into such items as salaries, rent and equipment, his thinking and his actions will be oriented along the same lines. In effect, there is a direct causal connection between the structure of the budget form and his budgetary behavior.

The extent to which the form of a budget influences budgetary behavior is affected by a number of factors. These may include the power of the organization requiring the form and the administrative sophistication of those responsible for preparing the budget. In general, however, administrative behavior follows form and it is a truly unique mental health executive who can satisfy the requirements of the object budget and at the same time, view his organization in program terms.

If behavior is significantly influenced by form, then a change in form may well be followed by a change in behavior. As Schick (1966) has indicated: ". . . the form in which information is classified and used governs the actions of budget makers, and, conversely, . . . alterations in form will produce desired changes in behavior."

While the relationship between form and behavior is less than precise, in mental health organizations it is likely that a change in budget form would be followed by a change in behavior, particularly if the change is required by a government funding source. A budget structure requiring the program approach and the use of program forms could significantly modify budgetary behavior. The current emphasis upon objects purchased and expenditure control could be shifted to a focus on program accomplishments, planning and decision making. In preparing his budget, the mental health executive would then be concerned with the following issues:

1. What are the objectives of this organization?
2. What programs are available to move toward these objectives?
3. What will each of these programs cost in human and material resources and what will each contribute toward accomplishing the desired objectives?
4. Which of these programs should be implemented and to what extent?
5. Do we have a feasible plan for implementing them?
6. Can we evaluate at appropriate times the relationship between the proposed and actual accomplishments?

These questions are very different from those that come up in current budgeting such as who will get paid how much next year, should a psychiatric social worker or psychologist be added to the budget and should we increase the budget for supplies by ten or fifteen percent. They can stimulate a meaningful approach to budgeting and result in a more adequate utilization of resources. The budget becomes instrumental in policy planning, encourages more rational decisions, prescribes the manner in which programs will be implemented and serves as a standard by which operations may be evaluated. By posing the important questions, the program budget can stimulate mental health executives to problem solve in a more meaningful and productive fashion.

Accountability and Control

The object budget minimizes the amount of discretion available to a mental health agency and ensures that its allocated funds are spent in the manner prescribed. In effect, mental health organizations are held accountable not for their accomplishments but rather for their orderliness in executing their budgets. While some State and local mental health authorities regularly collect quantitative data from the mental health agencies they fund, only rarely are these used to evaluate the amount of services provided with the funds expended, the efficiency with which mental health agencies are functioning and whether requests for additional funds are justified. In effect, the use of the object budget helps ensure a tight control over expenditures while ignoring the purposes for which the expenditures are made.

A program budget does not lessen the accountability of mental health agencies but instead changes the nature of this accountability. In program terms, accountability emphasizes the achievement of the objectives projected in the budget rather than the controlled expenditure of funds alone. A mental health agency becomes accountable not only for the integrity of its disbursements but for the provision of services to the extent contemplated by its budget. In program budgeting, funds are requested not for salaries and supplies alone but rather to provide a specified amount of service to a particular population over a given period of time. For example, funding may be requested to provide 500 additional direct service sessions for adolescents and their parents in a program designed to help control school drop outs. Accountability would then relate primarily to whether the amount of service originally budgeted was in fact provided and at what cost. To the extent measurable, the impact of the additional services on the drop out rate would constitute another measure of accountability.

In effect, this type of accountability adds the dimension of program performance to the emphasis upon expenditure control. It permits the mental health agency much greater flexibility in the use of its resources—it is responsible for the accomplishment of specific program objectives and can flexibly utilize the resources available to achieve these objectives.

The Development of a Program Budget

The first step in the development of a program budget is a formulation of the agency's objectives and an identification of those functions or programs which if implemented would lead toward the accomplishment of those objectives. In general, mental health service organizations are organized for the purpose of promoting mental health and preventing mental disorders. However noteworthy these objectives, they are not measurable and therefore must be sub-divided into their component parts. In essence, a series of operational objectives are formulated that are presumed to have a positive relationship with good mental health. These are developed on the basis of such factors as the needs of the area served, the expertise of the staff, the available financial support and the legal mandate. The specific factors that influence the determination of these operational objectives are indigenous to each setting. A community mental health center, for example, may have as one such objective a reduction in admissions to the State hospital for residents of the catchment area. Other objectives may include the provision of a specific amount of mental health services to a previously unserved group and the implementation of a consultation program in every school in the catchment area. The objectives formulated should be for the term of the budget period, generally one year.

In order to progress toward the achievement of these objectives, the center carries out certain functions or programs. In essence, "a program is a package which encompasses each and every one of the agency's efforts to achieve a particular objective . . ." (Greenhouse, 1966). The programs available to a community mental health center may include a treatment program, diagnostic program, consultation and education program, research program and others. Programs may be added or deleted depending upon the specific center—not every center has a research program, for example. While the designation of specific programs will vary between centers, in every center programs should be organized around specific objectives.

A program is thus an activity or group of activities designed to accomplish a particular objective. The treatment program, for example, might include individual psychotherapy and group psychotherapy with people of varying age groups and diagnoses. The consultation and education program might include consultation with schools, courts and social agencies and public education activities in the area of drug abuse. Elements of each of these programs are clustered around the particular objectives to which they relate and the programs are examined in relation to each other "so that the validity of each . . . may be assessed in terms of the overall approach . . . and costs may be compared with other competing programs potential or existing . . ." (Greenhouse, 1966). The program budget is designed to yield sufficient quantitative data around each of its objectives so that the costs and products of each may be compared to help make more rational decisions. In effect, the objectives and their component programs are competing with each other for the organization's resources.

Quantifiable Products

Following the establishment of objectives and the allocation of the various programs to these objectives, it is necessary to identify the criteria by which the utility of the programs can be measured. Program budgeting requires the identification of specific quantifiable products resulting from the operation of the programs. In a treatment program, for example, the number of treatment sessions provided is one example of a quantifiable product. The number of sessions can be subdivided into child, adolescent and adult components and these into specific treatment modalities such as group and individual therapy.

However, not every program within a mental health agency performs a function resulting in a quantifiable product. Where such a product is not identifiable, the program's performance is measured by activities instead. An activity is: "A specific and distinguishable line of work performed by one or more organizational components—. . . for the purpose of accomplishing a function for which the . . . unit is responsible" (Moak and Killian, 1963). In a research program, for example, the number of research projects completed during a period is obviously not a meaningful measure of its productivity for that period. A research program may be in process for several years until one particular year when several projects are completed. It is inappropriate to assess the program in the year of completion as being of significantly greater value than in the prior years when the major portion of the work may have been done.

Here, a description of the activities within the program would be more useful as an indicator of program productivity. The specific activities within the program will, to a great extent, be dependent upon the nature of the research carried out and its stage of development. In general, however, the activities would consist of a description of the actual work done during the period, (development of a study design, data collection, etc.) an assessment of the specific projects, their relative stages of development and their anticipated dates of completion.

In programs such as professional training and community mental health education, the product seems best measured by the number of the various services provided. In training, for example, the number of training sessions held and/or the number of people trained could be used. In community mental health consultation and education, the number of sessions provided, classified according to the nature of the recipient population, might constitute the most appropriate product.

Program Costs

To help evaluate the relative merits of the various programs, it is helpful to compare the costs and products of each. In a mental health program, program costs will include such factors as staff salaries, rent, supplies and other items of overhead with salaries as the major cost. Program costs may be direct or indirect—a direct cost is one which is clearly applicable to a specific program while an indirect cost applies to the agency as a whole and must be allocated on some appropriate basis to the various programs. The salary of a staff member working within the treatment program is one example of a direct treatment cost, while rent and other items of overhead constitute indirect costs.

The use of a program budget facilitates an understanding of the cost of each program in relation to its products as well as a comparison between the various programs. For a given period, it is possible to forecast for example, the cost of the treatment program and the number of treatment sessions to be provided. To accomplish this, all costs relevant to the treatment program must be allocated to it. In order to identify that portion of the agency's total staff salaries to be budgeted for the treatment program, the amount of staff time required to produce the desired number of treatment sessions must be estimated. If 1,000 hours of staff time will be required at an estimated unit cost of $10 per hour then the direct cost of the treatment program will be $10,000. Direct staff costs are allocated to the other programs in a similar fashion.

The allocation of indirect costs to the various programs in the budget is more difficult. Expenses such as rent, electric, telephone and similar items must be added to direct costs in order to project the full cost of the programs. In business, various methods are used to allocate indirect costs. For example, rent is frequently allocated to the various departments in a business based upon the proportionate amount of square feet each department occupies. If the rent is $10,000 per year for 10,000 square feet and there are four departments each occupying 2500 square feet, they would each be charged with 25 percent of the total rent expense or $2500 per year. Other indirect expenses may be allocated in a variety of ways depending upon the nature of the expense. For example, payroll taxes are frequently allocated to departments based upon the percentage of each departmental payroll to the total payroll while accounting expense may be allocated on the basis of the number of employees in each department to the total.

For the mental health agency, the allocation of indirect costs to its various programs is most appropriately based upon the percentage of staff hours to be spent within each program to total staff hours. For example, if the budget projects a total of 20,000 staff hours for the coming year and 10,000 of these hours will be spent in the treatment program, then this program will be charged in the budget with 50 percent of the indirect expenses. While it might be more technically correct to allocate rent and electricity, for example, on the basis of the square feet occupied by each program, the gain in accuracy would not generally warrant the additional complications. Staff time is the most significant factor in the delivery of mental health services. It bears a close if not direct relationship to actual productivity and is the largest item of expense.

The Program Audit

The use of a program budget adds a new dimension to the usual audit process. The traditional interest of the auditor in the accuracy of the financial records, the honesty of the personnel and the integrity of the expenditures is joined by an assessment of the relationship between agency costs, objectives and accomplishments. The audit addresses itself to whether the agency has accomplished its projected objectives and the costs involved. As Moak and Killian (1963) have indicated, "The primary objective of the post audit of performance is to discover the extent to which performance has matched the promise made at the time funds were being sought."

The program audit differs from the dollar audit in its emphasis on program productivity. The auditor reviews the records of each program to assess the program costs as well as the amounts of service actually provided. He checks expenditures to be certain that they have been allocated properly to the various programs. The basic objective of his audit is to determine the actual performance of the various programs as compared to the original budget.

The audit report contains the actual costs and productivity of each program and a comparison between these operating results and the original budget projections. It may further consider the factors contributing to any variances between the budgeted and actual operating results. If, for example, productivity has fallen below projections, the audit may include a consideration of this as it relates to the efficiency with which organizational resources have been utilized. This approach emphasizes the use of the audit as a management tool in addition to its more traditional role.

The Program Budget and the Board of Directors

The use of a program budget within a mental health agency can help restore the board of directors to a meaningful policy role. As discussed earlier, boards are generally uninvolved in the budget process and in the formulation of agency policy. They have relatively little impact on the size of a budget or its composition, spend very little time in budget discussions, and confine their involvement to issues of minor import.

However, when the budget is presented in program terms, a board member is able to question the advisability of a greater allocation of resources to one program instead of another. He can debate the need for an enlarged diagnostic program as compared to an expansion in community mental health education. He can dispute whether a given increase in expenditures on consultation warrants a proposed reduction in research.

Since the budget clearly and distinctly converts money into services, it becomes the vehicle through which the board can become involved in management issues. If the agency has provided significantly less service than has been budgeted, this becomes visible to the board and is a legitimate area of inquiry.

Budgetary Discretion

The use of a program structure materially affects the discretion available to the mental health executive. As indicated earlier, the object budget severely limits his discretion frequently to the extent that he is unable to make even minor shifts between expenditure lines without permission. With the emphasis upon programs rather than expenditures, the program budget permits a great deal of flexibility in the utilization of resources. What is at issue is not the nature of the expenditure but rather the achievement of prescribed ends. This implies that the agency has the freedom to accomplish these ends in the manner that seems most effective. The agency director becomes the designer and implementer of the methods through which agency goals are accomplished and is free to adapt and/or modify both human and material resources in his effort to optimally achieve its objectives.

The Program Budget and Evaluation

Criteria do not currently exist with which to evaluate the operating efficiency of mental health agencies. What quantity of human and material resources should be expended in the provision of services? How much should an outpatient session cost? A day of inpatient care? The *test of the market,* i.e. survival in a competitive economy, does not enforce efficiency in the nonprofit mental health field as it does in business. In the business enterprise, survival is the basic criterion of efficiency. "The more or less impersonal forces of the market will see to it that firms which operate unsuccessfully in terms of net profit will not survive. The market is the ultimate disciplining agency" (Burkhead, 1962). In mental health, there is no comparable market and and as a result, the survival of an agency is unrelated to considerations of efficency.

For mental health agencies, the program budget can help serve a function similar to that exercised for business by the competitive market economy. Together with an effective program audit, it can be used as a standard by which efficiency is evaluated. The program budget brings together in one document, data relating to projected program costs as well as outputs. At the end of the year, the program audit will indicate whether actual operations have attained the budgeted objectives and if not, the extent and nature of the variances. While it lacks the objectivity of the competitive market, the budget serves as a standard by which efficiency is judged. In quantitative terms, it assesses the extent to which the mental health agency has achieved its objectives in terms of costs as well as productivity. It also allows for comparisons over different periods of time. The number of treatment sessions provided last year and their cost may be compared with the results of the prior year and any significant changes will be highlighted.

For a mental health agency, however, the dimensions of success go far beyond considerations of efficiency. While quantitative accomplishments are important, they constitute only one limited measure of performance. Not only must a mental health agency render an appropriate amount of service at reasonable cost, but the service must be of high enough quality to benefit the recipient population. While a program budget can help enforce efficiency, it cannot determine the amount of mental health being purchased, the degree to which mental disorders are being prevented, or the impact of the program on the community. Other criteria relating to the effectiveness of mental health services must be used together with the program budget to adequately evaluate the total functioning of the mental health agency. The measurement of costs and productivity only facilitates judgments about efficiency rather than measuring effectiveness in any value sense.

Limitations of the Program Budget

Program budgeting is more complicated than the traditional object approach. It requires a grouping of all activities into functional programs that frequently cut across existing organizational lines. All expenditures must be allocated along these same program lines with indirect expenses apportioned on some equitable basis. Units of productivity must be identified, projected for each program and related to program costs. Obviously, the burdens on the management staff are increased and more manpower with specific training in budgeting may be required.

The resistance of professional staff members to the implementation of a program budget may be a problem. Some staff members may feel threatened by a system that examines the relationship between the time for which they are paid and their productivity in quantitative terms. The program budget with its emphasis upon the assessment of efficiency introduces a new element into the agency. Where there has been little concern about staff productivity in the past, this element may be a disturbing one.

Agency directors may be reluctant to adopt a program budget for similar reasons. They too may resist the type of accountability inherent in its use. With the object budget, their *success* is related to whether they spend the budgeted funds properly rather than their ability to produce a specific amount of service at a stated cost. While mental health executives may be unhappy about the inflexibility of the object budget, they may not welcome a substitute that makes the quality of their management far more visible.

Thus, both agency directors and professional staff may resist a system that focuses upon productivity and the relationship between costs and accomplishments as a criterion of satisfactory performance. To a great extent, the use of the object budget has insulated their functioning from appropriate scrutiny and evaluation. The visibility and accountability so inherent in the program budget may not be welcomed. As McKean and Anshen (1965) have indicated, the program budget may be seen "as a threat to existing, familiar, and manipulatable institutional arrangements." It may help to identify "overlapping and redundant activities" and assist in "the exposure of ineffective and inefficient employment of resources."

CONCLUSION

The need for mental health services greatly exceeds their availability. While the development of community programs represents a major advance, the imbalance between supply and demand will exist for a long time. As a result, it is essential that our mental health resources be used in the most efficient manner possible.

It is suggested that the adoption of program budgeting will enhance the efficiency of mental health programs through its emphasis on the amount of service provided in relation to costs. However, efficiency is only one of the variables to be considered in decisions about the allocation of resources. A number of other factors specific to each setting may affect the budget process. These include: (1) the experience, competence and desires of the staff; (2) the wishes of the board of directors; (3) the mandate from the funding sources; (4) the desires of groups within the community; (5) the perception of community needs and (6) investments in ongoing programs or sunk costs.

The program budget offers a language through which the mental health agency can become more visible and comprehensible to all of these parties to the budget process. It can enhance accountability and help prevent the continuance of mental health agencies as closed systems insulated from intelligible appraisal.

REFERENCES

Burkhead, Jesse: *Government Budgeting.* New York, Wiley, 1962.

Chamberlain, Neil W.: *The Firm: Microeconomic Planning and Action.* New York, McGraw-Hill, 1962.

Committee for Economic Development: *Budgeting for National Objectives.* New York, The Committee for Economic Development, 1966.

Dimock, Marshall E.; Dimock, Gladys O., and Koenig, Louis W.: *Public Administration.* New York, Rinehart, 1958.

Feldman, Saul: *The Outpatient Mental Health Center and Program Budgeting.* Unpublished Research, 1967.

Greenhouse, Samuel M.: The Planning–Programming–Budgeting System; Rationale, Language, and Idea-Relationships. *Public Administration Review, 26,* 273, 1966.

MacLeod, Roderick K.: Program Budgeting Works in Non-Profit Institutions. *Harvard Business Review,* Sept.-Oct., 1971.

McKean, Roland N. and Anshen, Melvin: Limitations, risks, and problems. In Novick, David (Ed.): *Program Budgeting.* Cambridge, Harvard University Press, 1965.

Moak, Lennox L. and Killian, Kathryn W.: *Operating Budget Manual.* Chicago, Municipal Finance Officers Association, 1963.

Public Administration Service: *Modernizing Government Budget Administration.* Washington, Agency for International Development, 1962.

Schick, Allen: The road to PPB: The stages of budget reform. *Public Administration Review, 26:*250-251, 1966.

Smithies, Arthur: Conceptual framework for the program budget. In Novick, David (Ed.): *Program Budgeting.* Cambridge, Harvard University Press, 1965.

Sord, Burnard H., and Welsch, Glenn A.: *Business Budgeting.* New York, The Controllership Foundation, 1958.

CHAPTER 3

PEOPLE MAKE PROGRAMS: PERSONNEL MANAGEMENT

H. G. WHITTINGTON

THE SUCCESS of any mental health administrator ultimately depends on the achievements of those working in his program. This is an insight that is hard to come by, since many mental health professionals, at the beginning of their careers, assume that it is their intellectual brilliance, their innovative program development, their grantsmanship, their ingenuity that will assure success. While these are necessary, they are not sufficient; since in the final analysis, all mental health programs are dependent upon staff performance for attainment of program goals.

Much of the director's time is spent dealing with staff. He characteristically goes through a series of phases, first seeing personnel problems as an annoyance which he would somehow like to be rid of; later translating clinical concepts to personnel management, and thereby seeing all of his staff as sick; and eventually, coming to a balanced understanding of the interplay between personal characteristics, system characteristics, and leadership style. Every mental health administrator initially hopes to develop a system that is self-sustaining, self-correcting, operates with efficiency and ease, and is—above all—logical and neat. That dream is never realized. No sooner is it approximated, than some totally unpredictable event, either intrinsic or external to the agency, upsets all the carefully laid plans.

Challenges in Mental Health Personnel Management

In the human services field, and especially in mental health agencies, the individual staff member operates with a high degree of autonomy and privacy, which defies the imposition of stereotyped, predictable behavior by any individual in a management position, or by any administrative or management system. The administrative arrangement for a mental health agency must be subtle and complex, and the leader must have well-developed sensitivity and flexibility.

At the moment the administrator recognizes that his main challenge is the management of staff, he faces a curious dilemma. He has seen himself as an expert in human behavior, by virtue of his training, experience, and demonstrated competence in modifying the disordered behavior of patients. He has committed himself, by his choice of life work, to the unique value of the individual human being. Usually his political affiliations have been with the party devoted to social betterment, and his identification with the concept of progress is correspondingly strong. And then he finds himself in charge of a mental health agency, endowed with money and ideas and vigor, and given the opportunity to implement his own unique values through a mental health organization. He often comes to feel, quickly, that the entire staff is dedicated to frustrating his aspirations, and blocking his legitimate exercise of authority. The management of staff is rendered even more difficult by the fact that there is no tangible product that can be inspected as it comes off the assembly line, so that the quantity and quality of the work effort is difficult to appraise. The total product of the mental health agency is dependent upon people, operating most of the time in confidential relationships with their clients. If the leader succumbs to temptation and regresses to authoritarian methods of control, he very quickly discovers what a fragile undertaking the mental health enterprise is; for we are asking staff to give something of themselves to their patients, to interact emotionally and humanly, not merely intellectually or technically. The relationship of therapist to patient is a delicate one, and is influenced by many forces, including the behavior of the leader, which impinge upon that relationship. While a surgeon may perform an operation with high technical competence, even though he feels that the leader of his program is autocratic, arbitrary, and derogates his importance, the mental health practitioner can rarely function with optimal efficiency if he has similar feelings about his leader. In every transaction with a patient, the management of the mental health center is an invisible but by no means silent partner.

Staff Expectations and Attitudes

The director of a mental health program has, at his disposal, some information concerning the perceptions, needs, and attitudes of mental health staff. Most recently, the study published by the Joint Information Service entitled, *The Staff of the Mental Health Center*, written by Raymond M. Glasscote and Jon E. Gudeman (1969), is a valuable background document. The chapter dealing with job satisfaction, dissatisfaction, and morale, is particularly useful to the mental health administrator.

First of all, if we examine the satisfactions reported by staff members, the largest percentage of staff reported that work with patients gave them the most satisfaction (59 percent). The next greatest source of satisfaction was staff associations (27 percent), followed closely by opportunity for new treatment approaches (22 percent), opportunity for learning experiences (21 percent), and community emphasis (20 percent).

A survey of dissatisfactions is likewise enlightening. The most frequently mentioned dissatisfaction is with the administration of the mental health center (60 percent). There is considerable reason to believe that in other types of mental health facilities, dissatisfaction with the administration would likewise score high. Interestingly enough, dissatisfaction with fellow staff members was mentioned second (31 percent); 23 percent of the staff reported that they were dissatisfied with treatment programs, while salary (13 percent), workload hours (13 percent), and communications (12 percent) came next in frequency. The study demonstrated that psychologists were the most dissatisfied with administration (88 percent), followed by social workers (84 percent), and psychiatrists (65 percent).

A consultant to the field study, Dr. Kent Miller, was quoted in the book as follows:

> Centers may be no worse than many other agencies, or even businesses, in terms of the quality of program administration, but what we have seen in these visits is in some respects discouraging. Even those centers that have several very bright people in central administration do not seem to be providing the necessary amount of ongoing and day-to-day direction. We heard sometimes of decisions being handed down from on high in arbitrary fashion, and at other times we heard of an atmosphere of *democracy* carried to such an extreme that the director finally had to move in such a manner that everyone lost. It may be that mental health centers, at least those of any size, need the same kind of administrative division of labor that occurs in universities—one man to *front* for the organization, representing it to the public, raising funds, and so on, as the university president does, another who develops programs and oversees the internal operation, as the vice-president for academic affairs does.

The authors of the book also state, "A significant factor influencing the staff's attitude towards the administration is its ability to make decisions in those areas that affect the non-administrative staff. When the administration is absorbed in fiscal and political matters or in long-range planning to the exclusion of providing leadership to and making decisions for the staff it administers, then morale suffers."

Subsequently, the authors of the study address themselves to the issue of how morale can be improved. They found, "Almost half of the suggestions fell into only two categories: improved communications, and clarify roles and responsibilities." The authors go on to state, "These complaints suggest once more that a number of professionals who come into community mental health centers because they are dissatisfied with the nature, emphasis, and outcome of the programs that they have been working in initially feel a great deal of attraction to 'doing their own thing,' but soon afterward begin to yearn for structure, definition, and clarification of role. Otherwise they feel abandoned and unsupported. A number of responses that we have placed in other categories carry elements of this need for the leaders to lead, for the managers to manage."

So there we have it: the staff of a sample of community mental health centers, at least, believe that personnel management is deficient in their center, and that improvement in the management of center staff, the meeting of their legitimate professional and personal needs, should have a high priority.

From this same study, some information is available concerning how staff in the community mental health center spend their time. While this profile would differ in various mental health agencies, it is fairly representative of trends in the utilization of professional time occurring in all mental health settings at the present time. The staff spend approximately 57 percent of their time in individual or group therapy or contacts with patients. In this major part of their work week, they function autonomously, privately, and in a manner that is quite different from the functioning of *employees* or *workers* in production, service, or sales organizations. The staff devotes 1 percent of the time to supervision, 2 percent to receiving training, and 16 percent to staff meetings. The administrator first coming into a mental health agency from some other setting, is always struck with the amount of time that mental health professionals devote to staff meetings and conferences of one type or another. The study would indicate that the average mental health professional spends about six and one-half hours a week in such group conferences, which become the main method of program control in the typical mental health agency.

Influence of Setting

While the study quoted has dealt with a sample of comprehensive community mental health centers, it should be borne in mind that the factors affecting the relationships between the mental health administrator and his staff are very complex and numerous. The social setting in which the center director operates will, and must inevitably, influence his administrative style and practices and his relationships with the mental health agency staff.

Size is a very important determinant. If the staff is small, the leader is visible, and his personal and professional characteristics can be well known. He can lead, then, by example and by directly teaching and encouraging staff. In a large mental health agency, this model of leadership is totally inappropriate, and if followed exclusively will result in the ruin of the agency.

Most mental health programs operate within a pre-defined personnel system, which has often been developed by a sponsoring agency previously. If the agency operates under governmental auspices, the career service structure, rules, and regulations will inevitably influence relationships between the management of the mental health agency and personnel. For example, in the Mental Health Center of Denver General Hospital, any mental health professional may be assigned responsibility for the leadership of an operating team. However, our personnel system is a nonpositional hierarchy, based upon professional training and experience, rather than upon functional assignment within the Mental Health Center. Therefore, a psychiatric nurse serving as a team leader will be paid as a nurse, while a psychiatrist serving as a team leader will be paid as a psychiatrist. This kind of an arrangement produces certain tensions between personnel and the leadership of a mental health program, because of the feelings that a team leader is a team leader is a team leader, and that there should be *like pay for like work*. If one has personnel who, on top of this feeling of discrimination on the basis of professional discipline, also feel discriminated against because of their sex and/or ethnicity, the setting is ripe for a major rupture in good relationships between the center director and certain of his key middle-management staff.

The type of staff employed clearly influences personnel management practices. The mental health professional comes to the agency with relatively predictable prior training, is usually licensed by the state (with resultant social control and legal regulatory mechanisms), and has accepted as a part of assuming professional status, conformance to a code of ethics ascribed to by his particular profession. It is assumed that standards of practice will be regulated largely by the internalized controls of the individual professional, and will not have to be taught or imposed by the management structure. To the extent that the staff of the mental health agency is made up of non-professionals, however, these assumptions may no longer hold. With such a personnel profile, the mental health professional becomes not only practitioner, but also supervisor and personnel manager in his own right. Most mental health professionals are totally unprepared for this role by training, and many are unsuited for it by interest and by personality. Only the psychiatrist and the psychiatric nurse have predictably had some training and prior experience in the supervision of personnel, and characteristically only the nurse has had experience in the supervision of non-professional staff.

The auspices of the agency clearly affect personnel management practices. If the agency is private, and hence dependent upon fee income for its survival, the emphasis in personnel management will be on optimizing productivity of the staff. If, on the other hand, the agency is in the public sector, and particularly if the salaries are low and the location not desirable, emphasis will be upon increasing staff satisfactions, as a way of retaining personnel. The philosophy, values, goals, and methods of the superordinate agency in which the mental health enterprise is lodged also have daily and vital effects upon personnel management. In the general hospital, for example, traditions of separate management systems for nursing and for psychiatric social work exist and must be dealt with in developing a rational and effective personnel management plan. If the emphasis is upon functional team organization, with unit control, the existence of these separate disciplinary supervisory lines causes serious problems. If the mental health agency is free-standing, the administration will generally have much more flexibility in determining what kind of social control and personnel management system is most likely to be effective, given the overall mandate of the organization, characteristics of the staff employed, auspices, and fiscal support system.

What Makes a Successful Mental Health Administrator

Up to this point, we have succeeded probably only in demonstrating that the issues involved in personnel management are so multiple and so complex, that no one should get involved in it! The reality is that many of us do, as we try to implement our personal values by attaining power in formal mental health organizations. Because mental health professionals are so often idealists and zealots, the leader often has great difficulty implementing his values. Each individual staff member has the power, in dozens of transactions each day, to either facilitate the policies of the agency, or to frustrate and divert them; to conform to the expectations of management, or to rebel against them. The typical mental health worker comes prepared to see the organization as his enemy, and to view it also as the enemy of the patient. For mental health personnel, more often than not, are private people, dedicated to the attainment of individual freedom for themselves and for their clients. Yet they often must interpret and enforce agency policies, if the superordinate goals of the agency are to be advanced. Since most mental health agencies are dependent upon fee collection for at least a part of their financial support, the ambivalence of staff members about money and fee collection usually surfaces quite early. Neglecting to send in billings, encouraging patients to understate their income to reduce their fee, requesting hardship consideration—these are a few of the ways in which the individual practitioner may effectively subvert agency goals.

Yet in spite of all these differences between agencies and situations, certain characteristics seem to differentiate the successful mental health administrator from the inadequate one. The successful leader has usually won his spurs as a competent mental health practitioner, prior to the assumption of leadership responsibilities. His staff is generally convinced of his involvement and concern, and see him as being available to them. The successful leader is usually proficient in defining the superordinate goals of the organization, in such a way as to facilitate conflict resolution, cooperation, and mutuality among the staff. He is a good communicator, both verbally and in writing; and whether he operates out of a model of consensual decision-making by staff, or follows essentially an authoritarian model, staff are informed about problems, solutions, program progress, future plans, and so forth. An important part of such a communication system is a consistent and rational reward system related to superordinate goals, so that personnel who behave in such a way as to facilitate achievement of the superordinate goals of the agency, receive tangible rewards in terms of salary increases, honorific appointments, paid professional trips, and personal recognition.

Most successful mental health administrators display a tolerance of diversity. They not only endure but actively encourage alternative and sometimes frankly experimental methods of trying to achieve program goals. They generally displace decision-making downward through the organizational hierarchy, encouraging staff at all levels to make independent decisions wherever possible, without recourse to higher authority. This would seem only rational in a mental health agency, when the individual practitioner in his clinical transaction often has life or death responsibility over a patient. Anomalously, in some agencies—usually troubled ones—the clinician is simultaneously given the responsibility to care for his patient in awesome solitude, while he is unable to decide how many pencils he may need in a week without recourse to higher authority. This kind of inconsistent communication results in a serious breakdown in respect and mutuality between the leadership and staff.

Mental Health Administration Is Different

Most of what has been said probably is characteristic of successful leadership in all sorts of organizations. Significant differences in personnel management do exist in mental health agencies, however:

1. The therapist frequently receives enormous ego-gratification from patients, who see him as all-powerful. It is difficult to move from a position of such great authority and status as a therapist, to a position as an employee of an agency. The mental health professional simply does not want to *fit into a system,* and his daily work with patients reinforces and encourages his strivings toward independence and special status.

2. Additionally, the personnel profile differs from that of the typical social institution. The mental health agency, particularly the newly developing community mental health centers, have a high ratio of professional personnel holding graduate degrees in

social work, nursing, psychology, psychiatry, etc. The mental health agency at times seems to be very much like the Italian Navy: there are more admirals than ships. These professional staff members have a highly developed need for status, independence, and autonomy. To have achieved such educational status in the American system, they necessarily have had to be competitive, energetic, and intellectually vigorous. A continuing need for growth and self-development characterizes their value systems. They suffer often from strong super-ego pressures, which demand a high degree of success in their treatment undertakings. When this need for success is frustrated by reality, they are prone to look for some external reason in order to dilute their own sense of personal and professional inadequacy: *the administration* is always an available and easy target.

3. The product in the mental health undertaking is ill-defined, so that productivity is difficult to determine and to reward consistently. This means that it is very easy for the mental health administrator to mistake conviviality for competence, obsequiousness for intelligence, and maliciousness for constructive criticism. The type of behavior that is rewarded within the system will, over time, come to be a predominant behavior among the staff. This realization should be foremost in the mind of the mental health leader at all times, as he engages in complex relationships with his staff.

4. There are special personnel problems within mental health agencies related to the characteristics of the various professions involved. Each of the major professions in a mental health program has developed from somewhat different historical roots, and each has its own sense of professional identity and social responsibility. Unlike some other professions, there is a high degree of overlap in the technical skills possessed by various disciplines such as psychiatry, clinical psychology, psychiatric social work, and psychiatric nursing. Since the technical repertoire of the mental health disciplines is not highly developed and greatly differentiated, jurisdictional problems, with status implications, are frequent in mental health agencies.

Rhetoric, also, is frequently often quite at odds with reality.

The emphasis in recent years has been upon expansion of the roles of all of the mental health disciplines, in order to achieve more comprehensive care for patients. At times this has also been referred to as role blurring. Regardless of the semantics, it is essentially recognition that the bulk of the activities of all mental health workers is generic. These activities involve the utilization of the practitioners' empathy and interpersonal and verbal skills in attempting to help a client adapt more effectively to his environment, and more completely achieve his personal goals. However, *salary blurring* has not followed. This predictably causes feelings of being treated unfairly on the part of many of the lower paid staff members. Resentment and conflict is sharpest between those disciplines whose pay and status most nearly approximate each other: between psychologists and psychiatrists, between social workers and nurses, and between social workers and indigenous nonprofessionals.

One principle of personnel administration that may go some way towards mitigating this sense of social injustice, is to establish a formal management and social control hierarchy that allows each of the disciplines to attain senior administrative rank by virtue of demonstrated competence. The reality remains, however, that the requirements of law and established social practice must be met, and that there will be differences not only in status but also in control capability, of certain disciplines. For example, National Institute of Mental Health regulations in the case of the community mental health center, specify,"Medical responsibility for each patient shall be vested in a physician." No matter what the rhetoric, this clearly delineates a special status and authority for the physician.

5. Community mental health centers, and many other mental health settings, are engaging in innovative program development at the present time. They are not pre-existing service delivery formats, deploying a known and standardized technology to a waiting body of consumers. Experimentation with service delivery formats, with techniques for treatment and prevention, and with governance and social regulation mechanisms, are prevalent in many mental health undertakings in the United States

today. The leader of a successful mental health program must, by definition, be an innovator, must be flexible in both ideas and behavior, and must embrace change as a way of life, rather than regarding it as an unwelcome disturbance.

6. The most rapidly growing category of personnel in community mental health centers is the indigenous non-professional. Similar developments are occurring in all mental health settings, as an attempt is made to provide services that are realistic in their cost, are psychologically and socially available to minority group persons, and have high social relevance. The characteristics of these personnel vary widely, depending upon the locale and setting within which they are employed. In many of the state hospitals, they are primarily white, rurally-oriented individuals, long-time residents of the locale of the state hospital. In urban mental health agencies, the non-professionals are more frequently from an ethnic minority background, and from an urbanized family. Likewise, the role assigned these individuals varies widely from agency to agency: from nursing assistant at the one extreme, to *ombudsman for the poor* at the other end. While the promise in utilizing such personnel is high, there is a corollary danger that service for the poor will come to be provided by individuals without professional training or clearly demonstrated competence, beyond the regulation of either law, ethics, or established standards of practice: that in effect, a system of *second-class care* will again be developed for the poor, with the best intentions and the most stirring rhetoric.

Mental Health Agency As a Social System

The mental health administrator must view his agency as a complex social system. He must ask himself, "How can this society be organized so as to increase the likelihood that the legitimate needs and wishes of the staff, of consumers, of the community, and of the governmental funding agencies, will be met or approximated?" Since the supplies available almost never equal the demand for mental health services, he must look to organizational strategies that will optimize the productivity of his staff, so that they will do more than is necessary or required. In order to accomplish this, he must develop a social system that maximizes ego-involvement, mutual communication, and effective conflict resolution. If the social system does not adequately subsume these goals, productivity will decrease as self-motivated, goal-oriented behavior decreases.

How may these goals of ego-involvement, communication, and conflict resolution be achieved? First, organizational units must be kept small. If a staff member is a part of a functional social group that exceeds 10 or 12 in size, he will tend to feel that his own individual behavior is less crucial to the group's productivity and success; and, group cohesiveness and peer control will also be vitiated. As with all *solutions* to life problems, small operating units in themselves engender new problems such as inter-team rivalry, potentiality of program fragmentation, and increased potential for inter-group conflict. Other social mechanisms, as will be discussed subsequently, must exist in order to prevent the development of operating units into closed, paranoid cliques.

The mission to be accomplished must be determined before deciding on the size and the composition of the organizational unit. From the mission, the administrator must move backwards to determine the processes and procedures that are necessary to achieve the mission. From this he should conceptualize the specific technical or operational skills that are required. Based on his knowledge of the attributes of the various professions and other personnel, he should then develop a staffing pattern for the operational unit. At that point, one comes to implementing plans in terms of real people, based upon who is available, and on their personal and professional attributes. The wise administrator pays a great deal of attention to his selection of the personnel who will serve together on a functional unit. There is no objective, quantifiable body of knowledge concerning the optimal composition of functional teams. We do know that certain characteristics have to obtain if the team is to be optimally functional:

1. The task or tasks must be clearly defined.
2. The leadership, and the responsibility and authority of leadership must be clearly spelled out.
3. The contingencies must be clear, so that the team members will

know the consequences of good or poor performance. There must be a consistent reward system for successful efforts directed towards the superordinate goals of the agency and the defined mission of the functional unit.

In large programs, the administrator must frequently decide whether to centralize his program—with the usual implications that there will be a large conglomeration of staff—or whether to decentralize it, in which case smaller staff units are more feasible. As an example, in Denver, the four generic, or neighborhood mental health teams, which constitute the main service delivery system for the comprehensive community mental health center, were not providing either quantitatively or qualitatively adequate services for alcoholics, addicts, and children with learning and behavior problems. We had to decide whether to establish centralized units to achieve those program goals, or whether to somehow modify personnel composition and functioning at the neighborhood mental health team level. In the case of the treatment of heroin addicts, the decision was made to establish a centralized treatment program for the following reasons: the number of patients to be served was relatively small, the skills required for a narcotic treatment program were not generally available among mental health professionals, and the degree of control and structure required for treating narcotic addicts was antithetical to the permissive and local control tradition of the neighborhood mental health teams.

In the case of services for school-age children, on the other hand, it was decided that relieving the neighborhood teams of responsibility for children would be bad program policy. On the other hand, the teams had clearly demonstrated over a five-year period their reluctance to commit significant staff resources to services for children, and to broaden the skills of team members into the psychoeducational area. Consequently, a psychoeducational specialist was assigned to each of the neighborhood mental health teams; however, he also related to a specialized mental health care for school-age children unit, which provided initial and continuing training and shared in the supervision of the psychoeducational specialist. Similar compromise arrangements have been made in such special areas as outpatient treatment of alcoholism and rehabilitation services.

Recruitment and Selection of Personnel

Recruitment and selection of personnel is a vital process to an effective organization. Personnel must be oriented to, and personally and professionally committed to, the goals of the particular kind of mental health agency by which they are being employed if high thrust and perseverance can be expected in the performance of their duties. It is a mistake to hire someone for a service program who wants to do research; or to hire someone who wants to *do his own thing* to work in a governmentally-sponsored, public program. Disillusionment, bitterness, and ineffectiveness are the inevitable consequences. As a part of the recruitment and selection process, it is important that a clear psychological contract be established with the new staff member before he is employed, so that he knows exactly what tasks he is being employed for, and how his effectiveness will be judged. The inexperienced mental health administrator, in his urgency to fill staff vacancies, and with the professional scarcity that exists, will often employ people who are not motivated for work in the particular kind of agency or position that is available, and will not define clearly his expectations to the individual, hoping that the new person will somehow *fit in*. That rarely happens.

Great care, then, must be given to the selection procedure. If the right personnel are selected for the jobs at hand, and assigned properly, the manager of the mental health agency stands a high chance of success. In the Mental Health Center of Denver General Hospital, we have adopted the following procedure over the years:

Initial inquiries usually are by correspondence. A letter goes out describing in a general way the program of the agency, emphasizing the goals of the program, its lodgement in the public service sector, and making clear that a process must be gone through before a decision may be reached about the employability of the specific individual. It is made clear in subsequent contacts that the decision that must be made is not simply whether the individual is a competent practitioner in his own particular discipline, but whether his unique combination of professional training, personality skills, motivations and interest are optimal for a vacant position within the mental health center. Every attempt is made, then, to stress that personnel selection is highly individualized, but operates within the context of choosing people for a public service agency. People are not employed to *do their own thing*. Rather, they are employed to be part of a complex social organization, because it is believed that they have a contribution to make to the work of that organization. We also make it clear that no one is employed on the basis of correspondence alone. Each applicant is expected to spend at least one day, and for those applying for more senior positions, two days, in being interviewed by and interviewing a representative cross-section of staff in the agency. Each interviewer is asked for his impression of the personal and professional strengths and weaknesses of the applicant, and is asked to assess the desirability of his employment. In general, the staff consensus has been quite high. While no one of us can say what attributes are required to function successfully in a community mental health program, an operational agreement does seem to have developed. It seems clear that energy, ideological commitment, personal effectiveness, and a high tolerance for ambiguity are some of the attributes that are identified by our staff as being necessary for work in our particular setting. We also make it clear that we expect the applicant to be trying to decide whether he wants to work in an agency like ours, with the kind of people that work there. This establishes the expectation that he is making a commitment to adapt himself to our existing social structure, and that he is not coming as a saviour or reformer.

The final decision concerning selection and employment rests with the management of the mental health center. Very rarely, the consensus of the group of interviewers will be overruled by management. Management also reserves the decision as to the assignment of the individual. We have agreed as an operating principle, however, never to assign an individual to an existing functional unit without the concurrence of the element leader. Likewise, we have agreed to give greater weight to the evaluation of the applicant's professional peers—that is, psychologists have a greater voice in determining the suitability of a psychologist, nurses in determining suitability of nurses, and so forth—in the decision about hiring.

During a recent period of rapid expansion, with massive Model Cities funding, these personnel selection procedures broke down. Individuals did not understand clearly the social contract being established between them and the mental health center. They did not understand what tasks they were to perform, and on what criteria they were to be judged. Insufficient attention was given to the suitability of the individuals for the tasks assigned. There was no systematic attention to attempting to compose new functional units with a combination of personality attributes that make successful work group coalescence likely. We have paid the price for this breakdown in great functional inefficiency, distorted and impaired communication, the development of paranoid sub-cliques, and general social turmoil.

Evaluation of Employees

The employee performance report is an instrument of personnel management. It is an important tool, but one which characteristically is disliked and disparaged by mental health professionals. This is often justified by the inapplicability of the employee performance forms that are utilized by personnel systems. The employment performance form should allow the supervisor to rate relevant areas of performance—such as responsibility for patients and clinical competence—rather than irrelevant areas—such as care of equipment and observance of safety rules. The importance of the personnel employee report must be demonstrated by the chief executive of the mental health agency, as he prepares and discusses these reports with his immediate subordinates. Despite a facade that often suggests the contrary, the typical mental health professional is intensely needy for approval, recognition, affection, and reward. This should not be underestimated, and if financial incentives are either not available nor utilized, it should be recognized that the employee performance report is a very valuable tool in rewarding effective behavior within the agency, and to some extent in punishing undesirable behavior.

A successful agency administrator must be prepared to discharge personnel. Within formal civil service systems, this is usually effected most easily during the probationary period, which customarily lasts for six months. Good personnel practice should make certain that there is a careful review of the performance of the new employee prior to the end of the probationary period, and if there is any question the probationary period should be extended. The administrator often fears the negative reaction of the staff if he discharges an ineffective employee. He should be more concerned instead about the lowering of morale and decreasing effectiveness of other personnel, if he allows an inadequate employee to continue on the payroll. There is no question that, over time, the maintenance of ineffective employees will lower the productivity of their colleagues. To some extent, small group organization makes the administrator's task more simple, since the group often exerts strong pressure on the underachieving worker; and if this is unsuccessful, the group frequently demands of the chief executive that the individual be discharged.

Policies and Procedures

Written personnel policies are often determined by the superordinate agency in which the mental health enterprise is lodged. The development of additional policies governing operations of the agency, and the development of procedure books, are of questionable usefulness. In settings where decisions must be made by persons with limited experience or minimal training, it seems clear that there is need for procedures to be written and to be readily available. However, there is an inexorable accretion of policies and procedures accumulated over the years, which come to have the force, first, of tradition, and then of immutable law. If management is to rely upon policies and procedures to govern the functioning of elements and personnel, there must be a representative and responsible system for the development of these policies and procedures; and this system must also regularly review, modify, and discard policies that become restrictive and impair the attainment of superordinate goals, rather than facilitating them.

Supervisory Practices

In maintaining high levels of ego-involvement and communication, it is important that the differences between supervision, consultation, and collaboration are recognized. In the case of fully trained and qualified professional persons, the concept of supervision has no relevance and should be abandoned. In reality, more effective quality control can usually be maintained by making consultation available, than by imposing supervision. This attitude of being a consultant and a collaborator, a peer rather than a superior, must be established by the top leadership of the mental health undertaking, so that it will be reflected at every level. The attitude that we all make mistakes, but that every person is responsible for continually improving the effectiveness of his professional or non-professional role, must be communicated verbally and non-verbally at every level of leadership. Collaborative undertakings, in which senior staff are willing to have their own inadequacies revealed to junior colleagues, are particularly important in developing this attitude of tolerance. If one adopts the idea that the administration should function as a super-ego, constantly criticizing and correcting the work of subordinates, a peculiar and disabling sickness afflicts the agency. In order to avoid failure, clinicians will avoid the most difficult cases, and will place heavy emphasis on *screening out unsuitable candidates* for therapy. By doing so, they will unconsciously be attempting to protect themselves from the criticism of their supervisors. Such an approach has no social utility, and should be eschewed.

There would appear to be a consensus among successful mental health administrators that an authoritarian administrative style does not optimally serve the superordinate goals of mental health agencies. There is less consensus as to the most successful alternatives to an authoritarian, stratified, hierarchical system of organization. What one mental health leader sees as democracy, might seem to another a rule of the proletariat, and be viewed by a third as anarchy. The basic goal is to optimize ego-involvement on the part of the staff, by insuring their participation in decision-making that affects their personal and professional futures, and the futures of their clients or prospective clients. It is not rational to insist that every staff member, regardless of training, competence, or prior experience, should be allowed to cast a vote on every management decision. It remains the proper responsibility and legitimate exercise of authority for the manager or director of a mental health agency to make decisions affecting the course of that agency, or determining its goals, policies, and procedures.

In this process, the wise and effective administrator will seek, weigh, and utilize the knowledge, experience, opinions, and recommendations of staff members. The leader will inevitably make decisions as to which staff members' opinions have the greatest relevance and validity; and in making these decisions, he will be vulnerable to all the hazards of personal preference, comfort-seeking, and idiosyncratic need-gratification. In consequence, if he is to maintain objectivity, he must also receive the opinions of representatives chosen by the staff through a democratic process, and not chosen or appointed by the administrator.

Role expansion is also an excellent way of increasing the ego-involvement of staff members who characteristically have held a lower status. Role expansion increases certain types of conflict, as the traditional professional boundaries are invaded by other professions or non-professional persons. This increases the importance of developing conflict resolution mechanisms, in order to prevent a decrease in staff effectiveness as a result of bickering and clique formation. The basic tool for conflict resolution is the same as that for effective family therapy: discussion between all involved participants, with the assistance of a non-judgmental and empathic person. To the extent the need for role expansion is clearly communicated and linked to the superordinate goals of the agency; to the extent that roles are expanded, rather than being diffused or blurred; to the extent that new gratifications are given professionals displaced from prior exclusive role functionings—conflict resolution will be less necessary.

However, it is the responsibility of the leader to make decisions, where they cannot be arrived at by consensus. The avoidance of authoritative decision-making when attempts to resolve difficulties by improved communication and the development of compromise or consensus have failed, can be extremely destructive to the functioning of the agency and to the credibility of the leader.

In a mental health agency, the conventional management tool of promotions and salary increases to shape the behavior of staff, become relatively less important. Punishments are particularly ineffective with mental health staff, and simply guarantee the increase of negativism and obstructionism on the part of affected personnel. The use of the positive rewards of recognition, status, and exceptional ability salary increases, hold far greater promise for increasing goal-synergistic behavior.

The Denver Experience

The author of this chapter writes from his experience for the last five-and-one-half years in the development and operation of a comprehensive community mental health center lodged in an urban department of health and hospitals. Our personnel management system has developed by trial and error, over time, and functions reasonably well. Some of the relevant mechanisms would perhaps bear some discussion:

The staff is formally organized in a number of ways. The medical staff, which includes Ph.D. psychologists, is composed as directed by the Joint Committee on Accreditation of Hospitals, since our mental health center is lodged in a department of health and hospitals, which includes a general hospital. The medical staff group provides a mechanism for professional monitoring of quality of patient care. Monthly departmental staff meetings are required, where the clinical work of the Division of Psychiatry is reviewed in a formal fashion. Members of the medical staff also participate in committee responsibilities of the general medical staff, including the Records and Audit Committee which examines each month a sample of clinical records and reports to the medical staff and to the operating units concerning the adequacy of these records; the Mortality and Morbidity Committee which reviews any suicides or other deaths, and any instances of unusual morbidity, and reports to the psychiatric staff at its monthly meeting; and the Psychiatric Training Committee which supervises and reports on the Psychiatric Internship and Residency Program operated by the Division of Psychiatric Services.

Each professional discipline has its own staff group, organized with a varying degree of formality. These groups meet at varying intervals: psychologists meet once a week, as do social workers; nurses meet approximately once a month, and psychiatrists meet at irregular intervals, usually every three or four months. The disciplinary groups consider matters of special relevance for the profession involved. The elected chairman of each group serves as an advocate for whatever vested interests may exist. The groups serve as an institutionalized affirmation that role expansion does not lead to dissolution or derogation of existing professional specialization.

There are a number of on-going groups that function as standing committees, in such areas as school liaison, training and education, volunteer services, etc. These committees serve as communication mechanisms around special interests of various staff members and also present recommendations to the management concerning needed programs, modifications, and so forth.

The formal management is structured by City Career Service as essentially a pyramidal, hierarchical, authoritarian system. However, mechanisms have been developed for insuring active staff participation:

The Management Advisory Committee meets each week to discuss and consult with the management of the mental health center concerning important program issues. The Management Advisory Committee consists of element and program leaders, and hence in itself represents and partly reaffirms the hierarchical structure of the organization.

In order to insure more genuine staff participation in important issues, the Management Advisory Committee appoints *ad hoc* study groups as special areas of concern come up. These study groups include members of the Management Advisory Committee (who are middle management) , and representatives from a

cross-section of affected elements, in order to assure wide disciplinary and status representation as well as provide needed special
competencies.

At least monthly, there is a general staff meeting, which has
an agenda partly structured by management, and partly open for
general staff discussion. During times of crisis, the frequency and
intensity of these general staff meetings increases, as a broad base
of staff understanding, participation, and assistance is sought.

Staff development activities have particular importance in any
mental health agency, and certainly in the Denver General Hospital Community Mental Health Center. Such activities not only
meet the personal and professional needs of individual staff
members, but also serve as a valuable mechanism to break down
boundaries between professions and between operating units and
cliques, through promoting communication and mutuality in
learning tasks. Attendance at special interest seminars is voluntary. Areas such as family therapy, child therapy, and mental
health consultation, have been foci of training groups lasting from
2 to 12 weeks. Special visitors from outside the agency are frequently utilized to give formal presentations and also to consult informally with small staff groups. This is a way of *repaying* staff for doing difficult work in the public sector, in a way that often has
greater meaning than financial rewards. Reimbursing staff for attendance at professional meetings and special institutes and
workshops also is a very important reward for behavior that advances superordinate goals of the agency. Joint publication ventures likewise have great value in increasing staff cohesiveness
and improving communication, as well as developing consensus
concerning means of pursuing superordinate goals.

Importantly, consultation services and community organization activities are a vital part of professional development. While
it is usually seen by the staff as being a service offered to other
agencies, the opportunity of meeting regularly with welfare
workers, visiting nurses, recreation workers, etc., has invaluable
educational benefit for the staff of the mental health center. It
offers the unique advantage of providing a learning experince in
which the staff member does not lose status by becoming a stu-

dent, but rather gains it by becoming a consultant. It provides real learning about the actual problems and concrete realities of the community, which after all any mental health endeavor is intended to address.

Leadership

Where does the leader fit into this complex social organization? Is there any role for leadership, if a democratic, consensual decision-making process exists? There is indeed. But there are many dilemmas.

The first, the whole issue of participatory democracy—such a hot and current topic in all social institutions at present—deserves some discussion. The staff of a mental health agency begins by occupying the psychological position that authoritarianism is bad. They tend to hold the conviction that participation is a transcendent good in itself, and that a democratic process is likely to bring positive moral good. There will be strong pressures from many staff, then, to expand the decision-making authority of both middle management and of the rank and file worker. The author of this chapter is in the midst of a very complex and troubling social process in his own agency, in which certain persuasive people within the staff have mounted considerable pressure to insist that all decisions must be made publicly, and that group process is inevitably more effective in arriving at decisions than might be the deliberations of a single individual.

Many decisions are fraught with pain and uncertainty. As an example, the leader must decide what course of action to take when there is evidence of failure of middle management personnel to achieve program goals. Let us say that a physician, a former alcoholic, has been chosen to develop an alcoholism treatment program in a mental health center. His dedication and vigor is without doubt, and his desire to do a good job is unquestioned. He is faced with great administrative problems within the agency, in terms of procuring needed facilities, resources, and personnel. Complex arrangements with other agencies such as the police and the courts must also be negotiated. In view of these mitigating circumstances, management does not become concerned about relative slowness in developing the program for several months time. However, it eventually becomes clear that the individual is not performing effectively in a leadership role. Attempts to modify his behavior result in alibis and evasions, coupled with evidence of mounting anxiety on a day-by-day basis. The program director must live with the clear certainty that continuing to increase pressure for performance on the individual is likely to result in a return of excessive drinking; on the other hand, his removal from the position is also likely to result in a return of symptomatic behavior. To allow him to continue unchanged in the position sacrifices vital program goals, and subjects other personnel to inadequate leadership. The comfort goal of the individual unit leader must, clearly, be sacrificed to the production goals of the agency.

As another example, a neighborhood mental health team undergoes a marked change in composition of personnel. Due to promotions and reassignments, the bulk of seasoned clinicians leave the team during a period of expansion, and are replaced by young professional personnel right out of training. The team leader continues to be an older professional person who has adapted well to the goals of a community mental health program, but yet continues to believe in the maintenance of professional supervision in order to insure quality of care. One of the holdover staff members, bitter because he has not been offered a team leadership position, begins to play upon the insecurities of the new staff members and to fan their anti-authoritarian attitudes. Over the objections of the team leader, the team decides that it is worthwhile to spend a considerable number of hours in order to have all team members trained in psychodrama. Similarly, there is the decision that the team should offer sensitivity training to the welfare workers, in lieu of mental health consultation. The team leader becomes progressively more uncertain, and begins to sense a loss of control and effective leadership capability over the team. The production goals of the team are clearly threatened as the team organizes to meet its own comfort goals, which have been rationalized and intellectualized. Again, the program director is faced with a delicate and painful problem, as he finds himself on the side of stability and control, in order to achieve the production goals of the agency. He also finds himself in the unpopular and uncomfortable position of being against *personal growth* and *self-realization* on the part of his staff members!

The leader's most important contribution is to help the staff articulate and reach agreement about the superordinate goals of the agency. The leader's role as an identity model for staff is irrefutable, even though many people in leadership positions are embarrassed when they hear their attitudes come out of the mouths of their staff, and see their characteristic behavior unconsciously mimicked by staff members. And yet it is a fact of life: when the leader grows a beard, beards sprout all over the place!

In all of the processes outlined above, the role of the leader in understanding the needs of the organization, and guiding social forces that bring about desired institutional processes is evident.

The leader is constantly caught between opposing goals. As mentioned, he must reconcile the comfort goals of the staff with the production goals of the community or funding agency. He must reconcile the antithetical goals of order versus freedom, of stability versus flexibility, of predictability versus creativity. He is the man in the middle, a conflict-resolver and problem-solver, continually compromising between the ideal and the feasible, continually espousing realism by living in the here-and-now while secretly harboring pessimism and cynical fears. It is these stresses that contribute to the pathology of leadership, resulting in rigidity, paranoid distrust, over-control, irrationality, and ineffectiveness.

The most important antidote for the development of such pathology of leadership is a social organization which allows the leader access to sufficiently valid, reliable information upon which to make his decisions. Many of the decisions of the leader are based on preconceived ideas stemming out of personal prejudice, prior experience, or ideological commitments. The effective leader must constantly attempt to add to these bases for decision-making rational, objective data. In this endeavor, a program evaluation operation is paramount. It is also important that the leader have direct access to an open communication between himself and a broad cross section of the staff, or the entire staff of the agency if this is feasible. To rely on intermediaries or informers exclusively, makes him vulnerable to misinterpretation and renders the system susceptible to the development of an informer or spy system.

The leader must constantly, through non-verbal and verbal behaviors, attempt to decrease status and hierarchy concerns, and increase task orientation. The mutual use of first names, an informal air, openness to comments and criticisms from the staff, participation in visible clinical and community service activities, a wide sharing of responsibility and authority—all are methods by which the leader can communicate his own personal value system, and put on display its effectiveness or ineffectiveness, so that the staff may judge whether to emulate or deviate from it.

Conflict Resolution

Within a complex mental health organization, many special groups have unique needs and pose special problems. The extreme competitiveness for status, and power hunger of psychiatrists is a problem which must be recognized and managed effectively. A cardinal rule of thumb should be that no part-time psychiatrist is given the directorship of any functional unit, in preference to a full-time member of any other professional group. To do so is to communicate a special value and status to the psychiatrist, which cannot help but be offensive and alienating to other staff members.

Psychologists, social workers, nurses, indigenous non-professionals, all have their special needs, pose their special problems, and offer their special contributions to an effective mental health program. The intent of this chapter does not allow a full exploration of all of these categories of personnel. However, the role of the secretary, who has great power in her lowly status, shoud receive brief comment. Too often, the secretary is left outside the flow of professional communication, support, and planning. To do so is unwise, for in most mental health agencies secretaries play crucial roles that determine not only the effectiveness of staff, but the effectiveness of the clinical program. Secretaries are required to answer questions and to respond behaviorly to a wide variety of patients and community representatives. If they are outside of the concerns and the social processes of the center, their behavior will be dilatory at best, surly and difficult at worst. The secretary must be included in planning, must receive rewards and recognition, and must be consciously included as a member of the professional team.

And finally, conflict resolution must be emphasized again, for this is an important function of the leader. The role can be performed successfully only if the leader recognizes that conflict is inevitable, often desirable, and will usually not simply *go away* or be resolved by itself. Just as conflict arises out of complex social processes, a social process to solve the conflict is necessary.

The exceptional conflict is centered between two individuals who have what is characteristically called a *personality difference*. These differences can usually be solved, or at least ameliorated, by discussion with both parties jointly. Or, in some instances one individual may decide to leave or will be asked to leave.

However, it should be recognized clearly that most such clashes between individuals are not true personality conflicts, but occur within a complex behavioral setting, and are usually only the overt manifestation of underlying social problems within the organization. It is all too easy, perhaps too tempting, to brush aside difficulties as based on individual personality clashes. The training of most mental health administrators and clinicians makes this a particularly tempting route to follow—but rarely a productive one. Just as difficulties between family members are usually indicative of breakdowns in communication and the existence of covert struggles which are expressed symptomatically in open conflict, so difficulties between staff members must be analyzed carefully within the context of organizational reality.

From this point of view a complex decision-making process must be undertaken which does not differ greatly from the diagnostic appraisal of family problems. The intrapsychic needs and conflicts of individual protagonists will, in such an analysis, emerge as much less important than the situational and interpersonal stresses, supports, and conflicts which play upon the individuals as they perform their day-by-day, demanding work as mental health personnel. Similarly, a plan for resolving such problems must look towards opening up communication between all of the affected individuals—which usually extends far beyond the two in overt conflict and to facilitate the exposure of unconscious or preconscious themes or aspirations. Conflict resolution should provide not only a medium for such discussion, but should also look to the reduction of situational stresses and the increase of situational supports. In such an endeavor, the understanding and cooperation of a significant number of staff personnel, at various levels in the administrative hierarchy, is usually required if a lasting solution which truly increases operational effectiveness is to be achieved.

A Point of View

It is clear from this discussion that the author believes firmly that administration is not a *technique* which can be *applied* to any system indiscriminately. An excellent administrator for a labor union may prove disastrous for a mental health operation; and the difficulty that medical and hospital administrators display in grasping the essential differences—both in problems and potential—of the mental health system is well known and frequently redemonstrated. However, the mental health professional has no inherent or divine right to administer a mental health program. If he wishes to do so, he must obtain the commensurate education and supervised experience in order to prepare himself for the task. To this end, there should and almost certainly will be expansion of programs to train the various mental health professionals in mental health administration, or else systems which stress parallel *professional* and *administrative* direction will certainly become the norm. The experience in the state hospitals in the past century would indicate that this has most undesirable consequences, as business and political goals take transcendence over patient and professional goals. Mental health agencies can be best administered by competent mental health professionals with special training and experience in administrative theory and practice. Nowhere is this more evident than in personnel management, upon which the success of the entire mental health program rests.

REFERENCES

Berlin, I. N.: Resistance to change in mental health professionals. *Am J Orthopsychiatry, 39*:109-115, 1969.

Brown, B. S. and Ishiyama, T.: The role of leaders in normal staff process. *Compr Psychiatry, 8*:217-226, 1967.

Glasscote, R. M., *et al.: The Staff of the Mental Health Center.* Washington, Joint Information Service, 1969.

Grunebaum, H., (Ed.) : *The Practice of Community Mental Health.* Boston, Little, Brown, 1970.

Maier, Norman R.: Assets and liabilities in group problem solving: The need for an integrative functioning. *Psychol Rev, 74*:239-248, 1967.

Reiff, R. and Riessman, F.: The indigenous nonprofessional: A strategy of change in community mental health programs. *Community Mental Health Journal,* Monograph No. 1, 1965.

Whittington, H. G.: *Psychiatry in the American Community.* New York, International Universities Press, 1966.

Whittington, H. G. (Ed.) : *The Development of an Urban Mental Health Center.* Springfield, Thomas, 1971.

CHAPTER 4

FINANCING MENTAL HEALTH SERVICES

ERNEST C. HARVEY

TRADITIONALLY IN THIS COUNTRY, the costs of providing mental health services have been borne primarily by the public sector. This is in sharp contrast to other areas of health care where government involvement has been quite limited. It has been estimated, for example, that only about 20 percent of all personal health care expenditures, including the military, are publicly financed; on the other hand, the comparable figure for mental health services is about 70 percent (Atwell, 1964).

There are many reasons for this extensive public involvement in the financing of mental health services. The most important of these appears to be cost, both to the individual and to society, as well as public attitudes toward the mentally ill. With respect to the individual, not only are expenditures for treatment burdensome but, if he is a wage earner, there is likely to be a considerable loss of income. Costs to society are multiple, reflecting an impact on the private sector in the form of loss of productivity, inefficiency, labor turnover, accidents, etc., and on various levels of government in the form of increased expenditures for social welfare, public protection, and other programs. Furthermore, the traditional rejection of the mentally ill by society stimulated the construction of large, expensive public institutions located some distance away from urban areas.

Limited data are available on the costs of mental illness in the United States. Annual expenditures for treatment have been estimated to range from $3.0 to $6.0 billion; loss of earnings to the mentally ill may exceed $1.5 billion annually; and the cost of mental illness to industry has been estimated at $3.0 to $10.0 billion annually. These estimates are very rough because of the difficulties in developing a rigorous definition of mental illness and in collecting uniform data. But, despite this lack of precision, the magnitude has been sufficient to encourage considerable public support for remedial programs, particularly programs more responsive to individual needs than those in the past.

In response to this support and federal efforts to speed the process, major changes have occurred during the past decade in treatment techniques and approaches to the delivery of services, particularly the development of community mental health programs. Sources of funding have also changed, although public support remains significant. This chapter is concerned primarily with the changing character of financial support and the resulting administrative problems in the context of today's approach to the delivery of mental health care. The chapter is divided into three sections. The first section provides historical information on the shifts that have occurred in the sources of financial support for mental health services. The second section discusses current funding characteristics, with emphasis on the funding of community mental health centers, and the last section concentrates on the administrative implications of these shifts in support.

SHIFTING SOURCES OF SUPPORT

The Early Years

Data on the sources of funds for mental health services have not been collected on a routine basis. A rough indication of the major shifts in support, however, can be provided by comparing the current pattern with that characterizing the early 1960's, before the enactment of Medicare and Medicaid and before major direct federal involvement in financing community mental health services.

Data for 1961-62 indicate that state and local government expenditures for mental health services totalled nearly $1.1 billion, with more than 90 percent going to public mental hospitals (U.S. Senate, 1963). Only $87 million was spent for community services, with 50 percent of that amount expended by three states (New York, California, and Illinois).

Most of the expenditures for mental health at that time were made by the states, since public mental health hospitals were for the most part state institutions and only twelve states required county contributions toward the cost of care provided their residents. Amounts spent varied widely among states, ranging from about 1 to 7 percent of total general fund revenues.

These expenditures included some private funds since many states levied charges on patients or their families. Policies regarding these charges varied widely among states as to the definition of responsible relatives, the maximum permissible charge, and the procedures for relating to the economic circumstances of the patient or his family. In many states, these charges did not appear as current receipts since they were allowed to accumulate as legal claims against the estate of the patient and frequently the estates of liable relatives.

In view of this extreme variability and the practice of accounting for these receipts as increments to the general fund rather than as offsets to program expenditures, the extent of the charges for service is unknown. It is estimated, however, that on the average less than 10 percent of the cost was reimbursed by patients or their relatives (Follman, 1970).

In addition to the $1.1 billion expenditure by state and local government, the federal government spent approximately $400 million in 1961-62. These funds were not generally available, however, since they were allocated primarily to specialized groups such as the Armed Forces, veterans, and federal prisoners.

Funds were also made available by the public sector for care of the mentally retarded and for special groups such as welfare recipients and school children. Most of the care for the mentally retarded, amounting to some $600 million annually, was provided in state and local institutions. Expenditures through school systems and public assistance programs were highly variable both among and within states; data are not available to indicate their magnitude but they are judged to have been relatively insignificant in the aggregate.

Expenditures by the private sector for treatment of mental disorders were estimated at about $220 million in 1960, (Follman, 1970), distributed roughly as follows:

	$ Millions
Private outpatient services	$100
Private psychiatric hospitals	79
Psychiatric care in general hospitals	40
Foundations	2
	$221

Sources of funds for these expenditures were principally from patients and their families, private insurance, and philanthropic contributions. The relative magnitude of these sources is not known either for the current time period or for the early 1960's. Then as now, private voluntary agencies providing mental health services were financed in part by philanthropic contributions but also by fees. Some labor unions had their own treatment facilities or negotiated insurance coverage for their members; a few employers also provided such coverage. But the comprehensiveness of this coverage or of that provided by private health insurance was highly variable, and the extent to which patients' or relatives' income and resources were required to make up the deficit is not known.

Given the hazards involved in analyzing the sources of funds for mental health services in the early 1960's, the following constitutes only a rough order-of-magnitude estimate:

	$ Billions
Public sector	
Federal	$0.4
State-local	1.0
Private Sector	
Payments to private sector	0.2
Payments to public sector*	0.1
Total	$1.7

*Payments by patients or their families for care provided in public facilities.

The New Emphasis

A number of new programs were initiated by Congressional action during the 1960's, each with a significant impact on the financing of mental health services. These included legislation making federal funds available for construction of community mental health centers (1963) and for staffing these centers (1965). In addition, the Medicare and Medicaid programs were enacted in 1965 as were the OEO and Model Cities programs.

President Kennedy's message to Congress in 1963 outlined a new federal approach to mental health services oriented toward the provision of services at the local level through community mental health centers. This new approach included a financing concept that extended beyond the use of government funds (Congressional Record, 1963).

> The services provided by these centers should be financed in the same way as other medical and hospital costs. . . Individual fees for service, individual and group insurance, other third-party payments, voluntary and private contributions, and state and local aid can now bear the continuing burden of these costs to the individual patient after these services are established. The success of this pattern of local and private financing will depend in large part upon the development of appropriate arrangements for health insurance, particularly in the private sector of our economy. Recent studies have indicated that mental health care—particularly the cost of diagnosis and short-term therapy, which would be major components of service in the new centers—is insurable at a moderate cost.

Although the financing concept as outlined above suggested that heavy private sector involvement was essential to the ultimate success of the new program, it was recognized in both the 1963 and the 1965 legislation that a high level of federal participation would be required to get the centers under way.

The 1965 legislation that provided for staffing grants, authorized federal support not exceeding 75 percent of eligible staff costs in the first fifteen months of operation, 60 percent in the next twelve months, 45 percent in the next, and 30 percent in the final year; a total period of fifty-one months. It is clear that the intent of Congress was to provide seed money to stimulate the initiation of centers that would, in a relatively short period of time, be supported entirely by funds from state and local governments and from the private sector. There had been considerable discussion of the need for staffing grants in 1963 when the community mental health centers construction legislation was authorized. Provision for such grants was made in the original legislation but was deleted in the final version.*

Current Patterns of Funding

Early analyses of the financial implications of the new program, however, cast considerable doubt on the ability of state and local governments and the private sector to provide adequate funding. It was estimated that construction expenditures of $1.3 billion would be required for a program consisting of one center for each 200,000 people (at an estimated construction cost of $1.3 million per center) (Connery, 1968). Since the average catchment area was likely to include less than 200,000 people,* a larger sum would result if a construction expenditure of this amount were required in every catchment area. On the other hand, to the extent that centers could be formed around existing agencies construction expenditure could be dispensed with or limited to renovations. It was apparent to those analyzing the new program, however, that large capital expenditures would be required for nationwide implementation.

Staffing costs were expected to constitute a more serious problem. A 1965 estimate placed them at $600,000 for a center serving 100,000 people, or about $1.2 billion annually, all but equal to the once-and-for all construction costs, if nationwide coverage were assumed. Serious doubts were raised regarding the likelihood that new revenues of this magnitude could be generated at the state and local level, particularly since this emphasis constituted a reversal of the general trend toward increased federal support of state and local programs that has become evident in recent years. The above estimate made no allowance for transfers of funds from other mental health programs, particularly from state

---

*See Robert H. Connery *et al., The Politics of Mental Health,* Columbia University Press, N.Y., 1968, for a discussion of the events leading to this new federal approach.
*The law provides for a range of 75,000 to 200,000 population.

hospitals, that could be expected if the community mental health program were successful. It was apparently assumed that the increased emphasis on outpatient and consultation and education services and the community orientation of the program would require significant infusions of new money.

What has in fact happened since the inception of the program? How rapidly have centers been established under the impetus provided by the federal government? How successful have those established been in adjusting to the decline in federal support?

As was indicated earlier, virtually no current data are available on private sector expenditures for mental health services. It would appear, however, that the bulk of such expenditures, as in the early 1960's, is for private psychiatric treatment, largely ambulatory, and for the care in nonpublic hospitals; the importance of general hospitals in the provision of such care is estimated to have increased (Follman, 1970).

Public expenditures for these services are estimated to have increased significantly during the 1960's, as shown in Table 4-I.

TABLE 4-1

ESTIMATED DISTRIBUTION OF PUBLIC EXPENDITURES FOR MENTAL HEALTH SERVICES

(Dollar amounts in thousands)

Public Expenditure Source	1960 Amount	1960 Percent	1968 Amount	1968 Percent
NIMH	$ 4,911	0.4	$ 49,336	2.0
Other federal	371,810	27.9	781,016	31.9
Public health service (ex. NIMH)	24,760	1.9	13,155	0.5
SSA (Medicare)	*	—	36,947	1.5
SRS	*	—	269,681	11.0
VA	320,888	24.0	385,983	15.8
Dept. of Defense	25,000	1.9	60,873	2.5
Justice Dept.	1,162	0.1	4,797	0.2
Federal other	—	—	9,580	0.4
Total federal	376,721	28.3	830,352	33.9
State and local	958,077	71.7	1,616,960	66.1
Total	$1,334,798	100.0	$2,447,312	100.0

*Not applicable
Source: NIMH

Total expenditures rose from $1.3 billion to $2.4 billion between 1960 and 1968, or 83 percent. In absolute terms, the increase in state and local expenditures was larger than that for the federal government in spite of the introduction of new federal programs such as Medicare, Medicaid, and the NIMH Community Mental Health Centers Program. However, in relative terms, state and local expenditures declined (from 72 to 66 percent of the total) while federal expenditures increased (from 28 to 34 percent).

It is not possible to estimate precisely the proportion of public expenditures allocated to the provision of community mental health services. Most of the ten-fold increase in NIMH expenditures represented such an allocation of funds as did some of the increase in other federal spending. State and local expenditures for this purposes have also increased, and in some states the number of state hospitals has declined as community services expanded. In 1970, about $188 million of public funds (including Medicare and Medicaid) were received by community mental health centers, probably amounting to 10 percent of total public expenditures for mental health services (see Table 4-II).

It is clear that the federal program stimulated considerable expansion of community mental health services. As of June 30, 1971, 452 centers had been funded, and over 300 were in operation; the catchment areas served by the operational centers included about 30 percent of the United States population. Although the revenue sources of these centers are diverse, government has remained the principal source of funding. Nearly 75 percent of total receipts consisted of direct government payments, largely for operating purposes; about 6 percent constituted Medicare and Medicaid payments; and some portion of other receipts from services would be transfers from units of government such as school districts, welfare departments, or other agencies.

The average data presented in Table 4-II mask wide interstate variations in the significance of the major sources of revenue, as indicated by Table 4-III.* In the case of federal staffing grants, the variation was from 8.5 to 63.5 percent; with respect to other sup-

---

*These data are based on a detailed analysis of information provided for 1969 by 172 centers; since this is not a statistical sample the percentages should be regarded only as indicative of the variation.

TABLE 4-II

ESTIMATED ANNUAL RECEIPTS DURING THE YEAR BY SOURCE
FEDERALLY FUNDED COMMUNITY MENTAL HEALTH CENTERS
UNITED STATES, 1970

Source of Funds	Amount	Percent
Total government funds	$175,066,819	73.6%
Federal funds	71,323,622	29.7
Federal staffing grants (PL 89-105)	55,440,303	23.1
Federal construction grants (PL 88-164)	7,782,846	3.3
Federal research and training funds	5,672,454	2.4
Other federal funds	2,428,019	1.0
State funds	76,242,813	32.5
Local government funds	25,381,508	10.5
Other government funds	2,118,876	0.9
Total receipts from services	54,569,157	23.0
Patient fees	18,724,154	7.9
Insurance (private and voluntary)	15,588,669	6.4
Medicare	4,049,480	1.7
Medicaid	8,940,893	3.9
Other receipts from services	7,265,961	3.2
Fund raising (campaigns, foundations, United Funds, gifts, etc.)	5,527,485	2.2
Other receipts	2,847,319	1.2
Total receipts from all sources	$238,010,780	100.0%

Source: NIMH

port, there was at least one state in which centers received no support from each of the listed sources. Even wider variation was observed in a study of funding sources of individual centers that was completed in 1970 (Harvey, 1970).

This study, which was funded by NIMH to ascertain the success of centers in obtaining funding to replace federal staffing grant support, indicated that, in general, the early centers had experienced considerable difficulty in moving towards the financing concept outlined in President Kennedy's 1963 message to Congress. Several had reached the point of operating virtually on a day-to-day basis, and others were considering significant program modifications. In view of the importance of the shift toward provision of mental health services on a community basis and the complex and variable funding characteristics of the program, a more detailed analysis of the financial experiences of the early

TABLE 4-III
VARIATION IN FUNDING SOURCES OF 172 COMMUNITY MENTAL
HEALTH CENTERS, 1969

Source	Range of Percent by State
Government	37.6 - 100.0%
Federal staffing	8.5 - 63.5
State	0.0 - 84.1
Local	0.0 - 59.5
Other federal	0.0 - 50.8
Other government	0.0 - 9.6
Fees and third party payments	0.0 - 62.4
Patient fees and insurance	0.0 - 54.5
Medicare and Medicaid	0.0 - 26.3
Other	0.0 - 13.6
Philanthropy	0.0 - 21.6
Other	0.0 - 31.3

Source: Computed from data provided by NIMH

centers is presented in the next section as background for a discussion of administrative implications.

The Experiences of Early Centers

The general characteristics of centers providing the basis for the analyses in this section are sumarized in Table 4-IV. Services were provided under a variety of auspices to populations ranging from rural to inner city. Program size varied from $0.2 to $3.5 million. As indicated in the table, these centers were established early in the program; most of them were breaking new ground and many faced problems that might not be replicated in newer centers.

However, a number of general insights can be obtained from an examination of the approaches used by the various center administrators to the problem of declining federal support, and of the factors limiting flexibility in financing. One of the difficulties experienced in conducting the study is indicative of a major financial problem as well: specific and precise data on sources of funds were not available from most centers. In general, account-

TABLE 4-IV

LOCATION AND GENERAL CHARACTERISTICS OF COMMUNITY
MENTAL HEALTH CENTERS INCLUDED IN THE SAMPLE

Center	Auspices	Type of Catchment Area*	Initial Staffing Grant Date of Award	Amount†	Estimated Size of Total Program FY 70 (millions of dollars)
1	Private	U,S,R,	1/67	$103,888	$0.3
2	Private	U,S,R,	9/66	148,014	0.6
3	County	U,S	8/66	136,575	2.0
4	City	I	8/66	140,350	1.2‡
5	§	U,S,R,	9/66	198,702	0.6
6	Private	U,S	2/67	113,314	0.2‡
7	State	U,S	8/66	510,080	1.0‡
8	Private	I,S	3/67	552,370	2.0
9	State	I	9/66	419,418	**
10	County	U,S,R	3/67	104,115	1.5
11	City	I	1/67	598,265	3.5
12	Private	I,S	1/67	285,499	1.6
13	††	U,S,R	8/66	51,249	0.2
14	Private	I	1/67	849,329	1.5
15	Private	I	9/66	718,826	0.6‡
16	Private	R	9/66	210,161	0.3

*Population served classified as follows: I,Inner City; S, Suburban; U, Urban; R, Rural.
†Includes first year supplements.
‡FY69
§Quasi-government: operated by an incorporated regional mental health-mental retardation board.
**This center serves as a state-designated catchment area of 31 counties; total program expenditures approximate $6.2 million. Estimates of expenditures in the catchment area covered by the staffing grant are not available.
††Quasi-government: operated jointly by the governing bodies of the catchment area counties through an appointive board of directors.

ing procedures were inadequate and there was an absence of financial planning beyond the next budget period.

Cost accounting systems appeared to be virtually nonexistent. In some cases, even relatively simple accounting techniques were not employed or were employed by only some of the units making up the center.* This lack of financial data is due largely to

*It should be pointed out that inadequate accounting systems are not limited to community mental health centers but characterize the medical care system in general.

the innovative character of the program and the associated problems of organization, administration, and recruiting. The initial emphasis was placed on program establishment; long range financial problems were regarded as secondary. By the time of the survey (third grant year), many of the organizational problems had been resolved and funding had become a critical issue.

PRINCIPAL FUNDING SOURCES FOR COMMUNITY MENTAL HEALTH CENTERS

Federal Support

NIMH Staffing Grants

In the third year of the original staffing grant, most of the centers in the study continued to depend heavily on federal support. Twelve of the sixteen centers surveyed received 20 percent or more of their revenues from this source and for six, the staffing grant constituted more than 40 percent of total revenues. Eleven centers received supplemental grants during their first three years of operation, and seven centers received growth grants.* At the time of the study, applications for growth grants had been made by three other centers. Additional funding, particularly in the form of growth grants, tended to postpone the effects of declining staffing grants. This factor helped contribute to the lack of long range financial planning that characterized most of the centers visited.

The federal staffing grant program imposes a number of specific requirements, several of which have significant financial implications. In the first place, matching funds sufficient to support a program consisting of at least five basic services must be provided, with prospects of rapid expansion to replace declining federal grants. To maximize the input of federal funds, therefore, rapid organization and staffing are necessary. Many of the centers studied were overly optimistic and lacked the administrative experience to organize rapidly. Since they were not able to expand as rapidly as expected, many received only a fraction of their

---

*Supplemental grants are available to cover additional positions within an existing program; growth grants cover staffing of new program activities.

grant entitlement during the first year; some had not fully used their staffing grants by the fourth grant year.

For some areas, the federal requirement that all five basic services be provided as a condition for receiving a grant may inhibit the extension of services to other catchment areas not already covered. The limited evidence suggests that this problem is likely to be most acute in densely populated urban regions where complete coverage by a comprehensive center for every area of 200,000 persons would overtax available financial resources. As indicated earlier, federal policy at the beginning of the program was to stimulate the rapid establishment of centers. Once several centers were established in urban areas, it may become increasingly difficult, because of funding requirements and the availability of qualified staff, to develop new centers in adjacent areas. Current policy is to support a relatively slow growth of services, and the Community Mental Health Centers Amendments of 1970 provide for phase-in of two of the five essential services over an 18-month period in poverty areas. Implementation of this policy should reduce, though not eliminate, this impact of the federal requirement.

A related aspect of the federal legislation that may aggravate financial problems is the definition of catchment area size, particularly the upper limit of 200,000 population. This maximum is said to have made the provision of services in some areas extremely difficult, even though exceptions to the maximum are permitted and centers are in any event not restricted to serving people only from their own catchment areas.

This problem also appears to be acute in high density urban areas where general health services may have been provided traditionally to larger population units. Expansion of mental health services to adjoining catchment areas could well be more rapid and less costly if existing centers could form the nucleus for such growth. Where centers are associated with hospitals, for example, there may be natural ties with a relatively large population that might be of value in the development of mental health services in addition to reducing capital investment requirements and permitting some operating efficiencies. However, programmatic concerns about accessibility, accountability, quality of service, and other factors must be considered in addition to economics in assessing a modification of the current requirements. It would appear desirable to add some additional flexibility to the law subject to specific, clearly defined constraints.

Given the existing characteristics of the federal requirements, therefore, the principal financial task for a proposed new center is an adequate matching fund base capable of expansion within eight years (under the 1970 amendments) to a level sufficient to support the entire program. As indicated above, this period may be extended through the use of growth grants. This suggests an optimal growth policy, at least from the fiscal point of view. The policy would consist of a minimum initial program, expanded through the growth grant mechanism as community support builds up and incorporating, if appropriate, some program shifts in the process. Such a policy might not be completely responsive to community needs, at least initially, and would be quite time consuming, but may be necessary if financial resources are limited.

Other Federal Support

Funding for community mental health services is potentially available from a variety of other federal sources such as research and training grants, the OEO neighborhood health center program, the Model Cities Program, and the narcotics and alcoholism programs. The terms and conditions of these programs are highly variable and will not be discussed here. The centers studied made limited use of these programs, primarily because of their complex interrelationships and the need for most centers to place emphasis on organizational and program development problems before seeking other federal support. As would be expected, newly organized centers are less likely to be able to generate such support than are established centers.

Some research and training grants are available only to teaching institutions, and may not be available to a center even if it is affiliated with such an institution; however, the center may benefit from the services of staff supported by grants, however, other research and training grants, such as those provided by NIMH and certain of those provided by the Department of Labor, are available to centers that are sufficiently well established to use them effectively.

One of the centers surveyed had developed a joint program with the Model Cities agency in its catchment area: Model Cities support, however, was confined to the provision of facilities and provided no direct replacement for declining federal funds. Another center was working with an inner city OEO community health center; for this center too, there was little likelihood of obtaining direct financial support.

Federal grants are also available to support drug and alcoholism programs. One center was treating narcotics under three programs of the Narcotic Addict Rehabilitation Act. Under two of these programs, aftercare was provided to addicts who had received treatment at a federal treatment center. The third program involved participation in a 10-year demonstration program to reduce heroin addiction.

The Comprehensive Alcohol Abuse and Alcoholism Prevention, Treatment, and Rehabilitation Act of 1970 provides staffing grants for approved programs. Many centers in the study were already treating persons with alcohol problems as a part of their ongoing programs or were planning to undertake such treatment. These grants will permit more rapid expansion or establishment of alcoholism programs but are subject to the same problem as the community mental health center staffing grants (need for matching funds initially and ability to generate nonfederal support for the program over a relatively short period). In some areas, treatment centers will be established as entities separate from the mental health center; in other areas, alcoholism treatment will be provided as a program within the center. In neither of these situations will the additional funding provide significant relief to existing financial difficulties. On the other hand, where alcoholism grants function as growth grants, some temporary relief can be expected, though with limitations on overall program flexibility.

Given the variety of federal programs that might provide

funds directly or indirectly to community mental health centers, considerable grantsmanship ability on the part of the center director is required. Recent work by NIMH in identifying potential sources of funds and disseminating information on these sources and on procedures for qualifying for such support has reduced this burden somewhat. However, significant amounts of time and effort are still required to meet the myriad requirements of these programs.

State and Local Government Support

As was pointed out earlier, extreme variability characterized both state and local government support of the community mental health centers studied. Four of the 37 states for which funding information was available provided no support to community mental health centers; in one, neither state nor local support was provided. However, in 26 states, state support was larger than local support, generally by a large margin; in only 10 states was local support larger than state support. These variations reflect differences in political philosophy regarding the operation and financing of locally-provided services and differences in the extent to which public support has been generated.

State Support

In many states, funding of community mental health centers is based on legislation enacted specifically for that purpose. Several reimbursement approaches are employed: state sharing of a portion of net costs, i.e. costs after deduction of fees and third party payments, federal staffing grants, and other revenues; state share equal to a portion of total expenditures; and per capita allocation of the total amount appropriated by the legislature. In all cases, however, state support is subject to the appropriation of sufficient funds, and the amounts authorized in the legislation are not guaranteed. A number of states allocate funds to counties or county boards, which in turn allot funds to centers within their jurisdictions; centers typically operate under contract with these units of government. This practice is followed, for example, in California, Kentucky, Michigan, New York, Pennsylvania, and Texas.

Where legislation has not been enacted to provide specifically for support of community mental health centers, allocations may be made through the appropriate state department. Centers in Massachusetts and Missouri, for example, are operated by the state. State appropriations are made directly to centers in New Mexico, and emergency funds have been provided to at least one center in West Virginia.

In general, states have much broader tax bases than do local governments, encompassing personal income taxes, excise taxes, and a variety of business taxes.* Furthermore, the state has traditionally provided mental health services, and, fiscal problems aside, local governments have been slow to participate financially in mental health programs. As indicated above, therefore, many states have provided significant support to the community mental health program, and appropriations for this purpose have increased rapidly in the last four years. However, none of the states visited have attempted a detailed study of the long term cost implications of this program, and a number of them are already feeling the fiscal pressure. Most states are experiencing difficulties in meeting the demands of other social programs, particularly education, and are faced with taxpayer resistance to higher taxes; this resistance has reached the point of a *taxpayers' revolt* in several states.

In some states, legislative leaders indicated that mental health programs have reached a plateau in terms of popularity and that further increases in appropriations would require a clear demonstration of effectiveness. Federal matching programs, particularly seed money programs, are being viewed with increasing suspicion by state legislators, a number of whom made it clear that the legislature was under no obligation to provide additional program funds merely because federally supported programs, whether they are labelled as seed money programs, demonstration programs, or new approaches to specific problems, become entrenched and federal support declines. In general, this reaction was not so much a result of experiences with specific programs as a response to the

*Not all states levy an income tax; in these states, questions of equity of the tax burden as well as adequacy of revenue have arisen in recent years.

increasing size and complexity of federal grant-in-aid programs and the resulting requirements for matching funds.

The prospects for increased state support in the future are not clear. On the one hand, some states such as California and Michigan have increased the state contribution rate, while other states such as Arkansas and West Virginia have recently provided support for the first time.* On the other hand, a number of states have pressed for increased local government participation; both Kentucky and North Dakota, for example, have passed enabling legislation to permit local property tax levies earmarked for mental health. The trend in many states, even where state support of community mental health programs is significant, is to strengthen the role of local governments in decisions regarding the allocation of funds. Initial budget submissions by mental health directors, with supporting program justifications, are to these units of government. However, a broader justification effort is also required in support of increased state appropriations for community mental health generally.

Local Government Support

The role of local governments in financing the community mental health centers studied was minimal because their flexibility in tax matters has typically been limited by statutory or state constitutional restrictions and because mental health has traditionally been a state function. Most local governments rely largely on property taxes and state grants-in-aid for revenue. Frequently, these grants-in-aid are earmarked for such special functions as education, roads, or welfare and are, therefore, not available for general government purposes.

Potential revenue from property taxes varies widely among local jurisdictions, depending primarily on the concentration of economic activities and, therefore, of the property tax base. Low income areas served by many centers have low tax bases that offer little revenue potential. Other areas are at their legal limits and

---

*Although California law was amended in 1968 to increase the state participation rate from 75 to 90 percent of net costs, a requirement was included for counties to pick up 10 percent of the cost of their residents in state hospitals. In the case of West Virginia, state support was provided on an emergency basis.

either cannot raise tax rates or must seek voter approval for an increase. In recent years, considerable taxpayer resistance to increases in assessment levels and tax rates have developed, and many students of local government agree that there is little likelihood of a significant increase in revenue from this source as currently structured. They also agree that because of its inequity and administrative complexity, increased reliance should not be placed on the property tax unless major reforms of the state-local tax structure are instituted at the same time.

A number of states are taking steps to reduce the tax burden on property owners. These include statutory reductions in the tax (through, for example, homowners' exemptions or elimination of the tax on personal property) ; increased grant-in-aid payments to local governments; assumption by the state of financial responsibility for programs that have traditionally, at least in part, been a local responsibility (e.g., welfare) ; and expansion of the taxing power of local jurisdictions. These approaches generate varying impacts on the ability of local governments to support a new and expanding program. In some states, statutory reductions have been made in the property tax without the provision of off-setting revenues by the state, thus compounding the local revenue problem.

Expansion of local taxing power through the use of income, sales, or utility taxes has been most common in large urban areas. However, the social and economic problems facing these areas are of such magnitude that, even with the broader tax base, they have continued to experience considerable fiscal difficulty.

In general, there appears to be little short term potential for significantly increased support of community mental health services by local governments. The few examples of shifts in this direction do not reflect a general trend; in fact, studies designed to provide solutions to the fiscal problems of local governments are under way in many states. To the extent that a trend can be discerned at this point, it appears to be in the direction of assumption of increased fiscal responsibility by states.

But, as was indicated above, allocation decisions are the responsibility of local government in many states where significant state support is provided. Where formal procedures have been established, the director of a mental health agency has to deal with only one local unit of government. His program, in competition with other local programs, typically receives a tentative allocation, subject to the receipt of adequate state funds by the local government unit. Some centers claim to have fared worse under this arrangement than when negotiations were conducted directly with the responsible state agency. But this trend is likely to persist where extensive center development is anticipated and a philosophy of local control is followed.

In states where formal procedures of this type have not been developed and where catchment areas are geographically large, the mental health center executive must frequently deal with a number of governmental units: centers located in rural areas may serve as many as 10 counties. Not only is it difficult to design and implement a program for such a dispersed population, but budget preparation and support may be onerous. So long as financial contributions to the center from the various local units of government are small, essentially token support, pressure for extensive fiscal justifications is typically not great. But if the use of special local property tax levies for mental health increases, this burden can be expected to consume significant amounts of staff time.

Fees and Third Party Payments

Fees and third party payments were relatively more important to the centers in the study operated under private auspices than to the publicly operated centers. This resulted from several factors, including variations in the ability to pay of the population served, different operating policies, and program emphases.

Patient Fees and Insurance*

Many centers serve low income populations, a reflection of the high priority placed on such populations for the provision of com-

---

*For most centers it is not possible to provide separate estimates of patient fees and insurance receipts because insurance payments are made directly to the center in some cases and to patients in others.

munity mental health services. The majority of the patients in these centers cannot afford to pay for care, nor are they covered by private insurance. This is particularly true of centers serving inner city areas but also applies to centers serving rural areas as well. Even in the case of centers serving populations with widely varying income levels and insurance coverages, case loads tend to be concentrated in middle or low income groups because of either center policies or patient choice. Some centers refer patients who are able to pay to private practitioners; in other areas, high income persons choose not to use center services.

Several of the centers in the study, because of fiscal pressure, have significantly increased their receipts from patient fees by improving management procedures and employing the staff necessary to implement fee collection policies, to the extent, in a few cases, of using collection agencies. Other centers, because of staff attitudes or lack of incentive, have not actively pursued these revenues. Staff in a number of the centers apparently feel that an aggressive fee collection program is not appropriate for a center that receives significant government or philanthropic support or that serves an area of low income. This is reported also to be the reaction of the general public, although extensive surveys of public opinion on this issue apparently have not been conducted. Furthermore, there is little incentive to collect fees (or third party payments, for that matter) where the revenues accrue to the state or local general fund rather than to the center, as is the case for centers operated directly by the state or another government unit.

Private insurance constituted a significant revenue source for relatively few centers in the study. In general, such coverage is provided by insurance carriers for major employers or unions. For the most part, inpatient hospital services appear to be covered adequately by many insurance policies, but coverage for outpatient and partial hospitalization services typically is either limed, subject to a deductible provision, or nonexistent. Mental health professionals and insurance companies appear to be having difficulty reaching agreement on suitable definitions for these services and on safeguards against abuse. Difficulties have also arisen regarding use of fee schedules. Some centers bill patients (who are covered by insurance) the full amount so that an insurance payment will be made, but collect the deductible portion from the patient according to a fee schedule; the practice has been opposed by some carriers.

Given the fiscal philosophy underlying the Community Mental Health Centers Program, it behooves the mental health executive to make every effort to increase receipts from fees and third party sources. As a minimum, a fee collection policy should be adopted and appropriate fee collection mechanisms instituted. Where centers serve populations with some insurance coverage, attempts should be made to broaden this coverage, by its extension to such services as partial hospitalization or by negotiating a per capita form of prepayment.

The latter approach allows more flexibility in the use of funds by the center than does the standard approach, and may be a possibility in areas where large group coverages already exist. Some experimentation will be necessary, however, in view of the general lack of experience data sufficient to determine prepayment requirements. The role of prepayment mechanisms in the improvement of health care delivery systems is currently receiving widespread attention as a result of federal encouragement and support of the development of Health Maintenance Organizations. Where such innovative changes are under consideration, mental health executives should participate in organizational studies and should encourage the inclusion of mental health services within the HMO.*

Medicare and Medicaid

Most of the early centers in the study received no revenue from Medicare because of limitations in coverage and because major program efforts of centers have generally been directed at younger age groups. The limitations of Medicare coverage for mental health care have received considerable attention in recent

---

*Some philosophical differences of opinion between professionals engaged in community mental health and private practitioners may be expected; receptivity to inclusion of center-oriented services will vary widely from area to area.

years (President's Task Force on the Aging, 1970; U. S. Social Security Administration, 1971). Coverage of outpatient mental health services is extremely limited and, unless a center is affiliated with a general or psychiatric hospital, certification as a Medicare provider is virtually impossible. Furthermore, some centers regard the expansion of services to children and adolescents as a higher priority need than the development of programs for the elderly. Only one of the centers included in the study on which this section is based was considering a program effort directed specifically at persons in the over-65 age group: provision of mental health services to nursing homes.

Although Medicare as a source of funding support has some potential, it is of little help as a substitute for other funds in centers where the program emphasis has been on other age groups. Furthermore, unless coverage is broadened, it is unlikely that program priorities will be modified.

Medicaid receipts also were not important for most of the early centers both because of limitations in the coverage, which varies from state to state, and because of certification problems. A number of states do not provide coverage for services provided by community mental health centers, others limit coverage to hospitalization, and others cover only the categorically needy or persons aged 65 or over. Since Medicaid has turned out to be extremely costly, the trend in a number of states appears to be toward limitation rather than extension of coverage. In any event, there is a considerable reassessment of Medicaid programs under way at this point, and future prospects of revenue from this source or from a substitute program, if one is legislated, are uncertain.

Other Fees for Service

Fees for services provided to other agencies or organizations were important sources of revenue in only a few of the early centers. Vocational rehabilitation was an important revenue source for some centers; the school system typically has not been a major contributor.

Most centers have not actively pursued contract revenues because of other pressures. A number of center directors believed that until a sound basic program has been developed, there would be little potential from contract services. Other directors have resisted this approach to revenue generation because of its potential program impact: staff would have to be committed to these services to the possible disadvantage of other services.

The significance of this source of revenue appears to vary from state to state depending on the *self-sufficiency* of the agencies involved and the philosophy of government in the particular state. In some states, non-mental health agencies employ their own psychologists, at least for routine testing and evaluation; others may contract for this service. A number of states do not permit any exchange of funds between agencies receiving state support.

While the development of agency contracts cannot be regarded as a short range solution to declining federal support, mental health executives should pursue this source of revenue with due regard to other program priorities. In any event, it is likely that pressure will come from the state level to increase the use of contractual arrangements as state officials become more aware of the magnitude of the funding requirements associated with declining federal support of existing centers and with the expansion of the community approach to provide statewide coverage.

Philanthropy

This source of revenue appears to be most important in areas where financial support from higher levels of government is least significant. United Funds or equivalent organizations often do not aid programs operated by government or receiving substantial amounts of government funding. Furthermore, if government support of a given center increases, there is likely to be pressure for a reduction of such philanthropic support as already exists.

Philanthropic organizations frequently require preparation of a comprehensive budget and detailed justification of program expenditures. In the case of one center, these requirements were more demanding than those imposed by the county that was also making a significant financial contribution. It is not uncommon

for the fiscal years of philanthropic organizations and government entities to differ, requiring maintenance of separate books
and adding to the administrative burden.

Philanthropic organizations are experiencing increasing difficulty in raising funds and, in most communities, are subject to
conflicting demands for support. Even in communities where the
United Fund has contributed to community mental health programs, it is apparent that support from this source cannot be expanded to fill the gap left by declining federal support.

Other Sources of Support

For the most part, sources of support other than those discussed above have been relatively insignificant in the centers
studied. In a number of cases where the center was affiliated with
a hospital, ancillary services were provided such as space and accounting and billing services. If the center is affiliated with a
medical school, uncompensated services may be received from
medical students, interns, residents, and faculty. Volunteers have
also been utilized in some centers. Although these services have
proven to be valuable in specific cases, they cannot be regarded as
a general solution to the funding problem.

Impact of Funding on Service Patterns

A change in the nature of the services provided by centers can
be expected if they are unable to generate sufficient revenue to
offset the decline in federal staffing grant support or if replacement funds are either limited in coverage (for example, private
insurance or Medicaid) or tied to specific functions (for example, contracts for specified services). While the patterns of
service in the centers studied do not seem to have been significantly influenced by the availability of funds, this is not likely to
continue. For example, if increasing reliance has to be placed on
fee payments for direct services, indirect activities may have to be
limited except where they can be provided under contract.
Again, partial hospitalization programs might be reduced and inpatient services increased if greater reliance is placed on insurance as currently written. Where rural centers serve large areas,

inadequate overall funding coupled with the need to provide at least minimal services throughout the entire area may force a heavy concentration on consultation and education services in the outlying portions of the catchment areas.

Shifts of this type were not observed in the programs of the centers studied due largely to the extent to which the states have entered the fiscal picture. An analysis of historical data for the sixteen early centers sampled indicated that in ten, the state was the major source of replacement revenue. State funds typically are not restricted as to use, and their substitution for federal funds would not be expected to affect patterns of service. Furthermore, centers that relied on increased fee-for-service income as replacement revenue either already had relatively diverse sources of support or were able to generate a wide range of fee-for-service arrangements. The net effect was not to impose major shifts in service emphasis.

The state is expected to remain the primary source of replacement revenue, and the use of these unrestricted funds should not affect service patterns. However, the magnitude of state support will be contingent upon the availability of funds, and there are no guarantees that allocations will be sufficient to meet the needs of specific centers. Furthermore, states may establish program priorities that could conflict with center objectives if aggregate funding is limited. In general, little planning has been done by centers to anticipate this possibility. The response of one center to a cut in the state allocation, for example, was to postpone plans for a growth grant and not to fill vacant positions pending a reassessment of program priorities.

In a few cases, local governments are expected to provide significantly increased support. Where multicounty catchment areas are involved, such as those served typically by rural centers, reliance on such support is likely to result in an increased emphasis on consultation and education services in outlying areas and the concentration of other services at one location. This emphasis, however, may reflect the geographic characteristics of the area as well as the exigencies of financing.

Where increased reliance is placed on fee-for-service income to replace federal funding, the impact on patterns of service is expected to be variable. It will depend on the extent of the fee income, the variety of contractual arrangements that can be negotiated, and the administrative and legal requirements of the programs involved. Some centers have been able to generate fee or contract income for most services; others have had limited success. In general, major efforts in this direction have only recently been initiated, and potential service impacts are not clear.

The requirement for replacement funds may be reduced by allowing a number of the positions funded under the original federal staffing grant to lapse or by shifting the responsibility for their financial support. Inpatient requirements were overestimated by several centers, and a shift in emphasis to other services is anticipated as a reflection of community demand. In some other centers, inpatient services will continue regardless of the availability of federal funds because affiliated hospitals have guaranteed their continuation. It is not clear in these cases whether there will be a change in the level of inpatient services, but as far as the center is concerned, the need for replacement funds is reduced.

It is expected that some centers will be forced to close their doors because of the unavailability of replacement revenues. However, the amendments contained in the 1970 legislation appear to have taken the immediate fiscal pressure off most of the early centers and have provided new centers with a longer period during which to obtain replacement revenue. With federal support at about a 30 percent level for the last three years of federal support, (or at higher levels in poverty areas) —it is likely that most early centers can continue their current program activities with few changes in service emphasis directly attributable to funding patterns. For new centers, the extended period of federal support permits the more careful planning of replacement revenue than was possible under the 1965 legislation, but does not obviate the necessity of such planning from the inception of the center.

ADMINISTRATIVE IMPLICATIONS OF
NEW FUNDING PATTERNS

It is clear that the implementation of the Community Mental Health Centers Program has resulted in a significant increase in the administrative burdens placed on mental health executives. Of course, any new program would be expected to impose burdens on administrators if only in the form of organization and staffing problems. But the Community Mental Health Centers Program is unique in a number of ways: its community orientation, the nature of the federal involvement, the organizational characteristics of centers, and the political interaction of state and local governments. These factors combine to increase the difficulty of some of the traditional tasks of mental health executives and to impose new requirements as well.

As long as treatment was provided largely in state hospitals, the principal financial procedure consisted of the annual budget preparation and the activities associated with securing appropriations. The state hospital program was well established in most states with a long history of state support, although at levels regarded by most mental health authorities as inadequate. Financial procedures were relatively well defined, and hospital staffs were organized to provide the necessary budgetary and support services.

The community program also entails budget preparation and justification activities, but of a more complex nature because of the innovative features of the program and the number of funding entities involved. Several specific tasks that relate directly to the financial viability of a center can be identified. Although they are interrelated, they are sufficiently important in their own right to be discussed separately.

Long Range Financial Planning

The federal program was clearly established to provide seed money rather than long term funding support. As was indicated earlier, the financing concept underlying the Community Mental Health Centers Program calls for the use of a variety of public and private funding sources, with federal construction and staffing grants providing the initial stimulus. The implication of this concept is that long range financial planning should be initiated concurrently with the establishment of a center. Although the initial application for a staffing grant under the federal program requires information on the historical funding sources of agencies participating in the center operation and on the sources projected to meet the anticipated cost of the first year's operation, there is no specific requirement for long range financial plans. Much of the initial effort of the early centers was devoted to organization and staffing, and little planning of this type was done. The result for most of them was a continuous search for funds, intensifying as the level of federal support declined.

In practice, the role the mental health administrator will be required to play in the area of financial planning can be expected to vary widely depending on the extent to which states or local governments assume responsibility for this function. For example, if centers in a given state are operated by a state agency, the financial planning responsibilities of the mental health executive will be similar to those applicable to an administrator in the state hospital program. Where centers are heavily supported but not directly administered by a state, responsibility for long range financial planning may be delegated to local units of government and assumed by an existing local department or by a newly established board or other organization. Here, too, the role of the center director may be quite limited.

On the other hand, where there is no formal delegation of authority or where state support is minimal, a major administrative task is to assure the availability of adequate funding for continued long term operation. Initially, the problem is to increase the level of nonfederal support as the federal contribution rate declines; but the planning must contemplate a comprehensive program supported largely without federal assistance. Even where states or local governments assume major responsibility for long range financial planning, there is likely to be pressure to develop other sources of revenue or resistance to new programs that are not largely self-supporting.

In other words, program planning must incorporate from the

beginning careful consideration of all potential sources of funding. The mental health executive, therefore, must become familiar with the terms and conditions of the various legislative programs, federal and state, under which financial support is provided, the characteristics of local programs and agencies that might provide direct or indirect support to the center, and the extent and character of third party coverages that are available to the population in his catchment area. He must also develop a strategy to maximize the financial support from these sources consistent with program growth and emphases.

Data and Record Keeping

The emphasis of the Community Mental Health Centers Program on maximum utilization of existing services and on multiple sources of funding requires the establishment of comprehensive and, in some cases, sophisticated record keeping systems. Many programs that were operating before the organization of a center had developed their own sources of support with considerable difficulty and were reluctant to be absorbed into a larger program without specific guarantees against diversion of funds. In some cases, specific sources of support were tied to programs serving specified clientele groups or specified geographical areas. Record keeping systems, therefore, need to be flexible enough to provide the necessary financial information for these groups or areas if required by the participating agencies.

Furthermore, these agencies may have accounting requirements of their own that further complicate the center's record keeping task. An affiliated hospital, for example, may not separate the costs of psychiatric and other inpatient treatment and may not allocate revenues to its various departments. In most cases, the costs and revenues associated with emergency and inpatient psychiatric services provided by such an affiliated agency can only be estimated. Equally difficult is a determination of the value of ancillary services such as billing and accounting or of free services by the staff of such agencies.

Furthermore, separate budget presentations, with supporting data, may be required by the various agencies providing financial support. Frequently, these agencies operate on different fiscal years, all of which may vary from the grant year used by the federal government. In practice, the center may be able to maintain one detailed set of books and provide the necessary budget information for agencies with different fiscal years by means of estimates. In any event, an extensive effort is required, and a comprehensive and flexible accounting system can be of great value.

As state support has accelerated, there are increasing requests for information to measure the program's effectiveness. Initially, the responsibility for demonstrating effectiveness in support of a budget request devolved largely on the center director, and most centers had developed at least minimal data systems to facilitate this task. Although this responsibility remains largely with the center director for local-level budget purposes and frequently for state budget presentations, many states have instituted data systems for center reporting and evaluation purposes. This trend will continue and these systems will be modified as progress is made in developing bases for measuring effectiveness.

The role of the mental health executive in this process will be variable. At a minimum, he will have to ensure that procedures are established to provide the required data inputs, no simple task where the center consists of several entities. In states that have not yet instituted data systems, he should develop measures of effectiveness and arrange for the collection of appropriate data to aid him in evaluating his program and supporting his budget requests. This is difficult both in concept and in practice, particularly if funding is tight and staff resources are limited.

Maintenance of Interorganizational Relationships

The federal program does not require all center services to be under one roof or even under a single sponsorship, but does require that administration of the center be adequate to provide continuity of care. There is, in fact, considerable variation in the organizational characteristics of centers because more than 85 percent of these currently operational were organized by bringing together two or more organizations that already existed in a community.

Because of the wide variation, it is difficult even to classify centers in a meaningful way. If they are classified on the basis of auspices of the applicant for federal funding, about one-half are under private auspices and the remainder under government or quasi-government auspices. However, services are frequently provided under contract, and *operational* auspices may well differ. For example, the services of one county mental health center included in the study were provided by a hospital district and another by a university. On the other hand, several private centers provided services for a government unit: two for counties and one for a tricounty board.

A primary task of the mental health executive is the maintenance of smooth working relationships between the organizations participating in the center operation, for both financial and program development reasons. The burden of this task can be expected to vary according to the complexity of the organizational arrangements and the consistency of the program objectives among these organizations. In any event, he will have to familiarize himself with the organizational structure of the center, the program objectives of the various entities and any unique local funding requirements that might affect the financial viability of the program.* This knowledge is essential ingredient to the long range planning function discussed earlier.

Understanding the Political Process

Because of the importance of government to the long term support of community mental health centers, it is essential that the mental health executive become familiar with the political processes and financing philosophy that affect his program. Several states participate in the funding of centers by absorbing a significant portion of the excess of their expenditures over their receipts from other sources. In other states, the importance of local government support is emphasized, by ensuring that appropriate taxing authority is granted to local jurisdictions.

In some parts of the country, states do not permit the ex-

---

*One center, for example, was organized as two separate legal entities because community chest support was not provided to hospitals.

change of funds between agencies receiving state support. In these cases, community mental health centers supported by state funds are expected to serve other public agencies, at least in a consulting capacity, free of charge. Even where permitted, success in tapping this source of support has been highly variable, at least for the early centers. Lack of success was due in part to the reluctance of established government agencies to utilize a new and untested program and in part to the limited efforts by some centers to explore this source of revenue. Once a strong basic program has been established, however, this source of support can become important if consistent with the state's financing policy. Any changes in this policy will be dependent upon legislative attitudes at the state capitol.

Some General Comments

It is apparent that this new concept of multiple financing for mental health services implies a significant role for the mental health executive in the area of financing. His role cannot be limited to program development and staffing; the extent to which he will have to participate in financing will depend to a considerable extent on the character, level, and permanence of the major sources of his center's financial support. He will have to familiarize himself with the financial details of the center and with the characteristics and needs of supporting agencies and organizations, so that he can defend his requests for funds to these agencies.

Program development and financing are closely related. If the use of funds from some sources is restricted to specific activities or clientele, programs may reflect the availability of funds rather than needs of the community, more broadly considered. The mental health executive needs to be alert to this danger and may, in many instances, be required to develop *grantsmanship* skills if he is to keep control of the variety and the extent of the center's programs. As a minimum, he needs to be familiar with the political process and skilled in the art of presenting his program to the public.

In sum, the financing requirements demand that he be an innovative and efficient manager, a long range financial planner, and a salesman with *grantmanship* ability. He can expect both frustration and satisfaction from this complex role.

REFERENCES

Atwell, Robert H.: *The Financing of Mental Health Services—A National View.* Paper prepared for delivery to the Task Force on Planning, National Commission on Community Health Services, Baltimore, September, 21, 1964.

Connery, Robert H., *et al.: The Politics of Mental Health.* New York, Columbia University Press, 1968.

Congressional Record. 88th Congress, 1st Session, Part 2, 1744-1749, 1963.

Follman, J. F., Jr.: *Insurance Coverage for Mental Illness.* New York, American Management Association, 1970.

Harvey, Ernest C.: *Sources of Funds of Community Mental Health Centers.* Menlo Park, Stanford Research Institute, 1970.

U. S. Senate, Subcommittee on Health of the Committee on Labor and Public Welfare. *Hearing on S.755 and 756,* 88th Congress, 1st Session, 1963.

U. S. Social Security Administration, Office of Research and Statistics: *Financing Mental Health Care Under Medicare and Medicaid.* Washington, U. S. Government Printing Office, 1971.

Toward a Brighter Future for the Elderly. The Report of the President's Task Force on the Aging. Washington, U. S. Government Printing Office, 1970.

CHAPTER 5

MANAGEMENT INFORMATION

JACK F. WILDER AND SUTHERLAND MILLER

LET US ASSUME THAT THE DIRECTOR of a community mental health center is urged by several members of his community advisory board to develop a methadone treatment program for narcotic addicts. Since the center maintains a continuous data file on the diagnoses of all active patients, the director is able to learn that twenty-two outpatients currently in treatment have a primary or secondary diagnosis of narcotics addiction. He checks with his community organizers and they report that narcotics addiction is a growing community problem. This impression is supported by a review of the nature of recent consultation and education requests to the center from community groups.

The director agrees to provide methadone to any outpatient who requests it and meets the clinical criteria for methadone treatment. He asks for a follow-up of those patients receiving methadone to determine the effectiveness of the program. In two months, he is pleased to learn that five addicts on methadone have returned to work. One month later, he receives complaints from his inpatient staff that the outpatient services will not make any new appointments for at least three weeks for any patients discharged from the hospital. This arrangement is directly counter to a stated goal of the organization, namely, to have immediate follow-up for discharged inpatients.

The director checks the diagnostic characteristics of new outpatients registered during the past three months and finds that eighty-five patients with a primary or secondary diagnosis of narcotics addiction are now in treatment. He checks with a central

120

addiction registry and learns that there are at least 1,500 addicts now living in the catchment area. Apparently, word has circulated in the community about the center's new drug program and the center's outpatient resources are being used much more frequently than ever before for new addict patients. This change in the allocation of scarce resources did not occur planfully. Apparently, it received a boost from several center staff members who felt that their major efforts should be directed toward drug addicts, and not toward other patients. As a result, less outpatient staff time is available for discharged patients.

Members of the outpatient staff become engaged in a disagreement about priorities and the time spent in trying to resolve their differences decreases even further the time available for discharged hospital patients. Faced with an escalating problem, the director conducts meetings with his service directors, the community advisory board, and representatives of the funding agencies. Agreement is reached that the center cannot provide direct services to meet all the mental health and social needs of the community. It is noted that another agency in the catchment area is actually charged with developing methadone programs and, in fact, has received funds to provide direct services. In contrast, the center's highest priority is direct services to psychiatric patients. A check with clinical transaction records reveals that the center is only providing minimal outpatient services to this target group. Any further reduction in outpatient care would compromise a basic purpose of the organization.

To resolve the problem, the director decides that the center will not accept any new patients with narcotics addiction as the primary diagnosis and within six months, all current patients with that diagnosis will be referred to the other community agency. The center will continue to accept new patients with the secondary diagnosis of narcotics addiction. Finally, the center agrees to seek special governmental funding to develop and educate a citizens group concerned about the drug problem.

In this example, the director got into trouble because he paid insufficient attention to obtaining careful planning information before he committed the center to the new program. He should have investigated thoroughly the feasibility and suitability of the center providing methadone treatment to any addict who met the clinical criteria for the treatment and who requested it. He initially should have obtained information related to questions such as the following: What is the size of the addiction problem in the catchment area? What is the current demand and potential demand for methadone treatment? What noncenter resources are available or could become available to meet the demand? What is the capacity of the center to mount a methadone program? And finally, what would be the impact on other programs in the center if resources were allocated to meet various levels of the expected demand for methadone treatment? If the director had obtained such planning information, he might not have started the program or he might have started a program with an identified maximum caseload or he might have sought new funding for an alternative narcotics program immediately.

The case example above illustrates the need for management information in the making of decisions. Mental health administrators, however, have given a low priority to the development of viable management information systems. At first glance, this comment seems inconsistent with the fact that many mental health organizations seem to be engaged almost endlessly in the gathering of data and in the writing of reports. The impetus for these efforts originates from sources both outside and inside the organization. Funding and governmental regulatory agencies want to know how many staff are employed, what their disciplines are, and how much they are paid. Sponsors also want to know how many new patients were seen and how many were hospitalized. Within the organization, the fiscal officer wants to know who should be billed and for what amount. The head of each unit wants statistics and anecdotes that will support his claim for a larger share of the budget. The clinician wants his charts to be in at least good enough form so that he will comply with legal and accreditation requirements. The researcher wants all the data he can collect in the hope that someday they will prove useful. Finally, the director himself wants enough information to prove to his board that he and his staff have been working.

While the data collected from the activities listed above are potentially worthwhile, if they are not related to clear organizational objectives, they are of little value. As a result, the organization is not asking the most important questions about its operation and the data generated do not help staff make decisions. Data gathering in itself is not an information system and it is not surprising that the data collected by mental health agencies are generally incomplete, often inaccurate, and the collection process is viewed as a burdensome chore. If, however, staff were more aware of the need for certain kinds of information in order to function effectively, they would be more likely to appreciate the importance of the information-gathering process.

Organization of Information Systems

A mental health program requires an information system for each of its major functions. For example, a community mental health center (CMHC) needs information pertaining to clinical care, consultation and education, research and development, and support services. Collectively the systems comprise a management

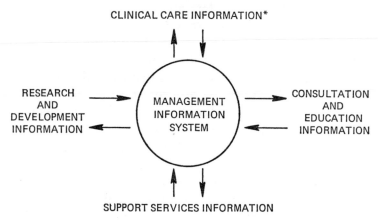

Functions Related To A Management Information System Of A Community Mental Health Center

*Based on Figure 1-1 (Krauss, 1970)

Figure 5-1.

information system; that is, they provide the information needed by administrators at all levels to make decisions.

Each system requires the definition, organization, collection, preparation and distribution of information. Within each system, data are collected for different levels of the organization, some primarily for an individual's use, other data for specific units, and some for the entire organization. Each system should be formalized, in contrast to the informal communication networks which usually exist. Furthermore, the information requirements of each system should be specified and built into the job responsibilities of each member of the organization.

One important consideration is the way in which the different information systems in a CMHC are related to each other. Let us look, for example, at the relationship of the management information system to the information systems designed for three of its functional components: clinical care, research and support services. In reality, each person in an administrative position in the CMHC will have decision-making responsibilities requiring information appropriate in kind and specificity to his job. For clarity of presentation, however, we will discuss only the management information needs of the top administrator of the CMHC, the director.

In the clinical care information system, most of the data the clinician collects is needed only by the clinician or his successor for dealing with individual cases. The director, however, is concerned with reaching goals involving many people, and has the responsibility for making decisions that affect the entire organization. For these reasons, the director will want selected aggregate information generated by the clinical information system.

Research personnel in a mental health organization also require data. The research can be labeled as either basic or applied. Basic research includes those activities directed toward increasing knowledge without concern for an obvious service application. The efforts expended in applied research are directed toward the solution of a specific problem. The information needs of the director include the findings of both basic and applied research conducted in the organization.

A diversified group of support functions assist the director in the operation of the CMHC. The specific assignment of support functions varies in different mental health centers, but generally includes at least accounting, billing, payroll, personnel, and inventory functions. The director of the CMHC will want reports of current aggregate information generated by the information system for support functions and access to additional information, if the need arises.

The director's information needs are not congruent with nor are they a simple extrapolation of the data from the clinical care, research, or support information systems. Staff in clinical care and support functions are engaged in a variety of daily transactions with patients, agencies, and each other, and it is very tempting to collect endless information without asking: *Why do we need it?* Requests for indiscriminate data also flourish in research units where the computer makes data gathering attractive, and the process of collection becomes more important than the purpose and the product. The director should not only obtain the information relevant to his needs, but should also avoid irrelevant information.

What Information Is Needed?

The primary goal of the administrator is to help the organization achieve its objectives. He accomplishes this goal through appropriate acts of decision-making which should take place in a continuous cycle. In general terms, the first phase of the cycle begins with planning; the second phase involves implementation; measuring and evaluation occur in the third phase; and finally, there is a return to the first phase of planning. Progression through such a basic cycle should be visible in the management activities of any administrator. The information needed by the administrator should be relevant to these three phases of the decision-making cycle. Information collected for the planning phase, for example, should answer several questions about the objectives of the organization.

Unfortunately, the cycle is often not evident in the management of mental health programs, at least in the public sector.

Programs are often initiated without specification of objectives and without concern for the congruence of the programs with organizational priorities and goals. Such programs are generally not subject to review and revision and appear to go on forever with few discernible changes.

Peter Drucker identifies key areas in which an organization should set objectives (Drucker, 1954, 1964). These areas are: market standing; innovation; productivity; physical and financial resources; profitability; manager performance and development; worker performance; and public responsibility. Setting objectives in these areas is as meaningful for mental health organizations as for any other kind of organization. For example, an objective in market standing for a mental health center might be to increase within one year the number of direct referrals of geriatric patients to the center by 50 percent, while decreasing the number referred to the State hospital by the same amount. Quantifying the objective provides a specific short-term goal whose attainment reinforces successful effort. This is especially helpful in mental health organizations where results are generally vague and incentives are few.

Objectives set in each of the areas cited by Drucker must be examined in the light of the following questions: (1) Is the objective worthwhile? (2) Does the organization have the necessary skilled manpower and physical resources to do the job? (3) Will the methods employed in the program produce the desired results? (4) Is the time right within and without the organization to introduce and carry out the program? and (5) After a reasonable period of time, will it be possible to determine if anything was achieved?

Since the decision to go ahead on a particular objective has been made, the implementation phase of the cycle has been reached. Management must determine: Who does what, to whom, when? This means that it must be clear how each individual and each part of the organization contribute to the overall goal. Identifying and monitoring this input are most critical in service organizations where the product seems intangible and cannot be inventoried. In other words, production and consumption occur simultaneously (Sloan, 1971).

The final phase of the decision-making cycle is measurement and evaluation. Information is required to ascertain progress in the achievement of objectives. One major problem that faces mental health service programs is the difficulty in demonstrating their effectiveness. One manifestation of this difficulty is the inability of mental health professionals to agree on criteria for assessing their effectiveness. Even when agreement can be reached on success criteria, they often feel that instruments sufficiently sensitive to identify causal factors and to measure change and progress do not exist. When agreement on success criteria and on evaluation instruments is reached, they may learn that their efforts are not productive, or worse, counterproductive.

Thus, it is understandable that mental health professionals believe little is to be gained to compensate for the burdens of paperwork in setting organizational goals and in monitoring their attainment. Rather than evaluating and possibly reformulating their goals, these professionals find fault with the management information system. They prefer to operate on hunches and biases and essentially to *do their own thing.* Yet, the organization is responsible for providing services to the people in its area. The administrator cannot wait for *final, definitive* answers, but must make decisions based in part on: *How are we doing?* He can look at how the program is doing in operational terms, for example, has the new service opened by the scheduled date? Or, he can evaluate progress in terms of the program's impact on its patients.

The decision-making cycle moves from the measurement and evaluation phase back to the planning phase. Based on the information from the third phase, the administrator should take corrective action. This could include continuing the program, modifying it, or abandoning it. The latter decision, unfortunately, is rare.

In all phases of the decision-making cycle, information should be simple, accurate, and timely. Since administrators are often confronted with more data, both relevant and irrelevant, than they can grasp, it is important to keep information brief, to-the-point, and in the language of the administrator. "All routine reports should be eliminated, unless they serve a specific purpose which can be served in no other way" (Krauss, 1970).

Every management information system should provide accurate information. However, while accuracy is important, it is equally important not to commit vast resources to time and manpower to collecting data at a level of accuracy beyond what is needed.

Finally, a management information system should provide timely information. Unless the data are available to management within a time period short enough to meet its specific needs, the so-called management information system is really a data collection system. A manager must not only specify *what* he must know to make his decisions, but also *when* he must know it. Time lags between asking for the data and getting them should be kept at a minimum.

Who Participates In The Information System?

If the top administrator in a mental health organization recognizes the need for a formal information system, he must decide who develops it, who administers it, and who contributes to it. The human factor is more important than the technical equipment in the development and operation of a system.

Administrators at all levels should be intimately involved in the development of the system. They are the key decision-makers in the organization and are in the best position to know their critical information needs. They can best appreciate the immediate benefits to be gained from the system in resolving day-to-day problems. Furthermore, they will be responsible for implementing the system; participating in its development will enhance their support for it. The top administrator must give continuing and enthusiastic backing to the project. He must realize that the system will take time to develop and to be implemented. Above all, he must not underestimate the resistance of the staff to anything new, especially when they feel *Big Brother is watching you.*

Generally, a mental health organization will not have within it all the expertise necessary to develop a management information system. It is important to avoid mistakes early in the project since it is very difficult to recover from a bad start. When an organization is considering the development of a system, it should become familiar with systems in comparable organizations and hire an experienced consultant. A consultant can help by identifying the requirements for a system that will meet the organization's unique needs.

In developing the system, a top-down approach should be used to analyze information needs. The top administrators are concerned with long-range planning and policy-making and their objectives will give the system a unifying theme. Other staff concerned with daily operations can identify any additional information needed solely at their levels and for their respective purposes.

Management information systems in mental health organizations run into trouble when the development and operation of the systems are assigned to research units because these units *collect data*. Research personnel often do not have the skills necessary to design information systems. Based on their own orientations, they are prone to collect data for future browsing. Their requests for excessive amounts of information engender resistance when meaningful data requests are made. Their training often leads them to seek a level of accuracy that is unwarranted for information used in decision making. As such, they may spend too much time tracking down *errors* and not enough time evaluating the available data. Line staff frequently resent data requests from researchers because they suspect that the data are *only being used to write papers*.

Above all, the research staff does not have the authority to implement the system. Management information is a line responsibility and should be under line supervision. The core personnel who man the system should be part of the functional units responsible for contributing the data and benefiting from them. Through this arrangement, the implementation of the system will have the full backing of administrative authority.

Just as it is not appropriate for the research staff to set the goals for the information system, so too, the technicians who run the system should not set the goals. Technicians who may be needed for in-house computer-based systems should only perform support functions. Systems often "fail when technicians, not management, are setting goals for computers" (Diebold, 1969).

The system should offer the contributors sufficient rewards to assure their cooperation. Anyone who has attempted to implement an information system in a mental health agency is well aware of the resistance of professionals to data gathering and organizational accountability (Beck, 1970). The professional traditionally feels accountable only to himself, or at best to a group of peers. Furthermore, he has rarely worked in an integrated system where success depends upon all the components relating well together.

The professional's resistance must be dealt with and this can be done in several ways. First, the staff must like the system. It should focus on a way to help them, such as cutting down on needless paper work or providing information much more quickly than is otherwise available. This is most important when the system is first implemented.

Second, the staff should be involved in the design of the system, particularly in designating what data are useful and the easiest way to get them. "In cases where the system has been thrust upon users, acceptance of the system is rare" (Krauss, 1970). An individual down the line in an organization is reluctant to contribute data if he receives no meaningful feedback. "Time and time again, it has been proved that the best systems are those that give the people who live with them some say in design and performance" (Krauss, 1970).

Third, if the professional staff's income is related to productivity and performance through an incentive system, and if the data have as one of their uses the determination of this productivity, then the staff is far more apt to cooperate in implementing the system. We have been impressed with the fact that professionals in other disciplines, lawyers who work in large organizations, for example, have far less resistance to collecting data about their work, presumably because their remuneration depends on it.

A final issue, particularly in community mental health programs, is the support of the agency's board and the community. The administrator of the program must consider their reactions and feelings about priorities. From the board's point of view, money spent for an information system might be better spent on a new program for children with reading disabilities. If the decision is based on a meaningful assessment of priorities, then the board is exercising its responsibility. If the decision is based on ignorance, then the administrator has not been successful in exercising his responsiblity to educate the board.

How Does The Information System Operate?

An information system should meet criteria of flexibility, economy, and confidentiality, and should employ data collection techniques appropriate to specific organizational needs.

A system should require minimum redesigning to meet anticipated or unexpected operational changes. It should be responsive to normal growth and programmatic shifts without requiring a major expenditure of money and time. "Of course it is impossible to visualize every future contingency, but if attention is given to flexibility during the stages of initial requirements, definition, and general design, it will usually pay for itself many times over in future operations" (Cohen, 1971). Given the fluid nature of mental health programs, the criterion of flexibility is essential.

The total cost of the system should be commensurate with its programmatic benefits over a given time period. This means that both developmental and operating costs should be considered. In determining costs, the biggest difficulties usually occur in estimating what is required to develop the system and to make it operational. To achieve a reasonable estimate, it is necessary to make a step by step analysis of what has to be done and to attach dollar signs to the steps. Operating costs include the expenses for equipment, the salaries of core staff who maintain the system, and the salaries of the line staff, prorated for the time they spend in contributing to the system.

Arriving at an estimate of the benefits is a much more difficult venture. In trying to answer the question: Will the organization save enough to cover the costs of the system, the system cannot be taken as a whole. Specific components must be examined individually. For example: How much will be saved by instituting a computerized billing system; how much will staff productivity be increased by providing them with feedback of their weekly productivity?

A more elusive issue is assessing how much benefit will be derived from the information system in terms of its contribution to general planning and program direction. No easy answer is available to the question of whether the system warrants the costs, but it is helpful to consider some specific issues. For example: How much does the system permit the organization to track and follow patients, determine utilization patterns, and assess the value of various interventions? With these issues resolved as best as possible, the organization can estimate what would happen without the data system, and make a final judgment about the expected benefits.

Whatever method for collecting data is selected, it should provide for confidentiality. For example, some people have claimed that the impersonal nature of a computerized system threatens a patient's privacy. With computers, however, it is easy to devise procedures to prevent unauthorized access to information about patients. In addition, most of the data an administrator needs are summary data. Data that are strictly confidential can be reported in a patient's individual chart. Entries in the computer regarding a specific patient can be coded for purposes of disguising identification. Finally, only selected personnel should have knowledge of the *key* to the computer.

Staff members, as well as patients, are concerned about the confidentiality of data referring to them in any information system. Personnel data that are in a management information system should be treated with the full restraints of confidentiality. Any individual report generated about the performance of a staff member should be given only to the staff member and his immediate supervisor, unless there is full knowledge by both parties that the information will be shared with others.

Three key questions arise concerning the methods of collecting data for information systems. First, when should sampling procedures be used and when should data be collected continuously? Second, should there be one system or several? And finally, when is it necessary to use a computer?

In manufacturing firms, it is said that when the paper work weighs as much as the product, a decision is made to ship the product. As noted earlier, a similar practice of collecting mounds of irrelevant and useless data is fashionable in many mental health organizations. To help with this problem, administrators can often employ sampling techniques to meet their information needs.* It works; the data can be sufficiently accurate. In fact, when the staff is very resistant to continuous data collection, sampling may yield more accurate data than a continuous system. Sampling has other advantages as well. It is economical; less time is expended on data collection, more time is available for data evaluation. It is timely; the feedback is generally quick. Finally, it lends itself to exploring an issue in depth.

Whether to choose a sampling or a continuous collecting procedure depends on the specific situation and the nature of the information system. For example, let us assume that to maintain the financial integrity of the organization, half of each clinician's time in the outpatient service should be devoted to billable patient hours. Administration has also set a guideline that no more than 25 percent of a clinician's time is to be spent in administrative and staff development conferences. The data required to meet these information needs could be obtained in several ways.

The data on billable patient hours could be extrapolated from a continuous billing system. It could be collected by receptionists alone, or in cooperation with clinicians who would complete a separate event-monitoring form for each substantive transaction with or about a patient. Another possibility is to get the information from a daily event record of each clinician's service activities. If the data are not required for billing, they could be collected by a sampling of monitored events or by a sampling of daily event records. In the work sampling approach, the clinician's daily activities could be sampled several days each month or during brief periods several times a year. In any case, gathering information on staff time spent in administrative and staff development conferences should be done through sampling techniques only. It is our impression that only a few, relatively small and well-managed mental health organizations can routinely collect information on the full activities of the staff.

Let us take another example. The organization is committed to providing equitable services to all socioeconomic groups and it

---

*We are indebted to Dr. Layle E. Weeks and Dr. Leonard Marhak for persuading us to appreciate this point of view.

appears that the disposition pattern in the 24-hour emergency room is one point in the system for assessing equity. The assumption is made that the criterion of equity is supported if the referral rates to state and community hospitals are comparable for all social classes. If the administration is concerned that its services are not being provided equitably, an ongoing monitoring system could be implemented. If continuous trouble-shooting is not required, it could be sufficient to have research assistants or clerical staff employ periodic checks.

The temptation to employ continuous data collection is greatest when routine data demands are made by funding agencies. For example, if a funding agency wants to know the source of referral for each patient, there is frequently a temptation to ask more about the source of referral than about the patient.

For many mental health organizations, a key question is whether it should have one information system or several. Currently, there is considerable debate in the management literature about this issue (Morrison, 1969). Generally, if the data processing routines (input, output, and editing) can be combined, it is most economical to have one data-base. For example, it is our experience that in a community mental health center, it is possible to collect data on the basis of transactions; e.g., ambulatory contacts, community contacts, hospital contacts, rehabilitation contacts, etc. This same data can be used for billing, assessing staff productivity, and identifying resource allocation. The use of a computer obviously increases the feasibility of a single data-base.

Finally, most mental health people assume that management information systems automatically imply computers. While it is not the province of this chapter to review the advantages and disadvantages of all the technological alternatives available for implementing a system, a few comments are in order.

A computer should be seen as making a necessary job easier and not harder. It should not be used as a status symbol (Feldman, 1970). Collecting unnecessary data because a computer is available can create exactly the opposite situation.

The degree to which the total system is computerized depends on a number of factors. Computers are able to store, analyze, and retrieve a great deal of information easily. If the organization is large and its information needs great, if data collection is repetitive, if data variables interact, if thorough analysis is wanted, and if speed in retrieval is needed, a computer may be indicated. Often, top-level administrators who are primarily concerned with policy-making have less need for a computer than do administrators who are responsible for operations.

Generally, time sharing can handle all the computer needs of a mental health organization, although the costs of any computer system can be deceiving. They must be separated into developmental costs which include planning, programming and debugging, and operational costs. It is our experience that computer firms are more likely to be inaccurate in their estimates of developmental costs than operational costs.

In any event, the entire system does not have to be implemented at once. By thinking it through in terms of modules it is possible to gradually build a complete system, integrating module after module into a whole. This approach permits greatly reduced start-up costs and some experimentation before moving ahead too rapidly. It also makes possible the selection of high priority areas that can be used to convince the staff of the benefits of the computer.

Once again it is wise to find a good management information consultant for assistance. Have him help select the company to use (other than his own). Another worthwhile investment is for the director of the program to take a brief course in computers so that he knows what they are capable of producing and how not to be confused by computer *experts.*

CONCLUSION

The growth of mental health systems parallels the changes in other service systems: services are delivered through organizations; organizations are big with significant budgets; providing and distributing services has become increasingly complicated. In one area, management, mental health has not kept pace.

A mental health administrator can no longer ignore the importance of basic management practices. Given an unlimited number of public health needs and a limited amount of money to be spent to meet these needs, mental health services will have to prove themselves to be effective and efficient. The advent of citizen participation in the planning and implementation of mental health programs and the rise of consumerism contribute to the increasing accountability of public services. A mental health administrator is expected to get results. His effectiveness will be reflected by his ability to make the right decisions. The complexity of present-day mental health organizations militates against decision-making by pure intuition. The need for sound information systems to help administrators attain objectives is urgent.

At first glance, the poor performance of current management information systems in the mental health field and the general resistance of professionals to participate in such systems are unexpected findings. Mental health professionals, especially psychiatrists, are carefully trained in the logical analysis of problems. It would be expected that such professionals would excel in the development of rational decision-making systems and that they would be ideal candidates for important administrative posts. In fact, the problem-solving method employed in medical diagnosis, treatment, and evaluation is cited in management texts as a model for management decision-making (Newman and Summer, 1963).

The problem is not that mental health professionals lack decision-making skills, but that they tend, by virtue of their training and credentials, to see themselves as individual enterpreneurs who need not be involved in organizational planning and who are not accountable for the achievement of organizational objectives. Since they tend not to see the need for planful decisions concerning the organization, they see little need for collecting information about the way the system operates. A management information system can be best developed and implemented in a mental health organization in which all workers identify with organizational objectives. This identification can only be accomplished by sound management in all areas of the organization. The management information system itself is solely a systematic process of putting facts together so that a top administrator can make intelligent decisions.

REFERENCES

Beck, James C.: Record-keeping and research. In Grunebaum, Henry (Ed.) : *The Practice of Community Mental Health*. Boston, Little, Brown, 1970.

Cohen, Burton J.: *Cost-Effective Information Systems*. New York, American Management Association, 1971.

Diebold, John: Bad decisions on computer use. *Harvard Business Review*, January-February, 1969.

Drucker, Peter F.: *The Practice of Management*. New York, Harper & Row, 1954.

Drucker, Peter F.: *Managing for Results*. New York, Harper & Row, 1964.

Feldman, Saul: The computer quandry. In Tulipan, A. and Heyder D. (Eds.) : *Outpatient Psychiatry in the 1970's*. New York, Brunner/Mazel, 1970.

Krauss, Leonard I.: *Computer-Based Management Information Systems*. New York, American Management Association, 1970.

Moore, Russell F. (Ed.) : *AMA Management Handbook*. New York, American Management Association, 1970.

Morrison, Edward J.: *Developing Computer-Based Employee Information Systems*. New York, American Management Association, 1969.

Newman, W. H., and Summer, C. E.: *The Process of Management*. Englewood Cliffs, Prentice-Hall, 1963.

Sloan, Frank A.: *Planning Public Expenditures on Mental Health Services Delivery*. New York, The New York City Rand Institute, 1971.

CHAPTER 6

THE SOCIOLOGY OF ORGANIZATIONS

David Mechanic

ORGANIZATIONS ARE SOCIAL groupings developed around the pursuit of specific goals. They can be characterized by a planned division of labor, distribution of powers and responsibilities, and lines of communication. They differ from families, tribes, and other social collectivities in the extent of their planning, the more limited scope of their goals, and the degree of substitutability of their personnel (Etzioni, 1964). Organizations as entities are social instruments that are less tied to particular individuals in contrast to other social collectivities, and appear to have an identity independent of their personnel who may change from one period to another. Thus, the identity of hospitals, corporations, universities, and government agencies transcends the individual orientations and characteristics of the doctors, businessmen, professors, and politicians who play a crucial part in shaping organizational activities.

It is not the purpose of this chapter to review basic concepts in organization theory. The reader who wishes to familiarize himself with these concepts will find a reading list at the end of this chapter which will provide some introduction to theoretical approaches to organizations and the variety of organizational research. It is noteworthy, however, that much of current thinking about organizations derives from the clash of two very different perspectives about organizations. The scientific management perspective has been concerned with the efficiency of organizations and has placed greatest emphasis on their formal characteristics. Constructed around the study of industrial organizations, scientific management emphasized the fit between man and machines, the most rational organization of tasks and their interrelationships, and the incentives that produced highest productivity. Much emphasis was given to the formal plans of organization, schemes for designating the hierarchy of authority, appropriate lines of communication, and the rules and procedures through which goal-directed tasks were to be performed.

As a response to this highly formalistic approach, the human relations perspective developed, which emphasized how noneconomic aspects of the work context profoundly influenced workers' orientations to their tasks, how subgroup formations developed, and how informal cultures became influential in affecting the motivation of workers. Particularly influential were the "Hawthorne" studies, a series of investigations carried out at the Western Electric Company's Hawthorne Works from 1927 to 1932 (Roethlisberger and Dickson, 1939). These studies began with various changes in lighting conditions, and it was assumed that improved lighting would increase worker productivity. The investigators were surprised to find that altering lighting—by increasing or decreasing it—had similar effects, and that the manner in which workers defined changes in working conditions was perhaps as important as the objective effects of the physical changes themselves. This led to a whole series of inquiries, which documented the variety of ways in which informal work groups developed and affected the conditions of work and rates of worker productivity. Thus, the human relations school emerged with an appreciation that human outcomes were the product of more than merely physical manipulations of the environment.

It was through the development of the human relations perspective that it became commonplace among sociologists and other social scientists to appreciate that activities in an organization frequently depart from the formal plan, that goals are pursued that may be irrelevant or even destructive to the major functions of organizations, and that an elaborate informal organization may develop which, in its operation, may significantly modify the aims and activities of organizational personnel. James Thompson (1967) has noted that:

Study of the *informal organization* constitutes one example of research in complex organizations using the natural-system approach. Here attention is focused on variables which are not included in any of the rational models—sentiments, cliques, social controls via informal norms, status and status striving, and so on. It is clear that students of informal organization regard these variables not as random deviations or error, but as patterned, adaptive responses of human beings in problematic situations . . . In this view the informal organization is a spontaneous and functional development, indeed a necessity, in complex organizations, permitting the system to adapt and survive.

Over the years, there has been a good deal of debate and interchange among proponents of each of the two perspectives I have described. The proponents, in pushing their own line of argument, have at times exaggerated the relative influence of the variables of major interest to them, but most organizational researchers borrow liberally from both perspectives, and current organizational thinking forms a synthesis of both points of view. With growing sophistication in the study of organizations, new problems have been given increasing attention, such as the relationship between organizations and the external environment, intra- and interorganizational linking and comparative organizational studies.

In considering organizations, researchers have usually classified them in terms of their particular functions, such as industrial organizations, schools, hospitals, prisons and the like. Such classification, however, fails to take into account the similarities and differences among organizations performing varying functions. A more ambitious classification was attempted by Etzioni (1964), who classified organizations by their compliance structures. He distinguished between predominantly coercive organizations, such as prisons, concentration camps and custodial mental hospitals; predominantly utilitarian organizations, such as white- and blue-collar industries; and predominantly normative organizations, such as religious organizations, hospitals, colleges and voluntary associations. Etzioni hypothesizes that clients in coercive organizations have an alienative affiliation, clients in utilitarian organizations have a calculative orientation, and clients in normative organizations have a moral orientation. He further argues that the use of power in these organizations will be related to client orientation.

Other students of organizations tend to focus on particular aspects, such as size, complexity, degree of centralization and the like. One of the most persistent problems in organizational theory and research concerns the growth of bureaucracy, and a great deal of attention has been directed to the theory of bureaucracy elaborated by the famous sociologist, Max Weber. Weber specified the following aspects of bureaucratic structure: (1) a continuous organization of official functions bound by rules; (2) specific spheres of competence; (3) the hierarchical organization of positions; (4) the technical specification of rules that regulate the conduct of positions; (5) separation of administration and ownership; (6) freedom from outside control and manipulation; and (7) the formulation of administrative acts, decisions, and rules in writing (Etzioni, 1961) . Many students of organizations have used these specifications as a guide in studying various types of organizations to see to what extent they approximated Weber's criteria, and in this way different descriptions of bureaucratic variations became elaborated. Weber's concept of bureaucracy was an *ideal-type,* a model which was not based on any particular reality, but which attempted to portray reality in an abstract sense* Weber believed that the *ideal-type* was a powerful model to use in studying organizational phenomena and, indeed, there are various studies, such as those of hospitals, indicating in what ways particular types of organizations deviated from Weber's specifications. In more recent years, a somewhat different approach to the study of organizations has become predominant, which emphasizes the empirical relationships among variables. Blau and Scott (1962) maintain that:

> To exploit Weber's insightful analysis, it is necessary, in our opinion, to discard his *misleading* concepts of the ideal type and to distinguish explicitly between the conceptual scheme and the hypotheses. The latter can then be tested and refined rather than left as mere *impres-*

---

*For a discussion of ideal types and alternate methodologies, see Mechanic, David, Some considerations in the methodology of organizational studies. In Leavitt, Harold (Ed.) : The Social Science of Organizations: Four Perspectives. Englewood Cliffs, Prentice Hall, pp. 139-182, 1963.

sionistic assertions. We can ask, for example: does tenure promote efficiency? Under what conditions does it have this effect, and under what conditions does it not? Only in this way can we hope to progress beyond Weber's *insights* to the building of systematic theory.

The Focus of This Chapter

At this point in time it is not terribly productive to summarize empirical propositions on the functioning of organizations that are relevant to the administration of mental health services, although we shall note such propositions when they are relevant. Instead, we will focus on the observation noted earlier that organizations frequently develop an elaborate informal organization that significantly affects the goals and directions of organizational activity. Although this observation may appear commonplace, it constitutes one of the major insights of organizational theory and offers the keen administrator an important focus from which to begin to understand his own activities. Like many generalizations, on the face of it, this observation appears to be of little pragmatic utility, but through an understanding of the conditions under which such organizational modifications develop and persist, one begins to grasp how people come to terms with the human problems that every worker must confront on the job in concrete form. Informal structures and culture frequently arise in adapting to such human problems.

Organizations, of course, will vary in the extent and importance of their informal structures. Professional organizations, and those in particular that are service oriented, tend to develop rather rich and varied informal networks that may be more indicative of daily activities than the usual descriptions of these organizations would suggest. This is not to imply that the formal organization has small impact or that administrative planning is futile. Administrative planning, however, must take place within the context of such considerations as the way in which the particular functions of the organization affect how people work, how professional norms and culture modify authority and other relationships, how interagency contacts require forms of relationships not specified by formal structures, and how outside social and political forces limit organizational activities.

Mental health agencies by their very character bring into sharp focus many of the complexities of organizations. The goals of such organizations—whether they be a hospital, mental health center, rehabilitation center, outpatient clinic, or some combination of these—are usually multifaceted and ambiguous. They normally encompass some concept of treatment, rehabilitation and consultation. They frequently combine such functions as providing service to clients, training of professionals and other personnel, and some research. In addition, they are ordinarily expected to perform various tasks for the community, such as the detention and evaluation of persons disruptive to the community, consultation with the courts and other community agencies, and a variety of other functions. Moreover, the organization may become involved in efforts directed toward community education, prevention and social amelioration.

These functions would be difficult enough under the best of circumstances, but problems are compounded at almost every point by the absence of agreed-upon technologies, by differences in ideologies among varying professional groups, by disagreements on basic intervention approaches, and by continuing situational pressures involving community support, funding, staffing, and the like. These problems and difficulties would ordinarily require considerable administrative direction and control, but the nature of professional organizations—and mental health agencies are dominated by professionals—confronts the administrator with personnel who are jealous of their rights, protective of their autonomy, and closely committed to particular ideologies about the nature of their work. The administrator thus must exercise his authority rather lightly, mediating jurisdictional and professional disputes, nurturing enthusiasm for new organizational directions, building commitment and loyalty to the organization's goals, and in general developing a sense of mission around some coherent set of viable functions. If an administrator wishes to have influence on anything more than the physical plant and financial aspects of his enterprise, he must have the capacity to command the loyalty and commitment of his personnel. But to the extent that he exercises authority rather than influences individuals to share his goals, he is unlikely to gain their loyalty or commitment, and may even have difficulty retaining them in the organization.

Mental health agencies require considerable discretion and flexibility on the part of their major personnel. In the absence of clear and effective technologies,* the worker must depend on his judgment and professional experience in dealing with the array of problems that he faces. The nature of these activities makes them almost impossible to control through formal mechanisms, and when such mechanisms are developed they are reasonably easily subverted or ignored. It is nearly impossible to effectively control a professional who offers a client service when there are limited criteria for evaluating the service and disagreement about how the service is most effectively delivered. To exercise controls only erodes the professional commitment and creativity of the worker, and may be conducive to making him a disgruntled member of the team (Scott 1969).

Conditions Affecting the Development of Informal Structures

Despite ideal definitions of organizational goals and the formal structures through which such goals are to be achieved, organizations must make continuing adaptations to the conditions of their environment—whether this be changing political demands, modifications of technology, scarcity of manpower or resources, changing interagency relationships or whatever.*† Moreover, in the area of human services it is inevitable that people in key roles will face problems or contingencies that have not been anticipated or for which there are no agreed-upon solutions. Or they may find

---

*Perrow, Charles: Hospitals: Technology, structure, and goals. In March, J. (Ed.): Handbook of Organizations. Chicago, Rand McNally, 1965. Perrow, in this paper, uses the concept of technology strictly excluding social devices which may have therapeutic effect. I see no good rationale to exclude social and educational interventions from the concept of technology. But Perrow's basic point—that in mental health work the interventions are for the most part of uncertain efficacy—still pertains.

*For a classic analysis of how organizations may respond to external constraints, see Selznick, Philip: TVA and the Grass Roots. Berkeley, University of California Press, 1949.

†For some view of what may happen to an organization in the face of a breakthrough in technology, see Sills, David, The Volunteers: Means and Ends in a National Organization. New York; Free Press, 1957.

that the prescribed solutions in the form of bureaucratic procedures are inadequate or ineffective, and these solutions will tend to be abandoned. Individual members of organizations may also work toward facilitating their own personal goals and aspirations, which may be more or less consonant with formally defined goals of the organization; and as organizations have multifaceted goals or ones that are intangible, it becomes easier for individuals to subsume their own goals within such diffuse organizational definitions (Warner and Havens, 1968).

Mental health agencies are particularly vulnerable to the incorporation of personal goals. Since the structures of such organizations tend to be new or changing, as in the community mental health centers, the possibilities for new role definitions of various workers abound. Indeed, with the growth of new types of mental health professionals, one can expect to find a great deal of role construction and modification going on.* Unlike more traditional hospital settings, mental health workers in community mental health centers are testing new relationships relative to clients and professionals, and since such roles are frequently not clearly defined, each of the professional groups attempts to stake out its work territory relative to other groups, new forms of cooperation, and new definitions of its scope of work, autonomy, and authority (Rushing 1964).

The manner in which such definitions develop is a relatively open process particularly in its early stages. Such factors as the personality and agressiveness of various workers, the nature of their training and professional experience, and the character of personal relationships within the organization all play a part. Although this process goes on as well in the mental hospital or in the more traditional mental health agency, authority relationships are more established, and the medical model prescribes the basic framework within which such adaptations will occur. But as the community mental health center moves away from the traditional

---

*The basic perspective taken here is outlined in greater detail in Strauss, Anselm: The hospital and its negotiated order. In Freidson, E. (Ed.): The Hospital in Modern Society. New York, Free Press, 1963, and Bucher, Rue and Stelling, Joan: Characteristics of professional organizations. *Journal of Health and Social Behavior,* 10:3-15, 1969.

medical model and involves a larger proportion of nonmedical and nonnursing personnel, an authority vacuum may develop that provides a wider field for attempts at role-construction and negotiations about the nature of work and relationships among workers. Such negotiations provide creative possibilities, but they also provide opportunities for chaos and conflict, and the particular outcome may very well depend upon the extent to which there is coherence of administrative perspective and the nature of power relationships in the community.

The provision of administrative coherence is difficult because of the various pressures acting on the organization that may modify its course in the implementation of its defined goals. The extent of such influences was not fully appreciated in organizational theory, since much of the early work on informal structure came from the study of industrial work groups who were faced with relatively well-defined work tasks. Even here it was observed that a system of social norms developed that defined the appropriate rate of work and controlled output (Roethlisberger and Dickson, 1939). Although these studies documented the presence of an elaborate informal system, the contexts studied involved sufficiently specific goals so that there was only limited opportunity for workers to pursue their own personal goals or external group goals within work contexts. They could pace work and control output if they wished, but they could not easily initiate changes in the assembly line or the manner in which work processes were performed.

In mental health agencies, as in human services generally, work tasks are not so closely prescribed, and the outcomes achieved are difficult to evaluate. Thus, individuals and subgroups in such organizations can initiate their own goals that may or may not be compatible with organizational goals, or their goals may be irrelevant to the organization's definition of its environment. The imposition of such subgoals may originate for a variety of personal reasons. In its most simple form, it may be the product of the participant's desire to achieve status, recognition or other rewards by working through his own professional framework and conforming to the values of his own professional group. Thus, many psychiatrists are reluctant to depart too drastically from what they perceive among their own peer group as the valued forms of treatment and treatment organization. Similarly, social workers may resist the establishment of a lay therapist program or other organizational modifications because it challenges their status position and presumption of expert skills. Whatever the circumstances, it is clear that innovations in organization are likely to threaten the autonomy or status of particular persons or groups, and such changes—if they are to be effectively implemented and if they are not to tear the organization apart internally—require considerable loyalty, assurance, and commitment on the part of organizational personnel.

The dispersion of goals can occur, of course, within the organization as well. Each of several organizational components may respond to its own situation, emphasize its own needs, and promote its own agenda independent of the needs of the whole. The personnel in each unit will come to see organizational goals in terms of the conditions they face without full awareness of the whole picture. For example, mental health centers may subdivide their staff into neighborhood teams, which are responsible for a selected population area. These teams then may *follow* their clients through all center services. This form of organization serves a closer relationship between services and population groups and continuity of care, but if the subunit comes to think of its work only in terms of the interests of its own population area, and not in terms of the larger population which the health center serves, conflict can easily develop between the subunits and the health center. Although there is much to be said for a subunit to serve as ombudsman for its clients, resources are inevitably limited, and if one subunit pushes too hard it may divert a reasonable and fair allocation of resources. Administrative direction is particularly crucial in decentralized units, for each unit only tends to see *a piece of the action* and may come to define the crucial issues and priorities on the basis of a distorted picture of the whole.

The difficulty of maintaining internal equilibrium often stems from the problem of controlling external pressures on the organization itself. The community often imposes demands on mental health agencies that are unrealistic in terms of time, resources, and available technology and knowledge. Thus, the community expects to turn to mental health agencies to manage community deviance and other problems which become manifest, independent of the demands that such agencies can realistically meet. Ideally, the agency would define its goals and its realistic limitations of knowledge and expertise, and expect support for its activities. But in competition for resources and community support, the agencies usually have to accept external definitions, and indeed they often encourage even more unrealistic expectations. Since such organizations usually seek to widen their scope of activities and the number of clients they deal with, organizational representatives are frequently unwilling to advertise their limitations and instead encourage further demands. One does not often find a mental health administrator—or for that matter any other kind of administrator—reporting to community funding agencies in detail his limitations of knowledge and efficacy. If anything, administrators tend to provide optimistic estimates of their accomplishments and possibilities for future contributions, since they see their budget and support dependent on such declarations. The competition for resources thus encourages a cycle of exaggeration and counterexaggeration that feeds public expectations and places such organizations under greater pressure to achieve the impossible. It is not surprising that personnel within the agency often tend to become cynical and come to develop roles for themselves which are comfortable and which they protect. Having been disillusioned too often, they resist innovation and seek to maintain the adjustments they have worked out for themselves.

The demand for particular kinds of task performance comes not only from clients and the public, but also from other community agencies that have formal and informal links with a particular organization. Regardless of how social organizations are defined legally and administratively, it is the nature of informal networks to encompass the regions within which work must be done rather than the formal boundaries of organizations. The activities of mental health agencies bring them into close contact with other community agencies and groups with whom they must deal on an ongoing basis, and an informal system develops that binds them together. Thus, mental hospitals, community mental health centers and the like become part of a particular social network that makes demands on them that cannot be ignored. These demands may come in the form of suggestions from Washington, influence from the County Board, pressures from a local judge, or complaints from the local police. Since the mental health agency must depend on all of these agencies for support and possible assistance, and is part of a larger system involving these agencies, social arrangements may develop that place considerable restraints on organizational work. Since these agencies must work together to facilitate their own efforts and goals, the failure to conform to informal arrangements may become costly.

Such arrangements are, of course, pervasive in the community, and would pose no special problem except that such external demands may come into conflict with the needs and interests of the client. Personnel responsible for therapeutic care may feel that a patient should be returned to the community, but the resistance of a local judge may pose problems for the agency. To the extent that the agency accedes to the judge's wishes, it may alienate its therapeutic staff who feel that political considerations are being given weight over the needs of the client; to the extent that the agency alienates the judge or other influential persons, it may be in for opposition in the future. Although sociologists have not made definitive studies mapping out such interorganizational linking, there are growing indications that social agencies that have public ideologies of protecting the client often become intimately linked with organizations that may have interests opposed to those of the agency's clients. For example, members of regulatory agencies tend to become more closely associated with the groups they regulate than with the groups they represent, and they come to share many of the attitudes and definitions of the regulated groups. Similarly, public defenders and parole and probation officers tend to become part of the court system, and on a day-to-day basis they must work more closely with district attorneys and judges than with civil liberties and rehabilitation groups (Sudnow, 1965 and Blumberg, 1967). This results in certain attitudes and behaviors that become necessary to sustain continuing cooperative relationships, which may be costly to certain clients. Since clients tend to pass through the organization —while agency relationships must persist through time—it is unusual to strain such relationships in the interests of particular clients except under very special circumstances. These quite typical processes raise grave issues as to who are the clients of mental health agencies, and what protection do patients have that their interests will not be abused.

The process of interorganizational linking described above have as their key element the principle of reciprocity. Favors done must be repaid by various forms of cooperation and a willingness to protect one's colleagues in related agencies. The informal networks that develop, therefore, not only facilitate some organizational tasks and the survival of the organization itself, but also may set up extraorganizational demands and expectations that organizational participants can violate from time to time, but not in any persistent fashion. Any continuing attempt to challenge such community relationships, to undermine the power of particular community groups, or to support one community group against others—whatever the merits of the case—will soon lead those responsible to be labelled as troublemakers and deviants. If they manage to survive at all, they will soon find it difficult to sustain sufficient cooperation to do their jobs.

I do not wish to imply that naturally occurring community processes are just; indeed, they tend to maintain existing power relationships and frequently are disadvantageous to particular community groups. The life of social agencies tends to be characterized by continuing transactions and negotiations, where various groups are allowed to define certain issues of crucial importance to them in return for allowing others similar privileges when their major interests are at stake. However reasonable such understandings may appear to be, the ability to play this particular game depends on what rewards one can mediate for others, and this, of course, depends on the distribution of power.* It

*For an elaboration of this point of view, see Thibaut, John and Kelley, Harold: The Social Psychology of Groups. New York, Wiley, 1959.

should be clear that there are constituencies who tend to be excluded from these understandings because they have no power. A
mental health agency that sees its mission as one involving a more
just distribution of power may develop procedures that build the
power potentialities of specific groups—as, for example, may occur
in developing mechanisms for community control. To some extent
this is possible to achieve on a modest scale in respect to the delivery of services, but it also involves dangers; and if the agency
comes to threaten seriously other community groups, they usually
have the power to destroy or reconstitute it. The potentialities of
community agencies are limited by the larger system of which they
are a part, and although they may take a leadership role, they
do not have the power by themselves to establish new priorities,
except in a very limited sphere.

As an interested community becomes conscious of how an
agency operates relative to its environment, the agency becomes
readily susceptible to the charge that it is corrupt and nonre-
sponsive to the needs of particular community groups. When the
larger conceptions and values are attacked—as they are by mili-
tants in battles involving community control—the organization is
then exposed to a variety of disputes that may threaten its existence. Critics may demand that rules and operating procedures be
explicit and standard, but at the same time they insist that flexibility and discretion be protected. They may demand more community involvement and cooperation, but in the process of the
confrontation, animosities and feelings may be so aggravated that
such cooperation becomes impossible. They may demand protection of individuals, but also insist on open meetings and dis-
closures that violate such protections. They may insist on a deep
examination of issues and priorities, but the context of such discussions often develops so that it becomes impossible for people
to feel they can speak honestly, and they may be attacked if they
do so. Unfortunately, these confrontations frequently become so
threatening that the organization becomes even less responsive to
disenfranchised groups.

Frequently, when administrators feel sufficiently threatened,
they tend to develop protective devices that make their organizations less accessible and less democratic. Pressures mount to abuse

discretionary privilege, to cover up administrative activities, to withhold information and engage in propaganda against opponents, and to engage in closed and informal decision-making. These pressures thus result in organizations departing more profoundly than ever from their ideals and usual operations, and such pressures feed the cycle of distrust and recriminations. Trust and legitimacy are the glue that holds organizations together; in its absence, administrators tend to place greater dependence on subterfuge and coercion, which in turn undermines the commitment of participants.*

Internal Adaptations To Problems Of Work

In a great variety of organizational contexts, people respond as much to the contingencies affecting their daily work as they do to matters of general public policy. The pressures of daily activities and the needs to overcome barriers to action lead to a variety of ingenious mechanisms through which organizational participants pursue their work. Organizational rules may be violated because participants often feel that the end result could be achieved as well or better through less time-consuming shortcuts. The violation of procedural norms tends to be justified in terms of work saved and other advantages.*

Such adaptations are particularly characteristic of professional workers who tend to resist bureaucratic regulations. Such workers have acquired particular professional orientations that emphasize autonomy and flexibility of decision, and they resent rules and regulations that close their options or require behavior that they do not see as goal-directed. In general, professional workers are more satisfied with tasks that maximize their flexibility; and

---

*For a theoretical discussion of the realtionships between forms of involvement and forms of control, see Etzioni, Amitai: A Comparative Analysis of Complex Organizations: On Power, Involvement, and Their Correlates. New York, Free Press, 1961.

*Various studies of the police illustrate these processes clearly. Police work has many similarities to community mental health. The policeman has great autonomy and discretion in dealing with various problems that he confronts, and it is particularly difficult to audit such encounters. See Skolnick, Jerome: Justice Without Trial. New York, Wiley, 1966; and Westley, William: Violence and the Police: A Sociological Study of Law, Custom, and Morality. Cambridge, The MIT Press, 1970.

militancy and independence of such workers tend to be associated with their degree of professionalism (Corwin, 1970).

Professional workers have strong commitments to their clients, and often resent legal restrictions or rules that interfere with what they regard as proper management in the clients' interests. They thus may readily violate regulations or make false certifications in respect to disability, indications for abortion, involuntary commitment, or in other matters in order to achieve *optimal outcome.**

Developing and Maintaining Direction in
Mental Health Agencies

Until very recently, mental health agencies have been characterized as rather dreary, routinized institutions—bereft of sufficient resources and staff to do an adequate job—and characterized by an atmosphere of hoplessness and apathy.* Typically, staff drifted into comfortable routines that made them reluctant to participate in innovations that would result in more work or disruptions in their established network of relationships. Administrators frequently found such institutions to be immovable and difficult to reorganize, and they either drifted away or also fell into a rather routinized existence. Such agencies often served the community more than the patients by isolating and detaining deviants whom the community did not wish to tolerate; the patients in these institutions deteriorated as much from institutional routines as from their problems.*

Since the middle 1950's, the situation has shown considerable improvement.* A variety of changes—including the introduction of psychoactive drugs, new administrative attitudes, growing community support for community care, and an infusion of funds

*For a discussion of the dynamics of such processes, see Mechanic, David: Mental Health and Social Policy. Englewood Cliffs, Prentice Hall, 1969, pp. 121-145.

*Belknap, Ivan: Human Problems of a State Mental Hospital. New York, McGraw Hill, 1956. Perhaps the most in.fluential treatment of this subject was Goffman, Erving: Asylums: Essays on the Social Situation of Mental Patients and Other Inmates. New York, Doubleday-Anchor, 1961, particularly pp. 3-124.

*For a review of such issues, see Mechanic, David: Medical Sociology: A Selective View. New York. Free Press, 1968, pp. 369-403.

*For an excellent review of recent developments in psychiatry and some future directions, see Hamburg, David: Psychiatry as a Behavioral Science. Englewood Cliffs, Prentice Hall, 1970.

from governmental sources—resulted in a growth of enthusiasm and confidence on the part of mental health personnel. With government support, considerable strides were made in the training of mental health professionals and in the building and staffing of community mental health centers as well as in the upgrading of state and county mental health institutions. There was also a wide appreciation that institutional living and prolonged inactivity could lead to a significant deterioration of skills and attitudes that made rehabilitation extremely difficult.

It will be argued for many years as to just which of the many components involved were most important in stimulating new attitudes and efforts. No doubt psychoactive drugs stimulated hope and confidence, encouraged changing administrative attitudes, and made it more possible to manage patients in the community. But there is also evidence that similar changes were noted prior to the introduction of psychoactive drugs in some English hospitals, where there was strong administrative leadership and encouragement for new forms of community treatment for the mentally ill. Whatever the specific impact of particular forces, it is reasonably clear from experience around the world, as well as in our own country, that the momentum of treatment institutions and the attitudes of personnel have a pervasive effect on the performance of patients. Whether we consider the history of moral treatment in psychiatry* or review the differential impact of the introduction of psychoactive drugs in hospitals where staff had varying attitudes toward them (Frank, 1961), it becomes clear that the communication of efficacy and hope is an indispensible aspect of an effective mental health facility. A major problem in all forms of therapy is the patient's poor self-image and history of failure, and if staff cannot communicate optimism to the client, it is difficult to see how the client can sustain it himself and persist

---

*For a brilliant historical analysis of the social forces affecting forms of treatment, see Grob, Gerald: The State and the Mentally Ill: A History of Worcester State Hospital in Massachusetts, 1830-1920. Chapel Hill, University of North Carolina Press, 1966; also see Bockoven, J. Sanbourne: Some relationships between cultural attitudes toward individuality and care of the mentally ill: An historical study. In Greenblatt, M., *et al.* (Eds.): The Patient and the Mental Hospital. New York, Free Press, 1957.

in attempting to cope with his problems and the external environment (Mechanic, 1967). Without hope he is likely to sink into a state of apathy and inactivity, and there is no better measure of failure than evidence that the patient is doing nothing and making no serious attempt to struggle against adversity.

In one of the few comparative studies of mental hospitals over time, Wing and Brown (1970) have traced the developments in three English mental hospitals between 1960 and 1968 and the effects of such changes on the clinical state and performance of schizophrenic patients. One of their most significant findings was that the most important factor associated with improvement of primary handicaps was the reduction of inactivity. In tracing the developments in these hospitals, Wing and Brown report considerable change in patient performance and clinical state following the implementation of modifications of hospital regimens and the initiation of a more developed rehabilitation perspective. Most improvement took place early in the study period, but by 1968 there was strong evidence in two of the three hospitals studied that the rate of improvement had declined as compared with the earlier period. In accounting for these changes, the investigators point out that there are several alternative explanations. It is possible, for example, that as patients get older, staff turn their attentions to younger and newer patients; but the researchers did not find sufficient age effects in their analyses to make this a very likely explanation. Moreover, the researchers do not believe that their study spurred staff on to greater efforts since staff knew relatively little about the details of the investigations. Still another hypothesis is that, with developing community care, a lesser proportion of clinical time was devoted to long-stay patients. In the context of our discussion, still another alternative that Wing and Brown offer merits attention:

> The second kind of explanation is, in some ways, more disheartening; that the therapists (doctors, nurses, occupational therapists and supervisors) began to feel, at different turning points in different hospitals, that they had done as much as they could; that expenditures of further time and energy would prejudice the chances of other patients, or simply enough was enough.

Wing and Brown speculate further that the loss of certain key administrators, who left these hospitals during the study period, would also have to be taken into account. For example, Dr. D. H. Bennett, who had done much to build up the rehabilitation and resettlement services at Netherne Hospital, left in June 1962 to become a consultant at the Maudsley. Anyone who has seen Dr. Bennett in action can appreciate his boundless energy and enthusiasm, his optimism and patience, and his abilities to nurture involvement and enthusiasm among the people who work with him. Although I am not a great believer in great-man theories of social organization, I have no doubt that these qualities are immensely significant in administrators who have as a prime responsibility the coordination of a network of services, and who must depend for success on a wide variety of therapeutic workers. Major aspects of the task include developing cohesiveness and a cooperative spirit, and underplaying the status and ideological differences that may separate such workers.

Community mental health centers and other mental health institutions operate in a great sea of uncertainty. In the presence of diffuse goals and the lack of clear standards of performance, it is not difficult to gravitate to traditional and familiar forms of delivering services to the least disabled and most attractive clients, thus neglecting those most difficult to work with and those most impaired. Similarly, it is easy to neglect the maintenance of a complex web of relationships that increase service potential or that allow flexibility in care. Moreover, it is not difficult to lose unattractive clients, to neglect those who appear less cooperative, or to pass them off on other agencies. In short, there is considerable incentive to fall into the patterns of old—following the easy routinized pattern of caring for those who most vigorously and agressively seek one's help, and of neglecting the rest. The major deterrents to falling into such patterns are a strong sense of commitment and mission, as well as an organizational network that can provide meaningful services to the more difficult and disabled patients.

How, then, does an organization ensure a continuing sense of mission? In part, one sets the conditions for enthusiasm by recruiting able and energetic personnel. Such personnel, if they have initiative, will wish to participate and share in policy formation and implementation, and will desire considerable autonomy in pursuing organizational tasks. To the extent directions and rules come from above without consultation, they will be resented and resisted. A major way of involving personnel in the goals of the organization is to make them feel a part of it and influential in its directions. This is inevitably time-consuming and may even be annoying, but it is usually a worthy investment. Administrators often become defensive and angry when the staffs they have recruited oppose them on particular decisions, but a staff that is first-rate will inevitably do so; and a successful administrator accepts such decisions in good grace. If he pushes decisions against the wishes of his staff, he will only alienate them, and he may very well find that his decisions are not being implemented anyway.

Frequently, *old hands* in organizations resist changes in procedures or insist that this or that innovation was tried in the past without success. Yet one will frequently find that new and younger personnel are committed to such change and wish to try it. They usually are not convinced by the advice of more experienced persons that all sorts of problems will become manifest, and that the innovation will not work as smoothly as imagined. The *old hands* may be technically correct, but to resist innovation when there are strong feelings in support can be extremely costly. There are many ways to pursue any particular goal, and more often than not the particular procedures followed have no great impact one way or the other. What does have impact is the involvement and enthusiasm of the staff; and if they have a sense of innovation and movement, it often encourages their energies and instills hope and enthusiasm in others as well. Mental health agencies probably help patients as much by instilling hope and confidence as in any other way, and a staff that is enthusiastic and hopeful is an invaluable asset. Maintaining this enthusiasm and movement is one of the major tasks facing a good administrator, and it is often the key to successful performance.

In pursuing innovation, initiation usually comes from professional staff; yet frequently modifications of procedures require other personnel—such as clerical workers, attendants and aides—

to assume new and perhaps more time-consuming tasks. Since such persons must often do the work, they frequently resent changes in their routines in which they have had no voice. Although such personnel can rarely initiate changes, they have the capabilities to resist and divert such changes and frustrate new programs (Mechanic, 1962). All workers, at whatever level, have a need to be appreciated and respected; and all workers resent changes that they feel are capricious or fail to take account of the difficulties they have in doing their jobs. Such workers have their own informal associations of freindship and work relations, and may do much to retard change if the administration fails to enlist their loyalty and to give them a sense that they are important to the success of the enterprise. An administrator who neglects his subordinates is bound to find himself in considerable difficulty (Scheff, 1961).

The Corrupting Effect of Rules

Bureaucracies tend to proliferate rules that standardize procedures throughout the organization. Such regulations are developed to ensure that certain standards of performance and functioning exist, and to protect against abuses and irregularities. Individual units of an organization and their personnel, however, have different functions, operate in varying environments, and face different needs. Rules that appear rational in general may pose real obstacles to individual departments. These departments will face the alternative of either subverting organizational rules or allowing efficient performance to suffer. Where performance is highly valued, rules are frequently violated, but in violating rules personnel feel vulnerable, and in being forced to do so their loyalty becomes eroded. Unfortunately, many large organizations invest greater resources in enforcing trivial rules than they could possibly lose through the termination of these rules. Rules serve a specific purpose and, like other investments, should be judged in terms of an overall cost-benefit assessment. Administrators too frequently fail to see the tremendous costs of unnecessary rules both in terms of resources and the commitment of organizational participants.

The enforcement of standardized rules that are not viewed as instrumental by those who are guided by them frequently leads to cynicism and tendencies toward violation of them. In the process both important and trivial rules tend to be violated, leading to an informal atmosphere of expediency. Many organizational participants come to recognize that, if they conscientiously conform to all the rules, they may achieve a certain security, but they know their performance will suffer. They thus violate rules, but in doing so they become vulnerable to criticisms that can later be used against them. There are some fearful persons who are extremely reluctant to violate rules and thus suffer in their work,* there are others who so liberally violate them that they call the integrity of the organization into question. Some administrators use rules as a device to control their personnel. William Westley (1968) has written about a police chief who elaborated a series of unreasonable regulations that he encouraged his men to violate. He could then use these to control his men when they became too enthusiastic in their duty in situations where the chief felt such action undesirable (arresting gamblers, for example).

The function of rules, of course, is to define expected behavior under ordinary circumstances, and they serve as deterrents to behavior that exploit the organization, its personnel, or its clients, or that compromise the organization's public stance. When problems arise, it is usually preferable to negotiate a resolution, and rules become part of the currency of such negotiations (Gouldner, 1954). It is preferable for organizations to operate on trust and informal resolution of disputes rather than on the formal invocation of rules. The major function of rules is not enforcement, but rather guidance and deterrence. When rules proliferate mindlessly and deal with every triviality, they tend to lose their power of guidance and may even encourage deviant and ineffective behavior. When persons are required to violate numerous rules to do their ordinary work, the rules themselves may become debased, and respect for rules is undermined. Moreover, rules that are

---

*For a discussion of the relationship between personality and bureaucratic behavior, see Merton, Robert: Bureaucratic structure and personality. In Merton, Robert: *Social Theory and Social Structure*. Rev. Ed., New York, Free Press, 1957.

often established as minimal standards come to be seen as standards of adequate performance and may even serve to encourage a low level of performance. It is always difficult to specify under what conditions rules are and are not necessary. A rule is a form of investment, and like other investments it must be evaluated in terms of what it can and cannot achieve. The positive gain as measured by likely deterrence or incentive must be weighed against the losses resulting from alienation, violation, disrespect for rules in general, and resulting limits on spontaneity and innovation.

The need to protect flexibility of response is sufficiently important in many activities that organizations frequently develop an informal code that protects rule-violators from external criticism. The unwillingness of professional organizations to take punitive action against their own members helps maintain an atmosphere where flexible action and risk-taking remain possible. Thus, for example, police departments are extremely reluctant to discipline their officers who violate due process, mental hospitals rarely punish nurses and attendants who illegally restrain patients, and organizations generally function by ignoring most rule violations. Since they must deal with rule violation selectively, they usually punish offenders when violations are clearly contrary to the welfare and goals of the organization, when the violator has incurred the wrath of others in the organization for other reasons, or when the violations become sufficiently visible to the community so the organization requires sacrificial lambs for its own survival. Rules just become one element of a complex negotiation process which involves consideration of the circumstances of rule violation, the *character* of the rule violator, and external pressures to respond in particular ways.

Professional organizations, because they give their personnel considerable discretion, often face external criticisms of alleged abuses. Increasingly, community organizations and clients insist on control mechanisms and review of professional work. In dealing with such external demands, such organizations frequently develop mechanisms that are recognized as ineffective by persons within the system, but which exist primarily to subdue criticism from outside and to protect discretion. Most medical societies, police departments, universities, hospitals and the like have disciplinary committees and procedures; but such measures are rarely strict or effective. They primarily function to assure outsiders that the organization has the will and the capacity to police itself. More recently, there has been growing awareness of the ineffectiveness of such controls, and there have been growing demands for stronger disciplinary procedures in professional organizations. Although protections against significant abuse are necessary, any mechanisms developed must protect a wide range of discretion if they are to facilitate innovation and constructive risk-taking.

Some Notes on Organizational Power

Power in organizations has its source in the ability to control persons, information and resources, and thus making others dependent on one's cooperation. Ordinarily, those having formal power also have considerable real power, because their formal position gives them ready access to control over these important elements of organizational life. However, persons with little formal power may also achieve access to information, persons and resources through their strategic location in the organizational structure, their expert information, the reliance of the organization on their skills and cooperation, and the like.

As long as organizational participants recognize the legitimacy of the rights and powers of those in formal positions of authority, power may operate as expected. However, in complex organizations where subunits are competing among themselves and share varying goals, organizational participants have opportunities for a variety of alliances, and they may use the advantages of their location in the organizational structure and their access to information and people to further one set of objectives or another. Although such participants may use what power they have to protect their own goals and patterns of work, they may also form coalitions to further particular organizational programs outside their own unit, or to retard particular policies they view as undesirable.

All organizations also have various groups that assume leadership on matters important to the organization. To be effective, these leadership groups must form alliances at various levels of the structure to ensure that policies developed will be translated into a true action potential. As persons in powerful positions have noted over and over again, it is one thing to give directions, and quite another to have them implemented. Each leadership group must seek from its possible constituency various persons among whom it can distribute tasks and privileges and from whom it can seek information and advice. Although theoretically the possible population from which such persons might be chosen is very large, in general those persons chosen are the ones the leaders have direct knowledge of or are aware of through their most trusted associates. Thus, within each leadership group there is a tendency for a *leadership circle* to emerge which may become intimately involved in the decision-making processes of the organization (Kadushin, 1968). As such persons prove themselves in performing certain tasks and come to be trusted by one another, they tend to seek each other's assistance as new tasks emerge.

There is a tendency for the *leadership circle* to perpetuate its influence in various aspects of organizational life since they have closest knowledge of members within their own social circle and tend to distribute tasks among them and share information. However, if the social circle from which participants are chosen is too limited or restricted to only one social segment of the organization, then the leadership group endangers itself since it is vulnerable to becoming isolated from main currents of organizational activities, information flow and personal transactions.

Defining a Coherent Mission

A mental health facility, like any effective organization, must have some sense of its priorities and commitments. Given the extent to which the term mental health comes to incorporate a vast spectrum of psychological, social, and even cultural problems, it should be reasonably clear that no single facility, or even a complex of facilities, can attack the entire array effectively. Many of these problems are manifestations of the dilemmas and contradictions in society generally, and are not amenable to effective intervention without vast modifications in the social and cultural fabric.

My own view is that priorities in the mental health field should be set in terms of criteria of need and assessment of the efficacy of intervention strategies. This implies that any mental health facility must have a population perspective that is alert to the manner in which disorders present themselves in the population and how they develop as well as those techniques that most effectively help manage such problems.* Such an agency must also be receptive to evaluation of its programs and must not become so committed to specific efforts so as to make assessment and change threatening to its personnel. This, of course, presents a dilemma since the process of nurturing enthusiasm and involvement also is likely to lead personnel to become committed to certain programs and protective of them. To the extent possible, administrators should nurture commitment to goals or outcomes as compared with processes, since the latter must change with the advance of knowledge and understanding.

One way of making priorities clear and salient is to develop a theory or set of perspectives about what the agency is supposed to be doing. It is helpful in constructing such models to develop understanding of the limitations and constraints under which the agency must work and what aspects of the problem are reasonably amenable to intervention. For example, in recent years growing interest has been evident in nonmedical approaches to mental patient care in the community. One such approach is the educational model which attempts to improve patients' coping capacities through retraining and rehabilitation experiences, or which make efforts to assist patients' significant others in helping the patient make an adequate adjustment to his life situation. In pursuing these goals, the agency may require a variety of services, among them partial hospitalization, transitional institutions such

---

*It is essential for any administrator to appreciate that the pathways into his facility or pattern of services are affected by a wide variety of cultural, social, psychological and situational variables, and that those who seek help may not be those most in need of the particular services available. For a review of this general literature, see Mechanic, David: Sociology: A Selective View. New York, Free Press, 1968, pp. 115-157.

as half-way houses, sheltered workshops, employment assistance, or whatever. The success of such ventures is likely to depend not only on the efficacy of the interventions, but the existing conditions in the community and the family. The efficacy of job training or retraining will depend on the job market; the success of family adjustment will depend on the attitudes of family members who may support or oppose the program of care. Mental health agencies, when they operate in the community, must work within a range of options which the community will at least tolerate if not accept, and they must be sensitive to the realities of what they can and cannot influence. Such realities are themselves changing, and the agency must be perceptive to such changes and to new opportunities as they present themselves. It is highly unlikely, as we noted earlier, that the formal definitions of relationships will be responsive to conditions as they change, and agency personnel must have the flexibility and opportunity to develop new patterns of service that are responsive to changing need.

As community mental health develops, services will increasingly occur outside the physical confines of any single facility, and such services will require significant coordination among various agencies. The concept of a community mental health center is basically a concept of an available array of services in special institutions and in the community, and by its very nature presents certain inconveniences to workers who, if they do their jobs well, cannot as easily settle into established routines as in some other kinds of service organizations. Yet, there is a strong tendency in all social organizations for people to attempt to develop a niche for themselves which presents them with a certain degree of predictability and security in their daily routines. When such needs become pervasive, coordination among agencies, coping with the complex and difficult client or the unresponsive family, or attack on the deeper and more resistant human problems may be compromised. It is my strong belief that when the task is not routine, and goals are uncertain or difficult to establish precisely, there is no force more important than a deep commitment to the job and a sense that one's agency has the capacity to do it. Established routines, rules, clear lines of authority and function, and other bureaucratic devices may help smooth the processes by which work in the organization is accomplished, but if they become too elaborate and deal with trivialities rather than instrumental needs, they may become significant barriers to successful performance. For in the final analysis, bureaucratic mechanisms are nothing more than instruments that facilitate desired performance; when they become ends in themselves, or take up large investments of time and effort, the organization can no longer maintain a mission or momentum.

REFERENCES

Barnard, Chester: *The Functions of the Executive*. Cambridge, Harvard University Press, 1938.

Blau, Peter and Scott, W. Richard: *Formal Organizations: A Comparative Approach*. San Francisco, Chandler, 1962.

Blumberg, Abraham: *Criminal Justice*. Chicago, Quadrangle, 1967.

Corwin, Ronald: *Militant Professionalism: A Study of Conflict in High Schools*. New York, Appleton-Century-Crofts, 1970.

Etzioni, Amitai: *Modern Organizations*. Englewood Cliffs, Prentice Hall, 1964.

Etzioni, Amitai: *A Comparative Analysis of Complex Organizations: On Power, Invlovement, and Their Correlates*. New York, Free Press, 1961.

Frank, Jerome: *Persuasion and Healing*. Baltimore, Johns Hopkins Press, 1961.

Goffman, Erving: *Asylums: Essays on the Social Situation of Mental Patients and Other Inmates*. New York, Doubleday-Anchor, 1961.

Gouldner, Alvin: *Patterns of Industrial Bureaucracy*. New York, Free Press, 1954.

Kadushin, Charles: Power, influence, and social circles: A new methodology for studying opinion makers. *Am Sociol Rev, 35*:685-699, 1968.

Katz, Daniel and Kahn, Robert L.: *The Social Psychology of Organizations*. New York, Wiley, 1966.

Mechanic, David: Sources of power of lower participants in complex organization. *Administrative Science Quarterly, 7*:349-364, 1962.

Mechanic, David: Therapeutic intervention: Issues in the care of the mentally ill. *Am J Orthopsychiatry, 37*:703-718, 1967.

Roethlisberger, Fritz, and Dickson, William: *Management and the Worker*. Cambridge, Harvard University Press, 1939.

Rushing, William: *The Psychiatric Professions: Power, Conflict, and Adaptation in a Psychiatric Hospital Staff*. Chapel Hill, University of North Carolina Press, 1964.

Scheff, Thomas J.: Control over policy by attendants in a mental hospital. *J Health Human Behav, 2:*93-105, 1961.

Scott, W. Richard: Professional employees in a bureaucratic structure: Social work. In Etzioni, Amitai (Ed.): *The Semi-Professions and Their Organization.* New York, Free Press, 1969.

Sudnow, David: Normal crimes: Sociological features of the penal code in a public defender office. *Social Problems, 12:*255-276, 1965.

Thompson, James: *Organizations in Action.* New York, McGraw Hill, 1967.

Warner, W. Keith, and Havens, Eugene: Goal displacement and the intangibility of organizational goals. *Administrative Science Quarterly, 12:*539-555, 1968.

Westley, William: The informal organization of the army: A sociological memoir. In Becker, Howard, *et al.* (Eds.): *Institutions and the Person.* Chicago, Aldine Atherton, 1968.

Wing, John K. and Brown, George W.: *Institutionalism and Schizophrenia: A Comparative Study of Three Mental Hospitals, 1960-1968.* Cambridge, Cambridge University Press, 1970.

CHAPTER 7

INTERORGANIZATIONAL RELATIONS

GREGORY M. ST. L. O'BRIEN

IN MENTAL HEALTH, particularly in community mental health programs, the pattern and climate of relationships between a caregiving facility and other organizations with which it interacts are crucial. Traditionally, it is through relationships with other organizations and caregivers, such as health and social agencies, courts and police departments, family physicians and clergy, that clients come to a mental health facility. The community mental health movement and recent legislation in community mental health and comprehensive health planning have stressed the importance of comprehensiveness and continuity in care delivery as well as the involvement of local groups in the planning process. In both of these areas, the interorganizational relationships of any caregiving organization play a major role.

The need for interorganizational coordination in mental health services has become increasingly evident as the demand grows for innovative community programs. In times of limited resources for service delivery, interorganizational coordination becomes an ever more immediate necessity. In the Community Mental Health Centers Program, for example, at the federal and possibly state and local levels, future funding will require greater interorganizational coordination. If an administrator fails to understand or to concern himself with interorganizational relationships, it could severely limit the growth and even possibly the continued functioning of programs with which he is affiliated.

The decentralization of mental health services including the establishment of community mental health centers, the geographic unitization of mental hospitals, and the identification of limited population areas for these decentralized units has coincided with a greater emphasis on maintaining the patient in his community setting. This emphasis has also facilitated interrelationships among a wide range of professionals in human service organizations serving the target catchment area. The tasks of patient care in the community may well depend upon the actions of a number of organizations. Focusing on a particular service area increases the interdependence of human service organizations, and increases the frequency and intensity of contact between them. As the size of the service area decreases, the number of care giving agencies decreases but the contact between them should increase.

To develop a maximally effective program will often require the establishment of collaborative relations with a wide range of public and private agencies. Such collaboration will be not only in areas of patient referral, but also in joint programs, shared staff and information needed by each organization for the assessment of its own effectiveness.

With even the most preliminary emphasis on preventive care, the need for collaboration with schools, churches, social clubs, and work organizations becomes imperative. This need stems from the broad acceptance by the community and the greater access to community groups which these existing organizations may have but a new community mental health program may lack.

The development and maintenance of positive interorganizational relations based on trust and mutual benefit is one of the primary tasks of the program administrator. Relationships, either by informal interchanges or more formalized contracts, cannot be once made and then forgotten. There are a range of different types of relationships in which a community based mental health program can, should, and even must be engaged. A constant awareness of the freedoms and limitations within these varied relationships will be a helpful tool to the administrator in maintaining open and collaborative communication lines. In turn, this will facilitate the effective, efficient and economic operation of his own program.

In addition to his own activities, the administrator must be aware of the full range of linkages in which other staff members are involved, since it is the full range that will determine the interorganizational climate.

The interorganizational environment of a mental health service program can influence not only the effectiveness of that particular program in reaching its goals, but even which goals will be selected. The climate of relationships between a focal organization and its environment can also have a major impact on the external organizational process of staff communication and morale. Thus, even where such collaboration does not directly result in the development of new programs, the range of organizational and environmental interaction that occurs will markedly affect how an organization operates.

This chapter will review some of the current conceptions regarding interorganizational relationships with particular reference to the ways in which a mental health program administrator may most effectively function under various conditions.

THE INTERACTION OF THE MENTAL HEALTH FACILITY AND ITS ENVIRONMENT

As open systems* organizations must engage in constant interchange of resources and information with their environment in order to survive. Relationships with the other organizations and individuals who make up an organization's environment are most often concerned with the input of resources (and information) or the output of the organization system's products (either resources

---

*The conception of an organization as an open system emphasizes that organizations in the processes of survival and goal achievement, draw resources from the environment which are the raw material for the *production* activities of the organizational system. These raw material resources are somehow changed—processed—by the organization system (conversion or technological processes) and these converted or processed resources are returned to the environment as an output. A steel mill takes (purchases) iron ore and coal from the environment. These are converted into steel (conversion process) and the resultant steel is returned (sold) to other elements in the mill's environment. In a hospital or other human service organization the raw materials might include patients, medicine, personnel, funds, etc. The conversion processes or technological processes would include prevention and treatment activities. The return of the patient to his family and his community would represent the output process.

or information). Since an organization depends upon these input and output transactions for survival, the members of the environment who engage in these exchanges exert considerable influence not only over an organization's processes (Simpson and Gulley, 1962) but even in the setting of organizational goals (Thompson and McEwen, 1958).

Organizational Boundaries

In conceiving of an organization as an open system, the concept of *system boundary* takes on unique importance. While the boundary of a system may be a territorial line or even a physical barrier, in social systems such as human service organizations, the boundary exists in terms of patterns of human interaction. Resources (patients, funds, staff, etc.) must be taken across the boundary into the system from the environment. After having gone through some conversion process these modified resources must be returned, across the system's boundary, to the environment. Likewise information needed to assess how well one's own organization is functioning is also gained through such transactions.

In a mental health program, cross-boundary transactions may involve such resources as funds, clients, staff, and information (for example: the opinions, guidelines, laws and evaluations by public and private groups and organizations concerned with mental health care). Most complex human service organizations will have a number of roles in which the primary functions are concerned with cross-boundary interactions.

The program administrator is in contact with citizen groups, legislative bodies, and mental health officials providing or taking in information. He (or she) is also involved in a variety of joint planning efforts and other exchanges with other direct service organizations. Key staff roles in service units such as intake, outpatient, and aftercare, geographically focused inpatient units, and staff departments such as social welfare and research also imply considerable cross-boundary transactions. Such transactions will involve contact with protective (police and courts) and service (hospitals and social agencies) organizations also involved in traversing organizational boundaries.

Many of the *boundary spanning* personnel of a community caregiving organization will have about as much contact with the staffs of other organizations as they will with their intra-organizational colleagues. Through such linkages, organizational role expectations (Baker and O'Brien, 1971) and organizational prestige (Levine and White, 1961) are communicated from the broader environment into the focal organization.

Organization Set

Each of these boundary spanning roles represents a different type of interchange among organizations, a different type of relationship between the focal organization and its environment. Evan (1966) has developed a conception for understanding the relationships between organization and environment. The term *organization set* has been used to delineate those organizations and individuals with whom the focal organization is most intensely concerned with regard to input and output transactions (called by Warren (1967) the Input and Output Constituencies). The members of the organization set can greatly influence the focal organization by means of supplying to it, or withholding from it, needed input resources and accepting, or refusing to accept the organization's outputs.

The types of influence which members of an organization set can exert on a focal organization vary with the types of interchange or transaction between them. Organizations which control the input resources for a focal organization (the suppliers of patients, as well as the suppliers of funds) will be able to influence organizational decision-making and goal selection (Baker and O'Brien, 1971). Likewise, patterns of making or not making referrals of patients with particular service needs can also influence the processes and organizational role definition within the agency itself and the organizational staff's own image of the role and status of their own organization (Baker, Schulberg, and O'Brien, 1969).

Just as a mental health organization receives resources from some members of its set, it also is a supplier of resources to other members. The allocation of patients and staff resources (shared personnel, decentralized location of outreach workers, etc.) and distribution of other resources which members of its set need, provide the mental health facility with means of influencing the organizations with which it relates.

Organizations, particularly organizations in the *business* of providing services to the community, depend upon information from local organizations and groups to assess how well they are meeting community needs and expectations. Feedback refers to such information which can be used by a system to assess and modify its functioning.

Usually information is drawn from a number of members from the focal organization's set allowing it to independently assess its own functioning. When one member of a focal organization's set is able to control all or almost all of the needed feedback information for the focal organization, a state of *feedback dependence* occurs.

If one organization is in a position to control the flow of needed information to a large number of the organizations with which it relates, that organization can exert considerable influence over the operation and goal selection of those organizations.

Chin and O'Brien (1970), in their study of the interorganizational relationships of a multi-purpose center for senior citizens, note that it was the potential for the development of feedback dependence relations across different organizational systems which prevented the development of a joint client information system for senior citizens in that city. All of the health and social agencies which dealt with the elderly agreed to the desirability of developing a centralized client information system. They could not, however, accept the high degree of control over information which would be implicit in setting up such a system to be located in any one agency (in this case the multi-purpose center would have operated the system). The resistance by many agencies to centralization (in one agency with which they all related) of control over information which they needed (for self-assessment—a condition of feedback dependence) prevented implementation of the information system.

Wechsler and Noble (1970) report a range of difficulties encountered in the establishment of an information system for a group of human service agencies and point to a similar phenomenon of reactions against feedback dependence in that effort. A climate of mutual trust and interdependence among a wide range of agencies can foster the most meaningful and open exchange of needed information. Such a positive climate will help to avoid the difficulties which can be encountered when feedback dependence does occur.

One of the major tasks for the administrator of a mental health service is to be aware of the variety of interchanges going on between his organization and its organization set. Different boundary spanning roles within an organization will cause the involvement of staff members with different types of organizations. The administrator must be aware of the various areas of interorganizational interaction as they affect financial, client, and staff resources as well as informational exchange.

Organizational records can provide a readily available source of information about the interorganizational transactions of a caregiving agency. By monitoring records as to those members of the organization set who provide and accept referrals, the input and output constituencies for patient exchange may be documented (and changes in them noted). By noting in which staff groupings and in what contexts references to other human service organizations occur in the minutes of staff and other organizational meetings, a picture of the total pattern of interorganizational exchanges may be readily achieved. This is of particular importance in documenting less formalized linkages. Evan (1966) pointed to the potential usefulness of such organizational documents in the description of the organization set. O'Brien (1970) compared the types of inter-agency references occurring in the executive policy level group meetings and specific problem level group meetings (operating professional staff) of a large coordinating organization. The different sub-systems of the organization were shown to deal with markedly different organization sets, with little or no cross reference to the different interrelationships ongoing simultaneously.

The concept of organization set points, again, to the two-way interaction between organization and environment. Organizations are influenced by and in turn can exert influence on the others with which they regularly deal. These influences can exert pressure not only on organizational processes, but also on the role a particular human service organization is to play in the total pattern of care.

Organizational Environments

Often the tone of relationships between a focal organization and the members of its set will be affected by the general climate of change within the larger interorganizational field* of which all members of the organization set are a part. A stable environment will allow for a more predictable interaction among caregiving organizations in any particular organization set. An environment of rapid change, however, will stimulate a greater degree of interorganizational action with less predictability.

Emery and Trist (1965) developed a fourfold typology of organizational environments. The first type of environment is a relatively unchanging *randomized environment* in which organizations encounter one another and need take one another into consideration only at random occasions. Planning in the long term is the same as short term decision-making, since trial and error represents the best tactic for such processes. Organizations are adaptive and function best in single small units.

---

*Warren (1967) introduces the term "interorganizational field" in order to identify the larger collectivity of organizations concerned in one way or another, with the provision of health, social, educational, or economic services which may be included under the term human services.

The concept of interorganizational field was developed, building on Evan's organization set concept, to stress that all the organizations involved in various activities such as funding, planning, evaluation, legislation, or service delivery may or may not fit into a single system. Such systems may not exist either in terms of single organizations or groups of organizations. The only commonality implied by the term *field* is all the organizations relating in one way or another to human services. Chin and O'Brien (1970) developed a similar conception in characterizing relationships between organizations as a general intersystem theory.

The second type of environment, a *placid clustered environment,* is also a relatively unchanging one. Here there is a larger number of organizations engaged in similar or complementary tasks; and they may more predictably work with one another toward the achievement of their respective goals. Since the environment is relatively unchanging, however, these relationships once developed can continue to exist without constant review. Because of the greater predictability, the organizations would also tend to be larger and more hierarchical in structure. The period of time between the growing popularity of the mental hygiene movement and the increased emphasis on technology of care brought about by the second World War may be characterized as such a placid clustered environment. Interorganizational relationships did exist, particularly among caregiving organizations. Such relationships were, however, of a relatively unchanging nature.

The latter two types of environments posited by Emery and Trist (1965) probably more closely characterize the interorganizational field of mental health and the broader interorganizational field of human services as they currently exist. A *disturbed reactive environment* is one in which the actions and goals of other organizations within the field represent the primary consideration in any single organization's planning. Change is ongoing in such fields, and it is through interorganizational collaboration that such changes are dealt with. In order to increase the predictability of the environment, interorganizational liaisons may often be more formalized and multi-organizations (large service delivery or planning bodies) may often develop. It is through these that more hierarchical decisions can be made. The actions and reactions of other organizations within the field become a primary concern. This is the type of environment in which many mental health agencies have found themselves for the past 15 years. Increasingly, with the development of a focus on decentralized mental health services in the community, the increasing pressure for new forms of interorganizational liaison have fostered a *disturbed reactive environment.* In such an environment, predictability can be maintained, but it is achieved primarily through the development and retention of interorganizational relationships.

Emery and Trist's fourth type of environment, *turbulent field,* is one in which not only are the relationships among members of the field changing but also the nature and defining characteristics of that field itself are undergoing rapid change. New legislation, the emergence of decentralized community mental health centers, the formation of very large centers of influence (through interorganizational merger or liaison) and the development of new technology for treatment may precipitate the development of turbulent field characteristics in mental health.

Although some have characterized the environment of mental health care as a "turbulent field" (Baker and Schulberg, 1970), it seems perhaps more accurate to state that at periods of rapid technological or sociological change within the interorganizational field of mental health, the environment becomes a turbulent field for a limited period of time and then returns to a "disturbed reactive environment" as described earlier.

In a turbulent field, predictability is at a minimum. New forces may develop which negate reasons for formulating already existing organizational liaisons. During such periods, a *shake up* seems to occur in that existing relationships may be severed or drastically altered and new relationships formed. By the actions of organizations during the turbulent field period, a return to a more predictable environment is eventually accomplished. The goals, status, and the patterns of service of many organizations may undergo a rapid change during such turbulent periods.

The decision by a large state hospital to decentralize its services for a metropolitan area may precipitate the emergence of a turbulent field in that area. During such a period of time, new arrangements among mental health caregivers may be formed. These new arrangements may in turn influence the larger hospital in the way it implements its decision to decentralize. As the decentralization process continues and new organizational relationships are formed, a greater predictability once again may return to the environment. Similarly, the development of a comprehensive health planning or mental health planning agency in a particular area may precipitate the formation of a turbulent environment. Once such planning bodies are formed and their internal processes are established, a greater predictability again returns to the environment. Since the Community Mental Health Centers Act of 1963, there have been repeated pressures on mental health care that have precipitated turbulent environments. In each case, new relationships are formed.

It is in a time of such transition that an administrator may be able to most fruitfully examine his current relationships to better meet the goals and needs of his own organization. In such analysis, it is vital to know not only the areas in which organizations currently depend on one another, but also areas of interorganizational autonomy.

Interdependence and Independence Among Caregivers

In the above discussion of organization set, a great deal of emphasis was placed on the potential of members of any set to influence one another. While patterns of mutual influence have been the major focus of interorganizational research carried out to date, in most cases of interorganizational relations there are aspects of interchange that imply independence as well as interdependence.

In reviewing the concept of boundary of an organizational system, it must be recalled that there are different types of exchanges or interaction that occur across the boundary. Interorganizational relations must focus primarily on these cross boundaries (or intersystem interchanges). These cross boundary transactions in turn affect (and are affected by) internal organizational processes.

Boundaries will be differentially permeable to different media of exchange. They may be permeable in one direction to one type of exchange and permeable or impermeable in the opposite direction for other types of exchanges. The relationships between organizational systems may differ quantitatively as well as qualitatively as a function of the types of interchanges that go on. Considering different media of exchange, there may be different degrees of interdependence. Organizations may have a great deal of interdependence in the area of information flow, but function separately from one another where financial resources are concerned (Chin and O'Brien, 1970). A voluntary health and welfare council and a publicly financed community mental health center may have a relationship where the CMHC participates in a large number of community-wide planning efforts but does so without specific financial involvement with the voluntary council.

When looking at the relationships among members of a particular field of caregivers, the assessment of these relationships may be analogous to examining the same sample of material under a microscope with different cross sectional slices. Using one type of cross sectional slice, certain components of this sample material (certain organizations within the field) may be closely linked with one another. Taking a cross section sliced from another angle (looking at a different type of exchange) the relationship between these same components (organizations) may be quite distant with no apparent interchange.

It is important to bear in mind the mixed nature of interdependence relationships among organizations, since it may often account for apparently unpredictable actions. The relationship between similarity of organizational goals and cooperation or competition among particular organizations has been a repeated area of investigation among interorganizational theorists (Levine and White, 1961; Baker and O'Brien, 1971; Litwak and Hylton, 1962; Evan, 1966). Some theorists have predicted that agencies with similar goals would develop cooperative relations while others predict that similarity of goals leads to competition. It seems that the best predictor of these alternative outcomes would be an examination of other areas of interaction and exchange that exist. Areas of interaction around funding, client exchange, information exchange, joint planning, etc., might each differentially affect the nature of cooperation between organizations with similar domains.

In general, different types of interchange will lead to differences of *trust, interaction,* and *the permeability of organization boundaries* in new areas of interchange. There seems to be a point, however, at which the greater the variety of types and quantity of interorganizational interactions that occur between two organizations, the greater the overall interdependence of these organizations.

When there are a large number of areas of interorganizational interchange and when these existing areas are of major importance for each participating organization to achieve its goals, then there will be a greater readiness on the part of both of those organizations to tolerate variations in the pattern of exchange. New areas of exchange can be more easily initiated and continuing areas of exchange may be changed within time limited periods. As an example of such interdependence, in their study of the multi-purpose center for senior citizens, Chin and O'Brien (1970) noted that the center was able to make more demands on the municipal hospital for accepting referred patients than it could on other hospitals, both public and private, in the city. The apparent reason for their ability to place a strain on this aspect of the exchange relationship with that particular organization was that other areas of interchange (joint staffing, similar funding sources, shared board members, etc.) already existed between them. Had these other linkages not stressed the interdependence between the multi-purpose center and the municipal hospital, the hospital could well have begun to refuse referrals of the type they would not ordinarily accept. This was a conscious aspect of the relationship on the part of the hospital staff and the MPC staff.

A TYPOLOGY OF INTERORGANIZATIONAL LINKAGES

Just as information exchange relations may be of major importance in linkages between a set of organizations and funding exchanges may not occur at all within this set, so too, the factors which precipitate the establishment of relations will often set the tone of trust, cooperation, and flexibility (or of distrust and avoidance). If an organization is forced into a relationship of resource exchange either (1) by law, (2) as a contingency for the receipt of financial resources, or (3) by hierarchical authority, the initial tone of that exchange relationship will be markedly different from the tone of relationships which are engaged in voluntarily for the mutual benefit of both organizations.

Increasingly, federal programs are developing such mandated relationships as a contingency for additional or continued funding in a wide range of health, mental health and other human service areas. To the extent that relationships between any two caregiving organizations are of a mandated type (as opposed to voluntary relationships), the tone of such relationships will be less trusting.

A second aspect of the typology was developed by Mott (1968) in the study of a state health planning organization. For Mott, managed coordination "is accomplished by deliberately organized instrumentalities such as coordinating councils and central budget agencies of which the principal types are coordination by council and coordination by hierarchy. Managed coordination is distinguished from *unmanaged* coordination which occurs in a rather self-regulating framework, as in a market place." We would suggest for our purposes that the concept of managed coordination be limited to situations in which there is some influence, even slight, allocated to the coordinating mechanisms. The mere fact that a group conducts meetings may not imply a truly managed coordinating mechanism.

These two dimensions, managed versus unmanaged coordination mechanisms and mandated versus voluntary relationships, may prove to be a useful scheme for the practitioner in the analysis of relevant conceptual models of interorganizational relations. Figure 7-1 shows four global types of relations among caregivers from within this board typology. To the extent that relationships between two organizations (or within an organization set) occur according to any one of these four types, the theoretical models most appropriate to this type of interorganizational interaction may prove particularly useful to an individual in a boundary spanning role. The wider the mixture of types that occur in any given set, the greater the variety of influence leverages the administrator will have in determining the tone of interorganizational relations.

Type I relationships represent free exchanges of resources and information mutually chosen by each participant as a means for achieving organizational goals.

Type II relationships indicate voluntary choice of linkages with efforts at the standardization of mechanisms of exchange by means of coordinating organizations or through contracts.

A TYPOLOGY OF INTERORGANIZATIONAL LINKAGES

Coordination Mechanism

Selection of Relationship	Unmanaged	Managed
Voluntary	Type I Voluntary Exchanges	Type II Voluntary Coordination and Contracts
Mandated	Type III Forced contract without decision mechanisms	Type IV Hierarchical Coordination

Figure 7-1.

Type III relationships include situations in which neither participant has any choice, but instead, the linkages are mandated. In this type of relationship no means for conflict resolution are specified, although they should be developed.

Type IV relationships are also created by mandate rather than by voluntary choice. However, mechanisms for conflict resolution and decision-making have been developed.

Type I—Voluntary Exchange Relationships

Type I relationships occur most often between organizations providing similar types of service (either direct service or indirect service such as planning agencies) rather than across levels. Here the nature of interdependency between any two organizations is a result of the judged mutual benefit of the interaction. The pattern of influence in Type I relationships is primarily a function of (a) the extent to which each organization needs (or desires) the resources or information of the other and (b) the extent (or lack of) alternative sources for the materials or information in the relationship.*

Voluntary Exchanges and Influence Patterns

If one organization were dependent upon another for a wide variety of specific resources, the overall dependency of the first organization on the other would probably be greater. However, it is of limited utility to consider a single degree of *overall dependence*. Just as exchanges may take on different patterns when different *media of interchange* are considered, so, too, power relationships will likewise vary with different media of interchange. In exchanging information, one organization may have a great deal of power over another. In another area such as personnel, the other agency may have greater influence. These two patterns of mutual influence may occur simultaneously (one organization influencing the second in one area of interchange, while the second is dominant in other areas).

Chin and O'Brien (1970) in their study of intersystems relations of a multi-purpose center cite an example of such differential interdependence between the municipal hospital and the focal multi-purpose center referring a number of clients to the hospital. At the same time, the hospital relied upon the center staff for interorganizational planning and programming for gerontological care. The patterns of influence between the two organizations were clearly reversed when those two types of interchange were considered.

Exchange Models of Interorganizational Relationships

Levine and White (1961) developed an exchange model for the analysis of interorganizational relations. Conceptually, their exchange approach best fits the voluntary-unmanaged (Type I) situation. According to them, exchange is defined as any type of activity in which organizations voluntarily engage with the intent of using the activity to fulfill their own organizational goals.

---

*Thibaut and Kelley (1959) in the elaboration of an exchange model for small group interaction, have developed the concepts of *Comparison Level* and *Comparison Level for Alternatives* paralleling factors (a) and (b) above.

In their study of patterns of patient referral and other free exchanges among health agencies, Levine, White, and Paul (1963) document that the direction of exchange was a function not only of their needs for specific resources (or lack of certain program capacities), but also of the "organizational domain consensus" among the agencies. Defining organizational domain in terms of target population, and the goals and services provided by the organizations, the authors noted a reluctance to enter exchanges when consensus was lacking.

Unless program administrators and other boundary spanning personnel are able to provide an assessment of their organization's domain that is generally agreed upon by members of the organization set, the ambiguities may prevent mutually beneficial exchanges. When the larger environment is in *turbulent field* conditions, consensus regarding organizational domain will be low and administrators and other key personnel should be sensitive to the ambiguities thus created and ways to reduce them.

It is important for the mental health administrator in voluntary-unmandated exchange relationships to carefully assess the value of multiple engagements. Given the transitory nature of many interorganizational exchanges (particularly in the exchange of information), and also considering the number of staff members who may be involved in such informal exchanges, criteria for decisions on entering relationships are difficult to set. It is wise, however, for the administrator to maintain some notion of the costs and benefits of the varied exchange relationships in which his organization is engaged.

There are a number of questions which may be helpful in reviewing exchange relationships. These questions can help diagnose the overall level of interdependence between two organizations. When interdependence is high, there will be a tendency to move toward more formal mechanisms for relationships (such as those in Types II, III, and IV). In general, the greatest organizational autonomy exists when exchange remains voluntary and unmanaged.

1. What are the costs and rewards of each particular type of interchange (money for service, influence for information, supplying

clients in order to relieve pressure from one's own caseload)?

2. If a large variety of interactions is ongoing, to what extent does the existence of one type of exchange affect other types of interactions? (Will altering the relationships with regard to shared information improve the possibility for new joint programs in areas of mutual need?)

3. Looking at all the exchanges, how fully (both in variety and extent) is either organization dependent on the other for needed resources and information?

4. Does interdependence imply an imbalance in exchanges which affect organizational autonomy? (And if so, are the rewards to be gained from the interdependence worth the reduction of autonomy?)

5. Are there alternative sources for the needed resource (material or information) if the interdependence is felt to be too extensive to maximize the effectiveness of each organization?

In general, the wider the exchanges, the greater the interdependence. Such interdependence may be beneficial to both agencies; on the other hand, decreased organizational autonomy may, in some situations, prevent organizational flexibility and innovation. These two factors must be assessed when the total pattern of interorganizational interdependence is reviewed.

If the organizational environment is one in which there is rapid change and prediction is difficult, a move to a Type II relationship (contractual and voluntary coordination) may be used to add predictability to the environment. Voluntary-unmandated relationships offer the possibility of greater organizational autonomy (given that there are sufficient and alternative resources for the choice of exchange relationships), but may be less functional for the organization in a turbulent environment. Such Type II relations will prove mutually beneficial only to the extent that Type I relations remain open and trusting in tone.

Type II—Voluntary but Managed Relationships

The second general type of relationship in this typology is a voluntary relationship in which some type of managed coordinating mechanism has been developed. In this case, the engagements between organizations are somewhat more formalized and the media of interchange are often of a more standardized nature. Membership in a community health and welfare council, Community Chest, or formal contracts might be characterized as Type II relationships. In voluntary-managed relationships, there is a greater degree of specificity of the areas of interdependence and of the overall balance of influence between participating organizations (at least within the limits of the contract).

Litwak and Hylton (1962) in their review of coordinating agencies noted that organizations with semi-autonomous constituencies (such as Federated Catholic and Jewish agencies) or with national rather than local constituencies (local chapters of Red Cross, Cancer Society, etc.) were able to exert more influence on the decision-making of coordinating agencies than could other member agencies lacking such identified constituencies. The conditional nature of their participation in local coordinating organizations illustrates the greater clarity and standardization of areas of influence in such voluntary-managed relationships. Jewish agencies could conduct separate fund-raising campaigns since part of the money thus raised would be used for national and international purposes. Catholic agencies, able to exist without membership in the Community Chest, could exert control over the eligibility of other organizations (such as Planned Parenthood) for membership in the larger coordination fund-raising body.

In contracts for services, the nature of the exchanges (services for dollars, shared staff for joint projects, etc.) is more specific. There will be additional (voluntary-unmanaged) interactions but they become less transitory and more predictable.

Litwak and Hylton (1962) hypothesized that "coordinating agencies will develop and continue in existence if formal organizations are partly interdependent; agencies are aware of the interdependence; and it can be defined in standardized units of action." The major stress of the Litwak and Hylton model then deals with diagnosing interdependence and standardizing the units of exchange within such interdependence.

In mental health care, such voluntary coordination may exist in relationships with referral resources such as nursing homes, back-up hospitals, etc. While a caregiving organization can withdraw from these relationships should the cost of participation become too high, participation helps to: (1) increase the predictability of the environment with regard to the provision of input (cases referred) and the acceptance of outputs (discharged cases referred) ; (2) standardize areas of interchange and thus more clearly delineate legitimate (in terms of the contractual or membership agreements) areas of interorganizational influence from areas not so legitimated.

The mental health center in establishing relationships with a back-up hospital may be able to specify the services to be received by patients they refer as a legitimate part of the exchange contract. It cannot, however, legitimately influence change in administrative staffing patterns within the larger organization.*

The principal benefits of engaging in contractual arrangements and other types of voluntary coordination is the greater stability it gives to a rapidly changing environment. The cost of reduced flexibility, however, must be weighed against this benefit. In *turbulent field* conditions, contracts and coordination can be a most helpful, and even necessary step.

In more stable environments, the principal question the administrator should ask when considering voluntary coordination is whether standardization in one area of exchange will allow needed flexibility in other areas. If the standardization helps to clarify the ranges and limitations of interorganizational influences, it is generally an advantage.

Voluntary contracts and standardized participation in coordinating bodies facilitate the movement of one's organizational environment from *turbulent field* conditions to the more predictable *disturbed reactive environment* conditions. This greater predictability may limit an organization's autonomy in some areas but by the same token may reinforce the autonomy of the organization in non-contractual areas.

Both Type I and Type II relationships represent voluntary participation on the part of the focal organization in a relationship for its own benefit. In areas of voluntary exchange, whether contractual or more transitory, each participating organization has the

---

*Influence on the basis of a new contract (or influence during periods of new contract negotiation—which corresponds to turbulent field situations) may be a means of influencing such changes in another organization.

choice to withdraw from the relationship should the cost become too high for participation. Such withdrawal may take more time in a contractual relationship but the option still exists.

The remaining two types of relationships, Types III and IV, represent mandated relationships. Within this category, the decision to enter the relationship is not left to the participating organizations but is specified by a third party. When two or more organizations are related by some external mandate, there will often exist or develop areas of exchange outside of the mandate which will more closely fulfill the conditions of voluntary relationships (Type I and Type II). The overall climate between two organizations will largely be a function of the free exchange which exists between them rather than their mandated relationships.

Type III—Mandated but Unmanaged Relationships

Coordination between existing service delivery facilities has increasingly become a precondition for the allocation of funds for new programs. Efforts to avoid duplication and overlap of services have resulted in the *mandate* of contact between organizations serving the same limited populations. These mandated relationships often do not specify: (1) the scope or limits around which contacts are to take place; (2) what benefits a participating organization may expect from the relationships; (3) the rewards or costs to be incurred by each participant (or third party) in carrying out its role; (4) any structure for the resolution of interorganizational conflict in areas where interests of participating organizations are not mutual.

A large state mental hospital, for example, may have to relate to a number of different primary caregiving mental health centers. The need for such arrangements may not only be the result of mandate by law, but also of physical or financial constraints requiring a reduction in the cost of patient care in a given area. Questions such as how many cases are to be referred and which organization has aftercare and case management responsibilities, are not specified when such relationships are mandated. Yet, the participating organizations must, by one means or another, resolve each of these issues. If they remain unresolved, the uncertainties will not only negatively affect the overall comprehensiveness of the program, but will also negatively affect the internal operations of each organization.

In such situations, there are no alternatives for the organization but to continue the relationship. Because of this lack of choice, the climate of other voluntary relationships plays a critical role. The pattern of the voluntary interorganizational exchanges, including the exchange of clients, information, staff, other joint programs, etc., will often be the most telling factor in the relationship between participants in mandated but unmanaged relationships.

Mandated but unmanaged relationships are essentially unstable. All the participating organizations feel the need for greater clarity about the freedoms and limitations of the relationships. In general, the administrator should help to specify either by informal agreement or by formal contract the nature of the relationship that will be developed. There will be a tendency for such relationships to become voluntary contractual if the pattern of the other relationships between the organizations is positive. It is likely to become a hierarchically arranged relationship if the other contacts between the organizations have been antagonistic, competitive, or nonexistent.

In his study of a state-wide governmental health planning council, Mott* (1968) points to the dependency on out-of-council treaties between organizations as the primary means for conflict resolution in the council. The council's existence was mandated but without specification of means for resolving conflict among participating members. The council served as a vehicle to identify areas of mutual interest or conflict and to allow such conflict to be settled by informal negotiations outside of the council chambers (voluntary unmandated exchanges). The mandated aspect of these relationships stimulated the creation of the other nonmandated exchanges and thus facilitated interorganizational

---

*Mott labelled this coordination by council as managed coordination differentiating it from free market types of unmanaged coordination. We might better characterize such mandated council relationships as mandated but unmanaged in the present typology.

collaboration. In reviewing comprehensive health planning patterns, Mott (1971) again points to the inability of such bodies to resolve conflict due to their mandated existence without the specification of financial or hierarchical mechanisms for settling conflicts.

An administrator's action within such mandated relationships is of crucial importance. By carefully evaluating areas of interdependence with other organizations with whom a mandated relationship exists, he may be able to set the tone for mutually beneficial relationships. If this is ignored by the administrator, the effect may be a reduction in the ability of his own organization to function effectively. In relationships where mandates exist but specified decision-making mechanisms do not, the administrator must play an active role. He has a greater latitude in the establishment of interorganizational relationships than is sometimes apparent.

Relationships in this category once resolved cannot be forgotten. With changes in legislation, innovations in care delivery, etc., the organizational environment from time to time takes on the characteristics of a turbulent field. Particularly at these times it is important for the administrator to be aware of and involved in the maintenance of trust and collaboration in interorganizational relationships. Once a climate of distrust sets in, communication decreases and the effectiveness of both organizations in reaching their goals will, no doubt, suffer. There will also be a tendency to move into more hierarchical arrangements where organizational autonomy will be centered in one party with a decrease in the autonomy of others.

Because of their ambiguity, Type III relationships may allow an innovative and active staff to become more effective. Their disadvantages stem from their instability. They offer an opportunity to establish new types of working relationships in areas of mutual interest but force other relationships which may not be of benefit.

In general, conditions of mandated but unmanaged relationships are not the *choice* of any of the participant parties but rather represent a situation in which each party must try to optimize the outcome and make the best of a given situation.

Type IV—Mandated and Managed Relationships

The most stringent type of relationship includes those where not only the establishment of patterns of interaction are dictated as a precondition for funding, but also certain aspects of inter-organizational decision-making are specified.

As local coordinating bodies take on increased responsibility for the delivery of comprehensive mental health services, such mandated and managed relationships become increasingly common. Here the concept of a comprehensive system of care delivery becomes possible with greater financial, informational and managerial functions located in one member of a highly integrated set. The analogy of such a set of caregivers as a single caregiving system, discussed by Baker and Schulberg (1970), may be fulfilled. Each participating organization has broad areas of interdependency with others. The organizations draw funds, most often from a limited financial pool and through the same funding body, thus reinforcing a high state of interdependency. In the public sector, many of the organizational functions such as identification of clients, information for organizational self-assessment and program design, may become centralized into large planning bodies of broader scope than any single organization. In local areas, a community mental health program may have responsibility for developing service contracts, providing information, and making decisions with regard to the delivery of mental health care in specific catchment areas, city-wide, and state-wide. Mental health planning agencies may take on the broader responsibilities for assessment of mental health needs and evaluating services from a broader perspective. Particularly as relationships become both mandated and managed, the autonomy of participating caregiving organizations may seem to be lessened. Here again, the fundamental question is how much autonomy is given up in return for a greater ability to fulfill organizational goals.

Within a unified (interorganizational) care delivery system with high interdependency, the boundaries of member organizations will generally become more permeable to exchanges and influence from other system members.*

Under mandated and managed conditions, it may be easier for an organization to establish new liaisons with other caregivers through third party interventions. While the tone of such relationships is still primarily a function of the voluntary interactions between them, the ability to identify and gain needed resources for new programs is facilitated. This is particularly true when new areas of collaboration are identified in conjunction with the centralized planning body.

For the individual administrator, the maintenance of a positive climate between his organization and other members of the mandated, managed caregiving system is most important. If distrust develops, information flow is decreased, and the ability of each organization to fulfill its own role will be lessened. Decision-making will become even more centralized, *outside of the realm of the individual organization,* since there will be fewer and fewer individuals with a full range of information available to them. By the maintenance of voluntary exchange relationships in non-mandated areas, a climate of interorganizational trust can be maintained.

Cooperation between organizations in a mandated and managed service system, may enable them to gain additional resources. To help in this process, the administrator must maintain individual contact with the other organizations.

Involvement in an integrated system for the delivery of comprehensive care can make new resources available to the mental health program from outside the usual mental health funding sources. A community mental health center, for example, may be able to increase the involvement of nursing homes, visiting nurse associations, family agencies, etc., in mental health as a result of its affiliation with other mental health programs that provide needed resources to those particular organizations.

---

*The example of relationships between a municipal multi-purpose center for senior citizens and a municipal hospital cited earlier illustrates the greater permeability of organizational boundaries within unified caregiving systems.

Use of the Typology

The typology presented above will hopefully aid the administrator in diagnosing the types of interdependencies in which his organization is engaged. Perhaps the greatest opportunity for him to affect interorganizational relations is in the areas of mandated unmanaged and voluntary interorganizational exchange. In both these areas, it is his willingness to explore a range of engagements that allows him to broaden his organization's scope or better fulfill its goals.

In managed relationships such as Types II and IV, the role and options of the administrator cannot be ignored. While both of these types are relatively standardized, other less regulated exchanges between the organizations must be maintained. The administrator cannot limit his interorganizational involvement to merely the fulfillment of contracts. It is only by attending to nonspecified areas of interaction that the administrator will be able to utilize interorganizational collaboration as a means of goal fulfillment.

As noted earlier, organizations are rarely involved in only one of these four types of collaboration. In reviewing all of a focal organization's relationships to members of its set, it is likely that all four of these relationships will exist. The administrator is faced with a mixed set of relationships, some voluntary, some managed, and many containing standardized as well as unstandardized interchanges. The administrator must identify those areas in which a unitary system of care seems to exist, and differentiate them from the larger interorganizational field in which many programs are involved but which relate only partially (or not at all) to each other.

GENERAL INTERSYSTEM AND MIXED ECONOMY MODELS OF INTERORGANIZATIONAL RELATIONS

To the extent that organizations interact as a single system of care in a given service area, the predictability of the environment for members of that system has increased. This predictability is, however, far less than perfect considering the human service activities within the area as a whole. When this wider range of caregiving, funding, planning, and service organizations is considered, and with new patterns constantly being developed, the conception of a single system of caregivers and the greater predictability to be expected from it become questionable (Baker and O'Brien, 1971). Since constant change is inevitable in the human services field, it is more of a constantly turbulent field than any individual sector of care, such as mental health or physical health.

Increasing attention has been paid to models and approaches to interorganizational relations that emphasize not only the continuity of these relations (such as the single system approaches described in Type IV), but also attempt to assess areas of discontinuity. These intersystems or mixed-economy approaches (Chin and O'Brien, 1970; Warren, 1967, 1970; Long, 1958) emphasize the autonomy as well as the interdependence of organizations within a broad field. It is through an examination of relationships between systems that gaps in continuity can be identified and understood.*

A Market Place Economy of Services

An illustration of the difference between single system and mixed-economy (or intersystem) approaches is the way overlapping organizational domains are considered in these two broad models. In reviewing the Levine and White (1961) exchange model, it was pointed out that organizations with similar domains will see each other as less cooperative (since they compete for the same clients). Most legislation which vests coordinating bodies with decision-making authority (Type IV relationships) stresses the elimination or at least the reduction of duplication. Where market place conditions prevail, the assumption is that if two organizations provide the same services to the same target population and each has a full complement of clients, they are both

---

*Long (1958), in a field study of social and political relations in Boston, characterized such interorganizational environments as an "Ecology of Games." In his model, it was shown that each organization or actor in an interorganizational field was involved in a variety of different interaction systems (games). Each game pursues different types of goals. While actions in one system (game) can affect goal achievement in other systems, the individual must be able to diagnose the nature and outcome of each game in which he is engaged.

needed. Where such services can exist independently from one another, the market model would imply that they should do so. This difference in models is elaborated by Reid (1970).

While the need for coordination to ensure a breadth of service (filling gaps in certain services and avoiding the duplication of others) is emphasized in a mixed-economy model, *redundancy* of service reinforces the adaptability of the interorganizational field to changes in service demands. It is assumed that when the *market* for such services is reduced, then the redundancy will also be reduced. In situations where clients have free choice among a range of redundant services, this type of model seems to have particular promise. In adoption, for example, where a number of agencies once served each community, there is a current trend to reduce the number of agencies providing adoptive services (this is more a function of a reduction in the supply of children rather than in the demand from prospective parents, but the model still seems to apply). Warren (1970) advocates the establishment of citizen-based service delivery agencies in order to act as a stimulus to more established agencies in meeting clients' needs for change in services. Competition would here be used as a stimulus to system change.

Intersystems and Mental Health Care

The applicability of a market place approach in mental health care is, of course, somewhat limited since the services are generally provided by means of referral from an agency rather than by self-referral of the patient. Also, mental health services carry more of a stigma than physical health or even income maintenance in many places.

For an individual caregiver, the intersystem approach is characterized by an emphasis on the identification of differing interorganizational relationships (with differing media of exchange) , that may include a variety of different caregiving systems. A mental health center may be part of a comprehensive community mental health caregiving system (in terms of funding and referral patterns for a given community, a Type IV relationship). At the same time, the center, with a group of other neighborhood service agencies, exchanges information on client flow (a Type I information exchange). The center may enter into a service contract for the provision of preventive and remedial mental health services for students and consultation for teachers in a local school (Type II relationship). The center may participate in a three state research project on the effects of methadone treatment as a contingency for receiving funds to implement a drug rehabilitation program (Type III relationship). Depending on the perspective, this center is a subsystem of other mental health caregivers, an independent agent engaging in voluntary exchange at the neighborhood level, a semi-autonomous participant in the provision of community educational services, etc.

While resource exchange may be expected to affect patterns of information flow and vice versa, the existence of one type of exchange does not necessarily imply that others will exist. A local mental health center must be sensitive to local demands for service which other members of a comprehensive community mental health caregiving system may not need to respond to. Only through the communication of, and legitimation of these demands by other members of its organization set will the center be able to avoid, or at least minimize, conflicting demands by organizational constituents. Such communication serves as a vehicle for the establishment of organizational goals and capacities. By the development of such a consensus, the administrator and other key staff can gain greater flexibility for individual action in the interorganizational realm.

Administrative Flexibility in Interorganizational Relationships

The typology of interorganizational relationships may help the administrator identify areas for analysis and action. It may be that there are fewer constraints on the actions of the administrator in the area of interorganizational relationships than there are on his intraorganizational roles.

Within an organization, the demands of administrative responsibility, salary-setting, hiring and firing, the actions of previous administrators, and the structures developed by organizational mandate or organizational history, all act to limit the options of the administrator. Within the realm of interorganizational relationships, however, the reverse seems to be the case. With the increased emphasis on the development of new patterns of interorganizational collaboration, many of these constraints do not exist. By analyzing the relationships between his organization and members of its set, and by a review of the patterns of interaction within the community's broader field of human services, the administrator can facilitate the achievement of his organization's goals. He may also be able to facilitate the achievement of a more comprehensive system of service delivery for the community.

It is also possible, at times, for an administrator to influence his own organization through his actions in the interorganizational field in situations where direct intervention on his part is not possible. The new director of a health and welfare council may not legitimately be able to influence the stand taken by the department of health within that council regarding local health planning. Through his relationships with the state health planning agency, he may, however, be able to get information to those staff members that might alter their opinions.

When interorganizational relationships take on the characteristics of a turbulent field, an administrator who can increase the predictability of that environment can play a most crucial role. Interorganizational analysis can help an innovative individual understand the leverage his organization has or which is available through third party interventions for the stabilization of the environment. It may be that such an analysis will suggest new areas for interorganizational cooperation which, when implemented, will provide at least some beginning structure around which a more stable environment can coalesce.

While the individual administrator can have a great deal of impact on the tenor of interorganizational relationships, such relationships are carried out by a variety of boundary-spanning individuals within an organization. An administrator must be able to communicate with his staff in order to gain and to share information on the interorganizational status of focal organizations.

This chapter has emphasized the review of an organization's voluntary exchange relationships in order to identify areas in which individual action may bring about system or intersystem change. Despite the type of relationships in which the organization is engaged, these voluntary and unmandated contacts tend to set the climate of trust and collaboration.

While voluntary unmandated relationships act as a primary vehicle for establishing the interorganizational climate, they also act as a primary area in which individual action can manifest a change in this climate.

The interpersonal contacts developed with other organizations through voluntary unmanaged relationships will set the tone of other types of interorganizational relationships. No amount of formalization, contracts, mandated authority, or hierarchical power will change an interpersonal climate from one of distrust to one of trust if the relationships between the actors in both organizations have developed negatively.

Bellin (1970) emphasized the ability of the administrators and key boundary personnel to work with members of other organizations as the prime factor in determining the success or failure of interorganizational collaboration, regardless of the structural relationships. Structures (the types of relationships or internal organizational structures) present limits or broadened possibilities for interorganizational collaboration but in and of themselves cannot determine an interorganizational climate. In order to help his organization have an impact during periods of relative turbulence, an administrator must thoroughly diagnose his own interorganizational capacities. Such a diagnosis includes a number of steps:

1. Identify the boundary-spanning personnel within his own organization and the organizational constituents with whom they deal.
2. Assess the rewards and costs of the voluntary exchange relationships in which his organization is currently engaged both from the perspective of his own organization as well as the others.
3. Assess areas of dissensus and consensus in organizational domain and organizational prestige, and note patterns of communication that operate in informal interorganizational relationships.

4. Maintain open communication between himself and other key boundary-spanning personnel (two-way communications to allow for information exchange on the changing nature of the interorganizational climate).

5. Identify areas of potential intervention, either direct or through third-party intervention, in order to increase the predictability of the interorganizational environment (for example, changing Type III relationships into a more stable set of formal and informal exchanges).

6. Attempt to formulate and communicate with his staff information on the relationship between their own organization and others.

7. Facilitate the opening of organizational boundaries to new interorganizational liaisons at all staff levels.

SUMMARY

The increasing demand for a comprehensive range of mental health services accessible at the local level has made even more important the development and maintenance of good interorganizational relationships. Broadened participation by local citizen groups in the decision-making process and the decentralization of both planning and services from the federal and state to the local level have emphasized this still more.

Building on the concepts of organization set and the relationships between a mental health facility and its changing environment, a typology of interorganizational relationships is developed. Emphasizing that different patterns of interorganizational independence and interdependence may exist when different media of exchange are considered, the typology considers (1) the *voluntary or mandated* nature of the relationships and (2) the nature of the coordinating mechanisms *(unmanaged versus managed)*.

The role of the mental health administrator and the latitude for innovation on the part of administrators and other key boundary spanning staff are discussed. Tentative steps to prepare an organization to function more effectively in bringing about intersystems change are presented.

REFERENCES

Baker, F. and O'Brien, G.: Intersystems relations and the coordination of human service organizations. *Am J Public Health, 61(1):*130-137, 1971.

Baker, F. and Schulberg, H.C.: Community health caregiving systems: Integration of interorganizational networks. In Sheldon, A., Baker, F., and McLaughlin, C. (Eds.): *Systems and Medical Care.* Cambridge, M.I.T. Press, 1970.

Baker, F.; Schulberg, H. C. and O'Brien, G.: The changing mental hospital —its perceived image and contact with the community. *Ment Hyg, 53:* 237-244, 1969.

Bellin, L. E.: Discussion of William S. Reid's paper "Interorganizational cooperation: A review and critique of current theory." In White, P. and Vlasak, G. J. (Eds.): *Interorganizational Research in Health: Conference Proceedings.* Rockville, National Center for Health Services Research and Development, U. S. Department of Health, Education, and Welfare, 1970.

Chin, R. and O'Brien, G.: General intersystem theory: The model and a case of practitioner application. In Sheldon A., Baker, F., and McLaughlin, C. (Eds.): *Systems and Medical Care.* Cambridge, M.I.T. Press, 1970.

Emery, S. E. and Trist, E. L.: The causal texture of organizational environments. *Human Relations, 18:* 21-32, 1965.

Evan, W. M.: The organization set: Toward a theory of interorganizational relations. In Thompson, J. D. (Ed.): *Approaches to Organizational Design.* Pittsburgh, University of Pittsburgh Press, 1966.

Levine, S. and White, P. E.: Exchange as a conceptual framework for the study of interorganizational relationships. *Administrative Science Quarterly, 5:* 583-601, 1961.

Levine, S.; White, P. E. and Paul, B. D.: Community interorganizational problems in providing medical care and social services. *Am J Public Health, 53:* 1183-1195, 1963.

Litwak, E. and Hylton, L. F.: Interorganizational analysis: A hypothesis on coordinating agencies. *Administrative Science Quarterly, 6:* 395-420, 1962.

Long, N.: The local community as an ecology of games. *Am J Sociol, 64:* 251-261, 1958.

Mott, B.: *Anatomy of a Coordinating Council.* Pittsburgh, University of Pittsburgh Press, 1968.

Mott, B.: *Citizen participation in comprehensive health planning.* A presentation at the Human Services Design Laboratory Colloquium, Cleveland, February 4, 1971.

O'Brien, G.: *Organizational constituency analysis: An approach for the analysis of the organization set of a changing health and welfare council.* Mimeographed. Harvard Medical School, The Laboratory of Community Psychiatry, 1970.

Reid, W. J.: Interorganizational cooperation: A review and critique of current theory. In White, P. E., and Vlasak, G. J.: *Interorganizational Research in Health*. Rockville, National Center for Health Services Research and Development, U. S. Department of Health, Education, and Welfare, 1970.

Simpson, R. L. and Gulley, W. H.: Goals, environmental pressures and organizational characteristics. *Am Sociol Rev, 27(3)*:344-351, 1962.

Thibaut, J. W. and Kelley, H. H.: *The Social Psychology of Groups*. New York, Wiley, 1959.

Thompson, J. D. and McEwen, W. J.: Organizational goals and environment: Goal-setting as an interaction process. *Am Sociol Rev. 23*:23-31, 1958.

Warren, R. L.: The interorganizational field as a focus of investigation. *Administrative Science Quarterly, 12:* 396-419, 1967.

Warren, R. L.: Alternative strategies of interagency planning. In White, P. E., and Vlasak, G. J. (Eds.) *Interorganizational Research in Health: Conference Proceedings*. Rockville, National Center for Health Services Research and Development, U. S. Department of Health, Education, and Welfare, 1970.

Wechsler, H. and Noble, J. H.: Obstacles to establishing community-wide information systems in health and welfare. *Welfare in Review, 8:(6)* 18-26, 1970.

CHAPTER 8

COMMUNITY PARTICIPATION

Seymour R. Kaplan

DURING A DISCUSSION of current issues in health services delivery, a member of the audience remarked that "community participation is community administration." He said this as much to himself as to the audience at large. Whatever else it communicated, equating community participation with the administration of health and mental health services was a dramatic way of emphasizing the importance of community participation to the achievement of organizational objectives. This point of view will prevail in this chapter.

THE PARAMETERS OF COMMUNITY PARTICIPATION

The term community participation is used to refer to a variety of contexts and settings. It may refer to informal or organized activities in communities. It may refer to activities that are unrelated to institutions or it may refer to activities specifically related to private or public institutions. A definition of community participation may be further complicated by the ascribed meaning of the words *community* and *participation,* each varying according to the user's frame of reference. Therefore, rather than attempt an explicit definition, it may be more useful to review the various direct or indirect references to community participation found in the literature and in the current rhetoric.

1. The Sociopolitical References

In the political context, the formal meaning of participation, to partake in common with others, refers to the democratic form of governance. When both a sociological and political context is inferred, community participation may connote the ideals of an egalitarian society. The sociological concept of community, in this reference, tends to be characterized by its social cohesiveness.

In addition to shared interests, facilities and cultural homogeneity, cohesiveness in a community requires a stable pattern of social relations conducive to a common psychological identification among its members. The multi-ethnic composition and high mobility of our urban populations and the lack of long range social planning has made communities, at least in this sense, a rarity. Partly for this reason, mandated community participation for programs in urban centers has not been established in identifiable *true communities*.

In the New York City public health and welfare programs, for example, the composition of the participating *communities* is defined by geography, usually based upon bureaucratic considerations. Community mental health center catchment areas defined as the communities to be served are determined by the boundaries of health areas, previously established by the New York City Health Department.

2. Other Parameters

Many references to community participation originate from historical developments and traditions as well as from a sociopolitical context. For example, there are a number of participant roles included within the parameters of community participation.

(a) Community Participant as Consumer

There are two aspects of the consumer role to which references are made in community participation. The consumer as a member of a community who uses free public services has a very different connotation from the consumer as a *customer,* who pays for his services (Roemer, 1962). However, the word consumer is currently applied to both situations and often used interchangeably with community. As third party payments become more widespread, the consumer, in the sense of customer, will become a much more significant participant in consumer-provider negotiations in the mental health field (Falk, 1966; Munts, 1967; Pollack, 1965).

(b) Community Participant as Volunteer

The role of the volunteer, until recently, is usually what has been meant by community participation in the programs of human service organizations (Seidel, 1960). The volunteer, individually or through organized groups, is an important manpower resource. The volunteer as a fund raiser, usually under community or national auspices, still adds significantly to the financial resources available to many human services organizations.

(c) Community Participant as Indigenous Nonprofessional

A major development of the past decade, community participation through the employment of indigenous nonprofessionals has been most prevalent in low-income areas, particularly among urban minority populations (Grosser, et al, 1969; Feldman, 1971). The nonprofessional as a new paid manpower resource is an extension of, and to some extent has supplanted, the volunteer in human services programs.

(d) Community Participant as Board Member

There are a variety of advisory and governing boards associated with public and private institutions whose members until recently have been almost exclusively appointed from volunteers prominent in business and professional affairs. A great deal of the recent attention to community participation has been focused upon board membership from among a cross section of the citizens of the geographical area served by the institution (Brieland, 1971; Galiher, et al, 1971; Piven, 1966). The role of community boards is discussed in detail below.

(e) Community Participant as Organizational Member

Another aspect of community participation refers to the large number of traditional organizations formed in relation to specific human service institutions, i.e., the Parent Teachers Associations. Citizen organizations such as the PTA have been the vehicle for major changes in the delivery of human services.

There are other important citizen organizations, too varied to review. They include such diverse groups as *watch dog* committees composed of prominent citizens that have influenced major social welfare legislation, and neighborhood groups such as *block associations*. These latter groups, in some instances, have been organized into citywide and national coalitions to form influential organizations such as the National Council of Welfare Committees.

HISTORICAL PERSPECTIVES AND CONCURRENT DEVELOPMENTS

The extent to which the roles enumerated above will continue as major vehicles of community participation will relate, in good measure, to the trends or movements from which they have emerged. This historical perspective, while frequently overlooked, is of great importance. Included within the parameters of community participation are developments reflecting both historical and current trends or movements. These trends include the volunteer and the nonprofessional movements, as well as the federal social reform movement, the consumer movement and the civil rights movement.

The Mental Health Volunteer Movement

The participation of volunteers in human service organizations is a tradition associated with the very origins of these institutions. Until the passage of federal social reform measures in the 1930's, many human service organizations depended upon private voluntary contributions for a considerable part of their funds and upon volunteers for needed additional manpower. To a significant extent, this is still true today.

Although health and mental health services, especially for children, have also benefited from volunteer participation, Greenblatt and Hinman (1970) date the beginning of a volunteer *movement* in mental health to post-World War II. This would correlate with the beginning of modern-day psychiatry, stimulated during the earlier post-war days by psychiatric services for veterans.

The volunteer movement described by Greenblatt and Hinman, at least in Massachusetts, primarily took root in the hospitals, particularly the state mental hospitals. The major population groups in Massachusetts contributing to the volunteer movement were the women of the Grey Ladies, hospital auxiliary groups and college students. "In Massachusetts alone in 1967, the number of volunteers giving service in hospitals and schools for retarded (13,300) approached the total number of employees in the entire Department of Mental Health (15,800). Recent survey data from the National Institute of Mental Health indicate that more than 7,000 student volunteers have been working in well over 100 mental institutions throughout the country."

Volunteers also serve on governing boards of public and private mental health organizations and have been the nucleus around which area and regional citizen boards are formed. The latter situation is the model for New York State in which volunteer citizen groups have established mental health programs by providing private funds to match federal and state grants. The extent to which private funds continue to be a factor in the financing of mental health services will influence the role and composition of community boards, particularly in regard to the involvement of citizens from low-income communities. Although the reliance upon private monies has decreased, the affluent board member still has a necessary role in maintaining the solvency of many of these institutions.

The volunteer, as a source of additional manpower, began to extend his role beyond the mental hospital toward participation in a vast array of innovative programs during the 1960's. The influence of the volunteer upon the nonprofessional mental health movement has been fundamental. Until the term began to assume the meaning we attribute to it today, the volunteer was the nonprofessional mental health worker. It is useful to keep this in mind since many of the critical issues we face today regarding the role of the paid indigenous nonprofessional are similar to those discussed in the past about the volunteer as a non-paid staff member. This analogy is often valid in the comparison between the low-income community board member and the prominent citizen board member.

The Mental Health Nonprofessional Movement

The role of the nonprofessional in mental health has been a particularly notable development in recent years and is intimately related to the evolution of community participation in mental health programs. The nonprofessional, for example, has been seen as a *bridge* to the community as well as an important new manpower resource. This *bridge* function is stressed by Hansell and associates (1968). Recently, however, the use of the indigenous nonprofessional has come to include roles other than those dependent upon membership in a particular class or stratum of society.

Riessman and Rieff (1964) distinguish the indigenous nonprofessional not on the basis of similarity to the client in background, language, and style, but on the basis of the services he performs. The authors describe three major jobs or roles for the indigenous nonprofessional: the direct service agent (homemaker, teacher's aide) ; the community organizer or neighborhood worker who functions to involve local residents in community planning and action; and the expediter or bridge man who serves to link clients with the agency providing the service. These three service functions describe the models that evolved from the work with the nonprofessional in the Neighborhood Service Center program of the Lincoln Hospital Mental Health Services, discussed by Hallowitz and Riessman (1967).

The Lincoln Hospital Neighborhood Service Center program was one of the first OEO sponsored demonstration projects granted to a health agency. The *service center* model was based on the experiences of the Mobilization for Youth program (Cloward and Elman, 1967; Weissman, 1969). The role models for nonprofessionals in mental health developed by the Lincoln program, along with the work done at Howard University by MacLennan et al. (1966) and in the California correctional system by Grant (1966), had a catalytic effect on the expansion of the nonprofessional movement.

However, there continues to be a need for definitive descriptions of the ways in which nonprofessionals function within established mental health organizations. Kaplan (1970) and associates have described some of the specific functions evolving from the use of the nonprofessional in the Lincoln program as they became integrated within both the direct service and community consultation and education programs. The development of specific job descriptions and standards for evaluation are necessary to establish certified training programs and for licensing. Without these, the *new careers* for this manpower resource will not become a permanent part of the mental health delivery system (Pearl and Riessman, 1965; Peck, et al, 1969; Southern Regional Education Board, 1969).

The Federal Social Reform Movement

(a) Federal Social Welfare Legislation

The recent emphasis upon community participation is in part the result of governmental legislation, particularly the federal programs initiated under the new frontiers of the Kennedy Administration. This legislation, in the spirit of Roosevelt's New Deal, included programs emanating from President Kennedy's Commission on Juvenile Delinquency.

Based on the *opportunity model*, a number of broadly experimental activities in ghetto areas were initiated, such as Mobilization for Youth in the Lower East Side and Haryou in Harlem, New York City. Although they were on a much smaller scale than the Office of Economic Opportunity and Model Cities programs that were to follow, they introduced a significant innovation. They provided for direct funding to local groups in an amount based upon an assessment of local need. These programs had a major influence upon both the expansion of neighborhood-based efforts and increased community participation in subsequent years (Graham, 1965).

The Economic Opportunity Act of 1964 was the first federal legislation to specifically require and support community participation. Although it did not define the term in a precise manner, it created a planning and programming environment in which the groups served could, in principle if not always in fact, play a decision-making role (Community Action Programs). However, the supporting documents and memoranda intended to implement this principle of consumer participation were issued with conflicting instructions and lack of precision as to purpose (Moynihan, 1969).

(b) Federal Health Care Legislation

The Economic Opportunity Act was preceded in 1963 by the Community Mental Health Centers Act, the beginning of major new health care legislation. During 1965, the 89th Congress passed the legislation establishing Medicare and Medicaid as well as the Regional Medical Program (Battistella, 1967; Komaroff, 1971; Myers, 1969). This "Health New Deal," as it is referred to, in conjunction with the other social welfare and public health laws of the 1960's also had a significant role in the development of community participation (Anderson, 1971; Dearing, 1966; Madison, 1969).

Although an assessment of the impact of recent federal legislation on health services requires its own extensive analysis, some general observations are indicated about its influence upon community participation in the health field. The OEO legislation initiated "maximum feasible participation" by members of the community in policy-making and program planning. The Community Action Agency is best known as that component of OEO which actively encouraged the participation of local residents, particularly in low income areas (Cahn and Passett, 1969; Clark, 1968; Zurcher, 1969).

The CAA programs, such as the Neighborhood Service Centers which emphasize the utilization of local citizens as staff members, indirectly influenced the development of community participation in the health field, particularly through the incorporation of these centers into health and mental health programs such as at Lincoln Hospital (Peck and Kaplan, 1968; Peck, Roman and Kaplan, 1967). The most direct influence of the OEO programs upon community participation in the health field is seen in the Neighborhood Health Center program (Geiger, 1967; Notkin and Notkin, 1970; Sparer, et al, 1970; Wise, 1970).

(c) The Community Mental Health Centers Act

The nature of public health legislation has been described by Hanlon (1964) as follows: "However thoughtfully a proposed (health) measure may be prepared by its framers, it has by the time it is enacted into law usually been so altered by ill-considered, hasty or prejudiced amendment as to have lost all semblance of its original form." If the Community Mental Health Centers Act was so altered, it is not evident from its impact upon local mental health programs. This impact has been so extraordinary that the observation by Yolles (1970) that it "caused a political ferment that involved not only traditional politics of politicians but also the politics of medicine, the politics of health facilities, and the politics of health purveyors" seems warranted.

The unusual nature of the Community Mental Health Centers Act is that it not only contains a comprehensive plan for a mental health delivery system but, on the basis of legislation passed in May 1964, it provides broad powers for the National Institute of Mental Health to directly implement the regulation of those programs contracted for under the Act. This enhanced authority of an administrative bureau has added to the impact of the law (Glasscote, et al, 1964, 1969; Kaplan and Roman, 1973).

The provisions require community mental health centers to serve a defined population contained within a specified area. The services include a comprehensive range intended to closely integrate acute hospital based services with outpatient programs based in the local community and to improve continuity of treatment. The centers are required to provide preventive programs and consultation and education to community organizations (Kaplan, 1970). Community involvement by residents of the catchment area is mandated (NIMH, Policy and Standards Manual, 1971).

The Community Mental Health Act is directed toward a redistribution of mental health care from hospital teaching centers and large custodial institutions to the local community and attempts to coordinate mental health with other human services needed in the care of the mentally ill. It combines funding resources with program mandates to a greater measure than ever before. While it has succeeded to an extent almost beyond expectation, there are still significant resistances to comprehensive planning in the health and mental health care fields that remain to be resolved (Battestella and Weil, 1969; Lewis, 1971).

The Consumer Movement

As the consumer movement has gained momentum in recent years, the word *community* is increasingly used synonymously with *consumer*. In order to combine the somewhat different though overlapping implications of the two words, Leopold (1971) uses the term "consumer community" for a population served by a consortium of health and mental health institutions in Philadelphia.

Reference to community members as consumers in recent years has also been influenced by the increasing percentage of third party payments for hospital care. The largest source of third party payments are government programs, particularly Medicare and Medicaid, which now provide well over 50 percent of the revenue for voluntary hospitals in New York City. Because public and private insurance plans are very deficient in their coverage of mental disorders, the community member as consumer has not had quite the same impact upon mental health as general health. This impact will become more evident in both health and mental health, as consumer attitudes become a major criterion in the evaluation of program effectiveness (Goldberg, 1967; Reuther, 1969; Wilder, 1971).

The Civil Rights Movement

The civil rights movement and the militancy of disadvantaged minority groups were major concurrent developments in the latter part of the 1960's that profoundly influenced community participation in human service programs. This participation has led to confrontation and institutional crises. Health and mental health programs in urban disadvantaged areas have experienced internal conflicts when they have employed significant numbers of minority group members. Although these disruptions have caused program setbacks, their effects must be measured against the overall positive influence of the civil rights movement upon the national social conscience.

The importance of attitudinal change can hardly be exaggerated. In his discussion of what has been learned about the delivery of health services to the ghetto, Silver (1969) has written, "There has been a reawakening of concern for the deprived, for the poor, for minority groups, and a reawakening of our consciences of what has been done and what our responsibilities are, as citizens and professionals . . . John Gardner pointed out that the times cry out for institutional change, and our institutions resist change with unholy stubbornness. Overcoming that resistance may be the most important lesson we have learned."

One of the contributions we can make is to take the lesson offered by Silver and attempt to learn from our own experiences. It is urgent that we search out the basic issues underlying the problems and dramatic events to which we are exposed and that we share our findings with openness and candor. There is, I believe, a noticeable effort toward this end. If this proves to be so, it will be one of the legacies that the past decade of accelerated change and conflict has left to us.

A GENERAL CLASSIFICATION OF COMMUNITY PARTICIPATION

While the literature contains a number of references pertinent to a classification of community participation, none are sufficiently comprehensive as yet to provide the basis for a taxonomy. In view of the variety of phenomena that have come to be associated with community participation, such a formal undertaking is probably premature.

Essentially, the references selected from the literature for this chapter describe the developments in community participation according to objectives or goals and the processes required to achieve these objectives. The references to goal achievement focus primarily upon the leadership groups in the community. One classification centers on the community group's formal relationship to the policy-making power structures of established organizations and the other focuses on the capacity of community groups to systematically organize themselves so as to become effectively involved in institutional policy issues.

1. According to Objectives

The objectives of community participation described in the literature fall within two broad categories. They are characterized according to whether the objectives are predominately addressed to service (organizational) issues or to political issues. This classification of objectives has been described in the Brandeis Reports (1969) on community participation.

> The organization dimension involves the direct participation of service users, or their representatives, in the making of policy and the administrative management of a community service organization . . . The objective of organizational participation by consumer groups is to maximize the provision of direct benefits from a particular organization to the user population.

> The political dimension of target area participation involves the relationship between traditional leaders and dominant interest groups in a local community, and those interest groups which have been historically excluded from community leadership . . . The intended objective of politically focused participation is not primarily to modify the detailed operations of a single service organization, but to bring about a realignment of power within the community in favor of those community interests which have been underrepresented in the past.

The participation of community groups is intended "to maximize the provision of direct benefits" by building trust and understanding among clients and potential clients. Through the participation of community groups in the identification of problems, issues and service goals, it is hoped that agency programs gain more community legitimacy. Since under-utilization of services is an issue for some health and mental health agencies, community participation is seen as a means of informing clients who are either unaware of the services or unwilling to seek them out.

The political objectives of community participation are addressed to the realignment of local community power. The specific services of an institution are seen as secondary to its potential as a vehicle for the achievement of political objectives. However, the application of these service and political objectives to mental health services must take into account the political and social realities of the specific community.

Experience indicates that there is not yet a significant enough mental health services constituency in most communities to pursue either the service or political objectives of community participation. With the exception of drug addiction, mental health is not an issue around which communities organize, when compared to other human problems as employment, housing, welfare and education. Rosen's (1971) review of the neighborhood health center movement during the first third of this century suggests that the decline in importance of health among the human services in the neighborhoods served was one of the factors in the demise of the movement. This of course does not mean that community members are uninterested in their health. Rather, it suggests that health and mental health *services* are not central issues around which a community will coalesce.

Nevertheless, the classification of community participation according to service and political objectives is useful, provided the political context is seen not only in terms of public politics but also in the politics of social change. The need for institutional change in the health and mental health field is becoming more pressing. It is important to bear in mind that social institutions undergoing change have political manifestations in common with each other apart from the specific nature of their social functions. Community participation has been a factor in changing human service institutions, either directly through the involvement of citizen groups or indirectly through their influence upon public attitudes.

2. According to the Policy-Making Process

Community participation usually implies a collective involvement by identifiable groupings of individuals rather than unrelated individual participation. The most important group formations to have emerged from low-income communities are boards or committees. Roman and Schmais (1972) have characterized community groups under five general types, according to their formal role in the policy-making process of the institutions to which they relate.

Viewed from the twin perspectives of legal requirements and program goals, there are five general types of community board models:

a) Incorporated Body Model
b) Delegated Authority Model
c) Shared Responsibility Model
d) Issue Delegation Model
e) Purely Advisory Model

The first two models are similar, and both are legally viable structures where the objective is maximum participation and control. In the incorporated body model—assuming, of course, effective community representation—the board may purchase the services of an administrative and professional staff. In the delegated authority model, the board would typically receive complete operating authority from a prime contractor which would, however, retain administrative and professional personnel on its own staff. The third model—shared responsibility—is based on legal responsibility being retained by the central affiliated institution but where administration and professionals are committed to working in agreement with the community board. In the fourth model, legal responsibility resides with the institutional staff, but decision authority on specifically delegated matters is in the hands of the board. In the final model, the community board holds neither legal nor de facto power of control over agency policy.

3. According to the Organization of the Community Groups

Sparer and associates (1970) evaluated the effectiveness of community groups, based on the extent of their involvement in the operational aspects of twenty-seven OEO Neighborhood Health Centers. They concluded that the effectiveness of the groups was positively correlated with the degree to which they were well organized. The criteria they used for evaluating good organization included clarity of committee structure and functions; completeness and availability of minutes; the status of by laws; and the adequacy of elections. The latter two criteria were considered to be most indicative of the overall organizational quality of the groups. The following summarizes their observations:

Of the 27 centers visited from 1967 to date, 7 are rated high in the degree of consumer involvement, 9 moderate, and 10 low. No pattern is apparent that would relate the administering agency to the degree of involvement. Hospitals, health departments, and community corporations appear in each group. Only three group practices and four medical schools are represented. The (formally designated) structure of the consumer group is not critical; two of the three consumer boards have a high degree of involvement but the third board rates low. Five of the seven high-rated groups have advisory functions only, yet actual function relative to program operational matters is indistinguishable from those two high-rated groups established as boards.

Another important criterion that Sparer and his associates correlated with the effectiveness of community groups is the presence of strong leadership favoring community participation. They noted this correlation whether the strong leader was a member of the consumer group or the health center. This latter observation was based on indications that a strong personality on the staff of the health organization positively oriented toward the consumer group, "sometimes may substitute for (consumer) group leadership."

Sparer and his associates supplement the observations of Roman and Schmais (1972) by noting that informal working agreements with a community group, which formally has an advisory role, may allow the group to exercise considerable de facto decision-making influence. It is the ability of the community group to organize itself to effectively exercise authority that Sparer and his associates stress. They also emphasize the distinction in decision-making between general program policy decisions made by governing bodies such as boards, and operational decisions, that implement policy and are concerned with daily functions. The classification by Roman and Schmais is primarily addressed to the former decision-making level and Sparer and his associates to the latter.

The lack of clarity about levels of decision-making and the specific issues about which decisions are made appears to be one of the main reasons for confusion about the role of community groups in the organizational decision-making process. This point will be discussed in more detail below since it is explicitly directed to the relationship of community participation to the administration of mental health organizations.

Sparer and his associates are of the opinion that community

groups can have their greatest impact upon health services by seeking to participate in operational decisions. They point out that when community groups seek to establish themselves as incorporated boards, in order to engage more effectively in operational decisions, they actually lose touch with the operations and become more involved in general policy-matters.

They refer to Michels' (1949) "iron law of oligarchy" which Blau (1970) defines as:

> The thesis underlying Michels' "iron law of oligarchy' is that administrative and political exigencies lead to bureaucratization in the form of centralization of authority even in organizations whose very purpose is to promote equality, such as socialist parties and unions.

This thesis may explain the tendency of governing bodies to relate to their organizations in a similar manner, whether they are composed of elected low-income community members or upper-income appointed members. If this observation is correct, it is an important factor to consider in the impact of community participation on the administration of mental health organizations.

ADMINISTRATIVE CHARACTERISTICS OF MENTAL HEALTH ORGANIZATIONS

1. The Policy-Making Body and Professional Tradition

While control over institutional governing bodies and policy-making processes is one of the major political objectives of community participation, the policy areas to which this control refers are usually not defined. In general, however, they include the selection of administrative and/or professional directors, the selection of nontechnical and some technical personnel, and decisions about program priorities and budgetary allocations. In effect, with the exception of hiring lower-level personnel, the expectations of community boards do not differ from those of less representative policy-making bodies. Their involvement does not ordinarily extend to the daily operations and functions of professionals in providing care to patients.

Conversely, professionals traditionally have not directly involved themselves in policy decisions. For example, it has not been the practice to consult or to include staff members of mental health agencies in the selection of their directors. Unlike organizational members in some other corporate enterprises, the mental health professional tends not to perceive himself as someone with a legitimate role in these matters. This also tends to characterize the professional staff's attitude in regard to the policy-making process and the establishment of program priorities. The professional rarely knows the composition of his Board of Trustees, or when there are any changes made.

The psychiatrist does not primarily identify himself with the organization in which he works but rather with his professional role and discipline (Friedson, 1970; Roemer and Friedman, 1971). He tends not to see any relationship between his professional self and organizational policy decisions on program priorities, and the selection of top executive and clinical staff. Although this attitude may not characterize the other mental health professionals to the same extent as physicians, I believe it is substantially similar.

Assuming the accuracy of the observation that there is no significant difference between the power of existing governing bodies and the powers to which true community boards aspire, and that changes in the composition of governing bodies would be of no special concern to the professional staff, what has all the fuss been about? Why the dissent among professionals and the disruption in some established programs over the issue of community participation or community control? Perhaps the dissent has *not* really been about community participation or control *per se*. The following description of the organizational and administrative characteristics of mental health organizations may help clarify this point.

2. The Policy-Making Process and Organizational Structures

For illustrative purposes, the Lincoln Hospital Mental Health Services program in 1968 will be used as a case example. Although some of the organizational arrangements are unique to its setting, the overall structure is relevant to most health and mental health organizations, particularly if they obtain a significant part of their support from public funds. A detailed description and exposition of these issues is described by Kaplan and Roman (1973) in, *The Organization and Delivery of Mental Health Services in the Ghetto: The Lincoln Hospital Experience.*

(a) The Multi-Authority Organizational Superstructure

All mental health organizations are subject to the direct or indirect authority of supraordinate bodies. An organization may have a supraordinate health facility of which it is a component; a supraordinate university structure with degree-granting and sanctioning powers legally chartered by the state: or a supraordinate professional body, such as a medical board or society, through which professional standard-setting and accreditation bodies exert influence.

If the organization receives public funds, there are contractual obligations which make it accountable to those governmental bodies responsible for the public purse. These may include local and state mental health authorities as well as federal agencies, such as the National Institute of Mental Health and the Office of Economic Opportunity. There are said to be over twenty federal departments and bureaus providing health or mental health funds.

Federal and state supraordinate bodies also have a major influence over private health and mental health programs through direct control over policies governing Medicare and Medicaid funds. Of potentially equal importance is the state's regulatory authority over reimbursement rates for private third party insurance carriers. Federal health planning agencies are another potentially significant superstructure.

Figure 8-1 shows the structural relationship of the Lincoln Hospital program in 1968 to some of these supraordinate bodies. It illustrates the susceptibility of the Lincoln program to extraordinarily complex constraints, limitations and sanctions. However, just as important as these multilevel structures themselves is the lack of defined procedures to coordinate them and to clarify, much less change, their influence upon the policy-making process within the Lincoln structure.

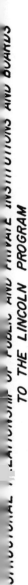
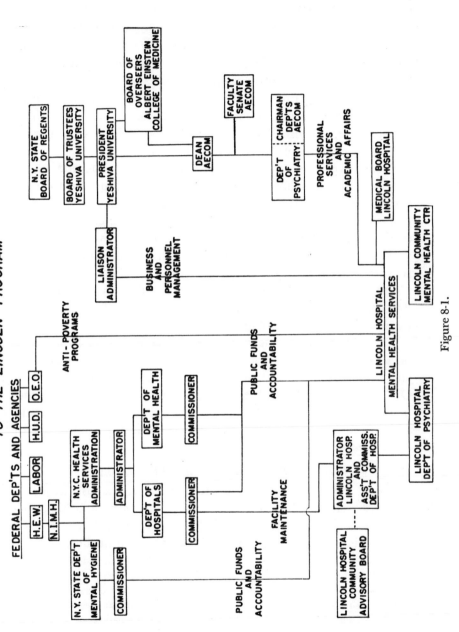

Figure 8-1.

(b) *The Lack of Interagency Coordinating Mechanisms*

The lack of any defined mechanisms for coordinating these multi-authority superstructures is a major factor in the governance of mental health organizations. The absence of coordination, aside from a problem of bureaucratic red-tape, presents obstacles to changes in organizational governance far beyond the issue of who sits on the governing body. Nevertheless, as apparent as these obstacles are, the disbelief that this situation in fact exists is widespread among both professionals and laymen.

The reasons for this disbelief are manifold but one major reason is that somehow these organizations do continue to function. One could, in fact, question how interorganizational programs can be implemented at all, considering the extraordinarily complex and contradictory policies regulating every aspect of them. Fortunately, the flexibility with which some administrative requirements can be interpreted allows for the coexistence of apparently contradictory supraordinate rules and regulations. Problems arise when attempts are made to formally change existing policies rather than to apply them flexibly.

The administrative leeway allowed by governmental agencies does permit innovation provided there is imaginative leadership and a convergence of events to which the leadership can respond. On the other hand, flexible regulations may by their very vagueness, compound the problems of interagency coordination and add to the confusion about the basis on which the authority of the organizational leadership rests.

(c) *The Absence of Formal Institutional Leadership*

Until the crisis in social institutions during the last decade, it was customary to think of these institutions as monolithic structures under unified leadership. That this belief has not been readily disabused, is reflected in this excerpt from Bucher, (1970).

> According to the ("students") statement, the (dean) asserted that "nobody in the university has the authority to negotiate with the students."
> "Obviously, somebody in the university makes policy decisions," the statement said, "and until an official body comes forward, we consider the present situation a refusal to negotiate our demands."
>
> Chicago *Sun-Times*,
> February 1, 1969

The above quotation reflects the plight of students and faculties throughout the nation during these times of student protest. It also cuts into the heart of our inquiry; what is the nature of power in an academic organization? Where is it located, how does it accrue, and how is it manifested? Above all, how are we to understand this apparently odd kind of formal organization? Student activists interpret as deviousness what is plain fact in many universities, namely that *nobody has the authority,* while harassed administrators cast about for the proper organizational forms to meet the student onslaught.

The experiences of professionals in health and mental health institutions is similar to that noted by Bucher (Roemer and Freedman, 1971). The multi-authority superstructures and lack of mechanisms for coordinating policy create confusion about leadership authority through the various organizational levels (Carnegie Report, 1970; Macy Report, 1969). For example, as Figure 8-1 indicates, the Lincoln program had a variety of structures to which it was accountable. Within the professional system, the Chairman of the Department of Psychiatry was the most tangible person to whom one could turn for program decisions and professional recruitment.

However, the Chairman's authority was informally delegated by the Dean, whose specific power was also unclear. This lack of clarity about the institutional authority in the College of Medicine is indicated by this excerpt from a meeting of the Faculty Senate.

In response to a question about the relationship of the Board of Overseers of the Albert Einstein College of Medicine to the Board of Trustees of Yeshiva University, the Dean stated, 'In 1954 the Board of Trustees of the University vested the authority for the management of the affairs of the medical school in the Board of Overseers—totally and unqualifiedly.' However, a faculty member noted that 'there is still confusion about whether the legal authority rests with the Board of Overseers, the Board of Trustees or with the President of the University.' (For example) when the President of the University recently met with the Committee to revise the Senate By Laws, the President stated that the legal authority rested with him and that he delegated authority to the Board of Overseers. . . (The Dean was asked) to explain who appoints members of the Board of Overseers and what the qualifications are for someone to become a member of the Board of Overseers. The Dean stated he didn't know how they were appointed.

ORGANIZATION FOR ACADEMIC AFFAIRS OF THE DEPARTMENT OF PSYCHIATRY,
ALBERT EINSTEIN COLLEGE OF MEDICINE (1968)

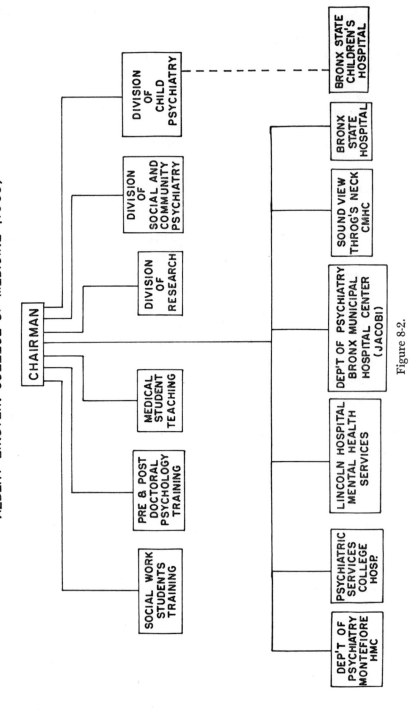

Figure 8-2.

The establishment of the Lincoln Hospital Community Mental Health Center as a component of the Lincoln Hospital Mental Health Services program further complicated the confusion about the formal authority structure. Although the arrangements for other grants and for service contracts were also uncertain, the administrative thrust behind the community mental health center concept heightened awareness of the uncertain legal structures under which the Lincoln program functioned. The problems associated with the community mental health center are noted by Curran (1970) :

> The term *community mental health center* has no particular legal significance. Most state legislation speaks of *programs* for community mental health, not *centers*. Many legal problems were added when federal legislation was adopted providing funds for such centers. The term *center* implies both a physical structure and an independent administrative organization. Yet many if not most of the community centers currently operating are not administratively or legally separate from their parent groups such as county governments or universities.

ADMINISTRATIVE CONSIDERATIONS IN RELATIONSHIP TO COMMUNITY BOARDS

The term Community Board, when capitalized, refers to the incorporated and delegated authority models, described by Roman and Schmais. This assumes that the board has sufficient representation on the governing body of the mental health organization so that it has a decisive or significant voice in policy. The term Community Advisory Board refers to a community group with no formal policy-making powers on the governing body of the mental health organization.

The structural relationship of a Community Board to a mental health organization is illustrated in Figure 8-3. This is a hypothetical organizational chart in which decentralization is a major characteristic. In Figure 8-1, discussed earlier, there is an illustration of the structural relationship between a Community Advisory Board and Lincoln Hospital. The dotted line reflects the lack of formal power in the Community Advisory Board.

1. The Formation of Community Boards

For illustrative purposes, the members of the Community Board in Figure 8-3 are presumed to be representative of their con-

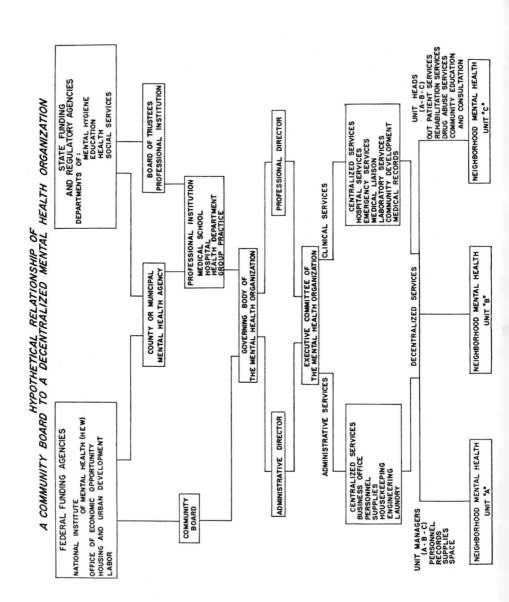

HYPOTHETICAL RELATIONSHIP OF
A COMMUNITY BOARD TO A DECENTRALIZED MENTAL HEALTH ORGANIZATION

stituency which is contained within a defined geographic area. This model also presumes that by whatever method membership on the Board is achieved, it is responsive to its constituency. These presumptions may be beyond what many would be willing to accept. The questions of *representativeness* and *responsiveness* of community boards to their constituencies are frequently unsettled issues that may generate strong political reverberations.

However, the purpose for stating the presumptions in this manner is not to avoid the difficulties that still remain to be resolved about this question. Rather it is to emphasize that it is not the responsibility of the mental health organization to initiate the formation of a Community Board nor to decide the legitimacy of its membership. The initiative must come from the citizens of the community. The governmental funding and regulatory bodies should assume responsibility for providing whatever fiscal support is needed for the formation of the Community Board and for monitoring its responsiveness.

The formation and the functions of Community Advisory Boards, however, may become the responsibility of those mental health organizations required by law to "involve the community in the planning, development and operation of the program." This quote from the NIMH Policy and Standards Manual for Community Mental Health Centers, goes on to state that "the exact form such involvement takes will vary from one center to another— (and) —may be formal or informal, and may include representation on policy and advisory boards." The guidelines, therefore, do not mandate the formation of community boards according to either of the models discussed above. However, where significant efforts have been made by mental health organizations to establish community boards, the prevailing model seems to be the Community Advisory Board. The reasons for this are inherent in both the resources required and the processes by which a community board is formed and developed.

2. The Formation of Community Boards—A Case Example

Sparer's observation that the key to the effectiveness of a community group is related to how well the group is organized is illustrated by a comparison of the formation of the community boards in the Lincoln Hospital program according to the "Hunts Point" model and the "Steering Committee" model. The initial plan called for the formation of three Community Advisory Boards each representing two of the six health areas composing the catchment area of the Lincoln Hospital Community Mental Health Center. Each of the Community Advisory Boards, representing a population of 50,000, would in turn form the Central Advisory Board.

The Hunts Point model refers to the agreement to accept, as one of the Community Advisory Boards, the community-elected members of the Executive Committee of the Neighborhood Multiservice Center of the Hunts Point Community Corporation, one of the Model Cities Neighborhood Demonstration Programs in New York City. The Multiservice Center was responsible for developing service programs for the population of its two health areas. However, although they had been funded to provide health services for the area, they did not have funds for a mental health program.

The Steering Committee model refers to efforts by staff members of the Lincoln program to establish, de novo, *grass roots* community participation to form a Community Advisory Board from the citizens who resided in two of the other health areas. The formation of an Advisory Board for the two remaining health areas was to follow.

Although at the outset the objective was the formation of Community Advisory Boards, the Executive Committee of the Hunts Point Multiservice Center Corporation demanded a Community Board for their area with the power and structure of an incorporated body. The directors of the Lincoln program concurred with this demand since integration with a Model Cities Multiservice Center was one of the planning objectives for the community mental health center at the time the grant was first conceptualized in 1966 (Peck and Kaplan, 1968). At that time, the Hunts Point Neighborhood Multiservice Center had not yet been formed, although discussions had been held with a subcommittee of the Community Corporation about the planning for the Lincoln Hospital Community Mental Health Center. NIMH (1971) guidelines require the endorsement of the Model Cities Agency when a community mental health center "impacts on or otherwise serves the residents of designated city demonstration areas." Special efforts had been made to have the boundaries of part of the Lincoln catchment area coterminous with the area that the Hunts Point Multiservice Center was expected to serve.

The ability of the Hunts Point Multiservice Center Corporation in 1968 to qualify as a fiscal agent for a component of the community mental health center attests to the sophistication of their organization. This arrangement required collaborative planning with the Office of Economic Opportunity, and the Departments of Health, Education, and Welfare, Housing and Urban Development and Labor. In addition to this unusual articulation between several Federal departments, it also required the planning of coterminous catchment areas several years in advance of the anticipated official boundaries through collaboration between the New York City Department of Mental Health and the directors of the Lincoln program.

The community-based group in the other area, however, had difficulties getting beyond the loosely organized arrangement of the Steering Committee. The process of this development is described in detail in *The Lincoln Hospital Experience*. The Steering Committee model illustrates, in contrast to the sophistication of the Hunts Point model, the lack of adequate planning to deal with the complex administrative issues encountered in the attempt to establish a community board with *grass roots* membership.

The overall differences in developing community boards according to the Hunts Point and Steering Committee models can be summarized in the following way; the former encountered the administrative problems of a complex bureaucracy, the latter suffered from the lack of a bureaucracy. Although it was legally incorporated and had been approved by New York State to operate a mental health service, the allocation of funds directly to the Hunts Point Multiservice Center created problems for some of the supraordinate government agencies. One problem was the legislative mandate of the Model Cities program itself, which formed the basis for the Multiservice Center. There were bitter local political struggles for control of the funds allocated to the Model Cities Program.

Another problem, illustrated in Figure 8-1, concerns the direct funding of part of the Lincoln program by OEO. At least in part, negotiations around this program as early as 1966 helped coordinate the program planning at Lincoln with other federal agencies and included discussions with a subcommittee of the Hunts Point Community Corporation. However, in 1968 when formal negotiations about the community mental health center began with the Hunts Point Multiservice Center, there were very few official guidelines to expedite the process. Although this allowed for administrative flexibility by the Federal and some of the local agencies involved, it created problems with the state and other local agencies responsible for allocating the matching funds for the federal grant. At that time, the state and municipal agencies were not familiar with the community mental health concept under traditional institutional auspices, much less under a community board. Adding to this problem, the nature of the entity to be formed was spawned by intergovernmental agreements for which there was limited precedent and no official regulations.

The Steering Committee approach, on the other hand, represented an entirely different set of complexities. There were no established public or private agencies to help maintain and give support to the potential membership from the community except from the staff and resources of the Lincoln program. In effect, the problem here was helping the community establish a committee to administer its own affairs and relate to the multi-government agencies as well as to the Lincoln program, without being overwhelmed by either. This proved to be an unrealistic objective since, among considerations, there was not sufficient time, funds, nor expertise to guide the process. On the average, it takes a minimum of two years for this type of citizen group to achieve a viable organizational structure.

Although it took a number of months, the Hunts Point Multiservice Center was allocated funds for the component of the Lincoln Hospital Community Mental Health Center it now operates in collaboration with the center. While Community Advisory Boards were established in the other two health areas, as Sparer's studies suggest, the Central Board tends to be dominated by the more sophisticated organizational capacities of the Hunts Point membership. While there were significant political issues involved in the competition between the local boards, due to conflict between Black and Puerto Rican leadership, the organizational experience of the established group was a major factor in its capacity to exert influence.

3. Relationship of Community Boards to Decentralization of Mental Health Services

In recent years, there has been a growing interest in the decentralization of mental health organizations. As with community participation, decentralization can contribute to the involvement of providers and consumers in the decision-making process and can foster personalized care. Whatever effect community participation may have upon changing the policy-making structures and processes of a mental health organization, alone it cannot significantly improve the quality of the relationship between the provider of mental health care and the consumer. A more fundamental change is required, such as the decentralization both of service structures and decision-making processes.

While structural rearrangements offer no assurance of increased effectiveness, decentralization accompanied by clearly defined structures increases the likelihood. In decentralization, it is important to distinguish between those functions that can be most effectively decentralized and those that cannot. In general, the greater the decentralization of services, the greater the need for some central administration. Because of this, some community planners caution that local community participation focused primarily on the decentralized services without a corresponding attention to the central level may actually decrease the influence of citizen participation upon the overall program.

4. The Community Board, Personnel Practices and
Labor-Management Relations

The relationship of community boards to personnel practices is an area of increasing importance, particularly in organizations where a significant number of employees belong to labor unions. While unionization is a relatively recent development in the mental health field, it is likely to accelerate in the future. The conflicts that emerged in New York City in 1968 around the decentralization of the public school system illustrate administrative issues quite similar to those in the mental health field.

New York City is divided into 31 decentralized school districts, involving over 900 public schools and about 60,000 teachers. Each district has a community-elected board with policy-making power over local program expenditures, according to the budget alloted to each district, as well as a voice in the selection of the district superintendent. The board also has a voice in the selection and placement of teachers, according to the policies established by the Central Board of Education through collective bargaining with the United Federation of Teachers. This latter arrangement was the source of bitter controversy, essentially concerning the respective power of the union and the community boards.

Prior to the passage of the legislation establishing the New York City school decentralization plan, there had been experimental decentralized school programs developed in some areas of New York City. In disadvantaged neighborhoods, where recruitment of qualified teachers is deficient, the local community boards of these experimental programs considered the power over the selection and placement of teachers essential to improve the quality of the teaching programs. This issue became one of the major controversies in the New York State Legislature over the decentralization plan, with the union taking the position that it could not adequately represent the teachers through separate collective bargaining arrangements with each of the districts. The union insisted that central management maintain the authority to negotiate the city-wide contract arrangements for the teachers. Since the union leaders and the teachers were predominately Jewish and the membership of the experimental community boards were predominately Black, very bitter racial attacks erupted over the controversy.

Of course the issues involved in the conflict are considerably more complex than this very brief summary indicates. In addition to the labor-management, ethnic and political issues there were basic unresolved questions about the learning process itself and the methods for evaluating the quality of education provided, whatever the personnel practices.

Although this type of controversy has not been widespread in the mental health system, a similar type of struggle has emerged in a few mental health programs particularly around the employment and use of mental health workers or indigenous non-professionals. However, one can anticipate increasing conflicts of this nature in the future. It is important for administrators of mental health organizations to implement labor-management policies effectively. Otherwise, the problems of implementation become the source of conflict obscuring the underlying issues and making their resolution extremely difficult. Considering the current state of affairs in the administration of mental health services, there is much to be done to achieve this limited objective.

5. Other Administrative Considerations

There are several practical issues that must be considered in relation to community boards. Mental health organizations must contend with money problems no different from those of other organizations. According to whether it is a private, non-profit or public organization, there are specific factors that are influenced by the composition of the governing body.

In nonprofit organizations, prominent businessmen among board members often continue to play a necessary role in the maintenance of financial solvency. Even though the amount of private contributions is comparatively small in the overall expenditures of mental health programs, they may be necessary to offset existing fiscal deficits. The influence of board members may also determine the availability of needed loans. For it should not be overlooked that health institutions can and do go bankrupt, not to mention the effect of a significant fiscal retrenchment to avoid bankruptcy on morale of the staff, an all too frequent occurrence these days.

In the public sector, the board membership of local community leaders influences the budget allocation process. This influence can be particularly effective during times of political change or during an election year. At the same time, it is important to recognize that local community board membership can also have a negative influence on budget allocations dependent upon the vicissitudes of their political role.

In addition to financial and political help, board members may also contribute needed professional expertise in legal, management, and other professional areas. Where this expertise does not exist, the training of community board members not skilled in these areas can compensate for this (Parker, 1970) and, equally important, the availability of funds to hire outside consultants can be a great help (Sunquist, and Davis, 1969).

FUTURE DEVELOPMENTS AND PAST HISTORY

We are entering the 1970's with the anticipation of basic changes in the health and mental health fields; partly in response to fiscal constraints and partly to the disappointments following a decade of expansion and experimentation (Somers, 1971). The same mistakes are likely to be made again if in attempting to change our institutions, we fail to learn from previous innovative efforts.

1. Innovation and Conflict

Innovative programs have encountered difficulties not necessarily as a consequence of their specific content but because they represent change (Coe, 1970; Dykens et al, 1964; Greenblatt et al, 1971). Institutions react to innovation with overt or covert resistances. The emergence of overt conflict between the members of an institution or between the institution and groups external to it depends upon many factors, which in turn help determine the constructive or negative resolution of the conflict. Seven of the consumer groups of the twenty-seven reported on by Sparer and his associates had identifiable conflicts. Their studies led them to conclude that conflict may have productive results. "Sometimes major strides in consumer movement and in project functioning have been an outcome of conflict."

However, it is much more difficult to constructively influence events when they reach crisis proportions. Once members become polarized during an institutional crisis, underlying issues become quickly obscured by the convergence of related and unrelated events. The polarization results in the formation of coalitions identified with formal or informal subgroups that existed before the crisis. In his review of the crisis in the community mental health center of the Temple University School of Medicine, Gardner (1971) refers to this reinforcement by power coalitions of preexisting subgroups during a crisis as the "polarization trap." Similar events are described in the *Lincoln Hospital Experience* and I have discussed the symbolic nature of the polarization that may occur during institutional change elsewhere (Kaplan, 1973).

2. The Distinction Between Events, Problems, and Basic Issues

It is difficult, if not impossible, in a time of conflict to distinguish the basic issues from among all of the other problems. The events are so encompassing that it is often only with hindsight that one can gain objectivity and attempt to search out the underlying issues. However, we are beginning to develop a body of experience, based upon retrospective study to help identify the nature of the problems associated with conflict. Cronkhite (1969) suggests, in relationship to conflict encountered in community health programs in ghetto areas, that "if one examines further the evaluation of the power structure and the decision-making apparatus of community health agencies, it becomes clear that further change takes place in a nearly predictable pattern."

However, we are far from reaching consensus about the basic issues. Although Gardner and Cronkhite refer to "universal forces" which they consider must account for developments in health programs, we are lacking the data upon which to base an analysis of fundamental causes. As Cronkhite implies, many of the problems stem from organizational and administrative issues.

However, there is a need for much more candor about these issues from many programs in order to obtain the necessary documentation. Detailed information on budgets and methods by which organizational rewards such as prestige and money are distributed is needed, at least to the same extent that this information is now required from stock corporations that sell shares to the public.

3. The Leadership Mystique and the Lack of Public Accountability

The lack of public accountability in human service programs, as well as in many other institutions, is paralleled by a mystique of leadership. We have become involved in ritualistic activities around the symbolic role of leaders as if their individual efforts will suffice to solve our problems. The ambivalence this generates has contributed to politicizing the role of the health and mental health executive and to "an epidemic of resignations" among professional mental health leaders (Greenbaum, 1968).

The basic difficulties do not lie in the quality of the leadership but rather in the attitudes of the followership. We have emphasized our differences rather than our similarities. Polarization is not the cause of conflict in our institutions but a dramatic symptom of existing subdivisions. Whatever new institutional arrangements we may wish to institute in the future to improve our health care structures, i.e., health maintenance organizations, group practices, neighborhood health centers, will run afoul, as resistances to change cause a deepening of already existing cleavages.

The problems we have encountered in mental health have not been caused by community participation or community control. To the contrary, they result from the lack of community control particularly as an instrument of public accountability. A measure of this state of affairs is indicated in this excerpt from an editorial in the New York Times (1972). "Careful program audits and independent evaluations are needed throughout the broad spectrum of municipal services . . . the Board of Estimate is right to seek such data now . . . (to) demand accountability (and to) insist on performance." Despite this declarative statement, the tone of the editorial was more wistful than affirmative and the Board of Estimate relented several days later.

Alinsky (1969) considers the organization of the overall community to be the essential determinant in effective community participation. Concerning the role of the community organization in bargaining with the establishment for health care services, Alinsky expresses this view:

> In order for citizens in any kind of society to be able to act, to have power, they must join together in organizations . . . Unless a people have organized so that their membership roster is open for public inspection, have met in convention, and agreed upon policy, programs, constitution, and elected officers, you do not have that necessary combination of circumstances from which legitimate, bona fide, accredited representation can be either selected or elected. . . . It matters not what kind of program is developed by the government, by private foundations, or by the medical profession, for so long as the citizens have a community lacking organization—meaning that they lack both the ability to act, or power, as well as the legitimate bona fide representation—then we do not have the essentials for collective bargaining, communication, equality partnership, call it what you will.

Citizen participation, as the meaningful involvement of individuals in significant organizational events, is not readily achieved. In our modern society, participation means a personal commitment of time and effort without guarantees of security. It requires training for ill defined functions by an educational process not geared to the task. It also requires an involvement in organizational relationships dependent upon traditions no longer as binding as they were and for which a new ethic has yet to evolve. New organizational structures are being proposed to take us "beyond bureaucracies" (Bennis, 1965). However, there is no substitute for ethical traditions as the basis for personal relationships between those who are served and those who serve, which in the final analysis defines the quality of human services.

REFERENCES

Alinsky, Saul: What is the role of community organization in bargaining with the establishment for health care services? In Normal, John (Ed.): *Medicine in the Ghetto*. New York, Appleton-Century-Crofts, 1969.

Anderson, Donna A. and Kerr, Markay: Citizen influence in health service programs. *Am J Public Health, 61*:1518, 1971.

Battistella, Roger M.: The course of regional health planning: Review and assessment of reecnt federal legislation. *Med Care, 3*:149, 1967.

Battistella, Roger M.; and Weil, Thomas P.: Comprehensive health care planning: New effort or redirected energy? *N Y State J Med, 69*:2351, 1969.

Bennis, Warren: Beyond bureaucracy. *Trans-Action, 2(5)*:31, 1965.

Blau, Peter: Decentralization in bureaucracies. In Zold, Mayer (Ed.): *Power in Organizations.* Nashville, Vanderbilt University Press, 1970.

Brandeis Reports: *Community Representation in Community Action Programs.* Reports Nos. 1-5, Florence Heller School for Advanced Studies in Social Welfare, Brandeis University, March, 1969.

Brieland, Donald: Community advisory boards and maximum feasible participation. *Am J Public Health, 61*:292, 1971.

Bucher, Rue: Social process and power in a medical school. In Zold, Mayer (Ed.): *Power in Organizations.* Nashville, Vanderbilt University Press, 1970.

Cahn, E. S. and Passett, B. A. (Eds.): *Citizen Participation.* New Jersey, New Jersey Community Action Training Institute, 1969.

Carnegie Commission on Higher Education: *Higher Education and the Nation's Health: Policies for Medical and Dental Education.* New York, McGraw-Hill, 1970.

Clark, K. (Ed.): *A Relevant War Against Poverty.* New York, Metropolitan Applied Research Center, 1968.

Cloward, R. and Elman, R.: The Storefront on Stanton Street: Advocacy in the ghetto. In Brager, G. A., and Purcell, F. P. (Eds.): *Community Action Against Poverty.* New Haven, College and University Press, 1967.

Coe, Rodney M.: *Planned Change in the Hospital.* New York, Praeger, 1970.

Cronkite, Leonard W.: What are the conflicts involved in community control? In Norman, John C. (Ed.): *Medicine in the Ghetto.* New York, Appleton Century, 1969.

Curran, William: Legal issues in establishment and operation. In Grunebaum, Henry (Ed.): *The Practice of Community Mental Health.* Boston, Little Brown, 1970.

Dearing, W.: Medicare—Its meaning to the consumer. *J Am Geriat Soc, 14*: 1087, 1966.

Dykens, James W.; Hyde, Robert W.; Orzack, Louis H., and York, Richard H.: *Strategies of Mental Hospital Change.* Boston, Commonwealth of Massachusetts, 1964.

Falk, Isidore S.: Labor unions and medical care. In DeGroot, Leslie, J. (Ed.): *Medical Care: Social and Organizational Aspects.* Springfield, Thomas, 1966.

Feldman, Saul: Ideals and issues in community mental health. *Hosp Community Psychiatry, 22:*325, 1971.

Fishman, Jay: *Training Nonprofessional Workers for Human Services, A Manual of Organization and Process.* Washington, Howard University, 1966.

Friedson, Eliot: *Professional Dominance: The Social Structure of Medical Care.* New York, Atherton, 1970.

Galiher, Claudia B.; Medleman, Jack, and Role, Anne J.: Consumer participation. *HSMHA Health Report, 86:*99, 1971.

Gardner, Elmer A. and Gardner, Mary L.: A community mental health center case study: Innovations and issues. *Seminars in Psychiatry, 3:*172, 1971.

Geiger, Jack: The neighborhood health center. *Arch Environ Health, 14:*912, 1967.

Glasscote, R.; Sanders, D.; Forstenzer, H. and Foley, A.: *The Community Mental Health Center: An Analysis of Existing Centers.* Washington, Joint Information Service, 1964.

Glasscote, R.; Sussex, J.; Cumming, E. and Smith, L.: *The Community Mental Health Center: An Interim Appraisal.* Washington, Joint Information Service, 1969.

Goldberg, Theodore: A consumer looks at medical care. *Med Care, 5:*9, 1967.

Graham, E.: Poverty and the legislative process. In Seligman, Ben B. (Ed.): *Poverty as a Public Issue.* Glencoe, The Free Press, 1965.

Grant, Douglas: *A Strategy for California's Use of Training Resources in the Development of New Careers for the Poor.* Sacramento, Institute for the Study of Crime and Delinquency, 1966.

Greenbaum, Marvin: Resignations among professional mental health leaders: study of a mild epidemic. *Archives of General Psychiatry, 19:*266, 1968.

Greenblatt, Milton and Hinman, Frederick J.: Citizen participation in community mental health and retardation programs. In Grunebaum, Henry (Ed.): *The Practice of Community Mental Health.* Boston, Little Brown, 1970.

Greenblatt, Milton; Sharaf, Myron R. and Stone, Evelyn M.: *Dynamics of Institutional Change.* Pittsburgh, University of Pittsburgh Press, 1971.

Grosser, Charles; Williams, Henry, and Kelly, James: *Nonprofessionals in the Human Services.* San Francisco, Josey-Bass, 1969.

Hallowitz, E. and Riessman, F.: The role of the indigenous nonprofessional in a community mental health neighborhood service center program. *Am J Orthopsychiatry, 37:*766, 1967.

Hanlon, John: *Principles of Public Health Administration.* St. Louis, Mosby, 1964.

Hansell, N.; Wodarczyk, M. and Visotsky, H.: The mental health expediter. *Archives of General Psychiatry, 18:*392, 1968.

Kaplan, Seymour R.: Teaching of community psychiatry in psychiatric residency training programs. In Lidz, T., and Edelson, M. (Eds.): *Training*

Tomorrow's Psychiatrists. New Haven, Yale University Press, 1970.

Kaplan, Seymour R.: Characteristic phases of development in mental health organizations. In Goldman, G., and Millman, D. (Eds.): *Group Process Today: Evaluation and Perspective.* Springfield, Thomas, 1973.

Kaplan, S.; Boyjian, L. and Meltzer, B.: The role of the nonprofessional. In Grunebaum, H. (Ed.): *The Practice of Community Mental Health.* Boston, Little Brown, 1970.

Kaplan, Seymour and Roman, Melvin: *The Organization and Delivery of Mental Health Services in the Ghetto: The Lincoln Experience.* New York, Praeger, 1973.

Komaroff, Anthony L.: Regional medical programs in search of a mission. *N Engl J Med, 284:758,* 1971.

Leopold, Robert: Process report on the West Philadelphia Community Mental Health Consortium. *Seminars in Psychiatry, 3:245,* 1971.

Lewis, Irving: Government investment in heatlh care. *Sci Am, 224(4):17-25,* 1971.

Macy Report: *Report of the Commission for the Study of the Governance of the Academic Medical Center.* New York, Josiah Macy Foundation, 1969.

MacLennan, B. W.; Klein, W. L.; Pearl, A. and Fishman, J.: Training for new careers. *Community Mental Health Journal, 2:135,* 1966.

Madison, Donald L.: Organized health care and the poor. *Medical Care Review, 26:1,* 1969.

Michels, Robert: *Political Parties,* Glencoe, Free Press, 1949.

Mobilization for Youth. *A Proposal for the Prevention and Control of Delinquency by Expanding Opportunities.* New York, 1961.

Moynihan, Daniel: *Maximum Feasible Misunderstanding. Community Action in the War on Poverty.* Glencoe, Free Press, 1969.

Munts, Raymond: *Bargaining for Health: Labor Unions, Health Insurance, and Medical Care.* Milwaukee, University of Wisconsin Press, 1967.

Myers, Robert: *Medicare.* Homewood, Richard D. Irwin, 1969.

National Institute of Mental Health, Community Mental Health Center Program, Operating Handbook, Part 1: Policy and Standards Manual. Washington, U. S. Department of Health, Education, and Welfare, 1971.

New York Times Editorial: Demands for Accountability, March 12, 1972.

Notkin, Herbert and Notkin, Marilyn S.: Community participation in health services: A review article. *Medical Care Review, 27:*1178, 1970.

Parker, Alberta: The consumer as a policy-maker-issues of training, *Am J Public Health, 60*(11), 1970.

Pearl, A. and Riessman, F.: *New Careers for the Poor.* New York, Free Press, 1965.

Peck, H. and Kaplan, S.: A Mental Health Program for the Urban Multiservice Center. In Shore, Milton, and Mannino, Fortune (Eds.): *Mental*

Health and the Community: Problems, Programs and Strategies. New York, Behavioral Publications, 1968.

Peck, H.; Levin, T. and Roman, M.: The health careers institute: A mental health strategy for an urban community. *Am J Psychiatry, 125(9):* 1969.

Peck, H.; Roman, M. and Kaplan, S.: Community action programs and the comprehensive mental health center. In Greenblatt, M.; Emery, P., and Glueck, Jr., A. (Eds.): *Poverty and Mental Health.* Washington, American Psychiatric Association, 1967.

Piven, F.: Participation of residents in neighborhood community action programs. *Social Work, 11:*73, 1966.

Pollack, Jerome: The voice of the consumer: cost quality, and organization of medical services. In Knowles, John H. (Ed.): *Hospitals, Doctors, and the Public Interest.* Cambridge, Harvard University Press, 1965.

Reuther, Walter P.: The health care crisis: where do we go from here? *Am J Public Health, 59:*12, 1969.

Riessman, F. and Rieff, R.: *The Indigenous Non-Professional: A Strategy of Change in Community Action and Community Mental Health Programs.* New York, National Institute of Labor Education, 1964.

Roemer, Milton I.: On paying the doctor and the implications of different methods. *J Health Hum Behav, 3(4),* 1962.

Roemer, Milton I. and Freedman, Jay W.: *Doctors in Hospitals.* Baltimore, The Johns Hopkins Press, 1971.

Roman, Melvin and Schmais, Aaron: Consumer participation and control: a conceptual overview. In Bellak, Leopold, and Bartin, Harvey (Eds.): *Progress in Community Mental Health.* New York, Bruner, 1972.

Rosen, George: History and analysis of the first neighborhood health center movement in the early 1900's, implications for the present. *Am J Public Health, 61:*1620, 1971.

Seidel, Victor: The citizen volunteer in historical perspective. In Cohen, N. (Ed.): *The Citizen Volunteer: His Responsibilities, Role, and Opportunity in Modern Society.* New York, Harper, 1960.

Silver, George: What has been learned about the delivery of health care services to the ghetto? In Norman, John (Ed.): *Medicine in the Ghetto.* New York, Appleton-Century-Crofts, 1969.

Somers, Anne R.: *Health Care in Transition: Directions for the Future.* Chicago, Hospital Research and Educational Trust, 1971.

Southern Regional Educational Board: *Roles and Functions for Different Levels of Mental Health Workers; A Report of a Symposium in Manpower Utilization for Mental Health.* Atlanta, 1969.

Sparer, Gerald; Dines, George and Smith, Daniel: Consumer participation in OEO—assisted neighborhood health centers. *Am J Public Health, 60(6),* 1970.

Sunquist, James L. and Davis, David W.: *Making Federalism Work.* Washington, The Brookings Institution, 1969.

U. S. Office of Economic Opportunity: Organizing Communities for Action; Community Action Programs. Washington, U. S. Government Printing Office, 1967.

Weissman, Harold: Priorities in social service for the slum neighborhood. In Shore, Milton, and Mannino, Fortune (Eds.): *Mental Health and the Community: Problems, Programs and Strategies.* New York, Behavioral Publications, 1969.

Wilder, Jack: *Consumer Evaluation of Mental Health Services.* Keynote Address, Region 2 Annual Conference of National Council of Mental Health Centers, Rochester, New York, October, 1971.

Wise, Harold B.: Physicians and health centers, *Postgrad Med, 47*:130, 1970.

Yolles, Stanley: The community mental health center in national perspective. In Grunebaum, Henry (Ed.): *The Practice of Community Mental Health.* Boston, Little Brown, 1970.

Zurcher, Louis: Implementing a community action agency. In Shore, Milton, and Mannino, Fortune (Eds.): *Mental Health and the Community: Problems, Programs and Strategies.* New York, Behavioral Publications, 1969.

CHAPTER 9

THE GOVERNMENTAL SYSTEM

John A. Morgan, Jr. and Robert H. Connery

THE PROVISION of mental health services is essentially a public program involving federal, state, and local governments and a host of sometimes related, sometimes uncoordinated, activities and agencies. As a consequence, what has and what has not been done to date, and what can and will be done in the future, are largely functions of the complicated governmental/political context within which mental health services and other public programs are developed and administered. In the United States, this context is immensely complex, and change, in whatever direction, typically occurs as the result of a "continuing process of bargaining, pressuring, inducing, bribing, supervising, demonstrating, harassing, encouraging, and publicizing, (Connery, 1968*)."

The degree to which mental health administrators understand and are able to manipulate the governmental/political environment within which they must operate will largely determine both the nature and quality of the programs they manage.

Unlike most areas of health care, mental health services have long been largely publicly provided. The current level of government involvement merely continues a trend (albeit snowballing in recent years) established very early in the Nation's history. The first public asylum for the mentally ill was built by Virginia in 1773 at Williamsburg. Although five decades elapsed before another was opened, during the mid-nineteenth century several

---

*Much of the discussion of the history of public mental health programs that follows is drawn from this work, especially chapters II and III.

additional state institutions were opened and after the Civil War the number and variety of state hospitals increased rapidly. Although other types of services were also developing, particularly after 1946, there were 284 state and county mental hospitals in operation by 1963. Employing almost 200,000 people, the operating costs of these institutions totalled $1,142,841,000, almost two-thirds of all the public expenditures for mental health in the United States.

Federal participation on any significant scale is of much more recent origin. While there had been some limited activities directed primarily toward a restricted clientele (most notably services for veterans provided by the Veterans Administration), it was not until the National Mental Health Act of 1946 that the national government began to treat mental health as a general public health problem. That Act created the National Institute of Mental Health (NIMH) and the National Advisory Mental Health Council and authorized a number of research, training, and service activities. Among these were research grants to universities, hospitals, laboratories, and other public or private institutions; grants for training, instruction, and demonstrations; and, most significantly, direct aid to states for the development of their mental health services. Importantly, the federal aid authorized was not intended to subsidize the operating costs of mental hospitals. Rather, the purpose was to stimulate a new form of community mental health activity. The major objective was to make it possible to treat a patient in his normal environment rather than in a mental hospital by providing a network of out-patient psychiatric clinics.

In the years following the passage of the National Mental Health Act, the federal government's role expanded rapidly. From a modest beginning in the 1948 fiscal year with a budget of $4.5 million, NIMH activities grew steadily. Total expenditures in the fiscal year ending June 30, 1965, were $186 million and during this period there was notable progress toward the objectives of the 1946 Act.

Although confinement in mental hospitals continued to be the principal method of state care for the mentally ill, both in terms of the number of patients treated and the extent of financial support, the beginnings of change were readily apparent. Admissions to these hospitals more than doubled during the period 1946-1965, but while admissions rose, so did separations; and 1955 marked the beginning of a steady annual decline in the resident population. In less than a decade, hospital personnel more than doubled, producing a far more favorable patient-staff ratio; and expenditures for operating costs quadrupled.

At the same time, the availability of other services was increasing. After the passage of the National Mental Health Act of 1946, the increase in the number of outpatient psychiatric clinics was remarkable. In 1945 there were approximately 450 clinics in operation; at the end of 1954 there were 1,234; and by 1965 the number had risen to 2007. In 1945, fifteen states had no facilities of this kind; in 1965, every state had at least three clinics in operation. The grants-in-aid to states authorized by the 1946 Act had been intended to stimulate a greater interest in community mental health services. And over the years there was a great increase in state and local expenditures for community mental health purposes, a development attributable in large part to the availability of federal funds. While federal grant-in-aid expenditures rose from $1,653,000 in fiscal 1948 to $6,675,000 in fiscal 1965, state and local expenditures during the same period increased from $2.4 million to approximately $120 million.

During this period of increasing federal involvement, the governmental organization of mental health services was being further complicated by the re-emergence of local governments as significant participants. With the gradual assumption by the states of responsibility for the care and treatment of the mentally ill in the closing decades of the nineteenth century, what little local governmental activity there had been was largely supplanted. Apart from a few states where county mental hospitals continued to operate, local governmental efforts all but disappeared. But the increasing emphasis on the importance of treating the mentally ill in their own communities led to a renewed interest in locally based facilities and an increasing tendency to decentralize responsibility for at least some kinds of mental health services from the state level to the local community. In 1954, New York became the first state to enact a community mental health law that permitted counties or groups of counties, municipalities of specific size, and in some instances other governmental jurisdictions to operate mental health clinics. Others followed, and by 1965 twenty-four states had provided for sharing the operating costs of these mental health clinics with local governments. As a consequence of the community mental health acts and varied programs of local assistance in other states, the rapid growth of outpatient psychiatric clinics was accompanied by a growing involvement of local government in the provision of mental health services.

Despite the intensified efforts of the late forties and fifties and the notable progress that resulted, mental health services remained a comparatively neglected public program. In 1962 the average daily number of resident patients in the country's institutions for the mentally ill was approximately 600,000, with well over a million receiving treatment at some time during the year. Yet, public expenditures for all mental health services totalled only $1.8 billion, with the average expenditure per resident patient about four dollars a day. And despite the multiplication of outpatient psychiatric clinics and the greatly increased expenditures for community services, the Director of NIMH summed up the situation in 1961 as follows: "There probably is no ideal community mental health program in the United States today. The integration of mental health services into community health and welfare programs is a task for the decade ahead" (Felix, 1961).

In its report to Congress submitted on the last day of 1960, the Joint Commission on Mental Illness and Health (1961) recommended that expenditures for public mental health services be doubled in the next five years and triple in the next ten. Only by this magnitude of expenditure could the typical state institutions be made in fact what currently they were in name only—hospitals for mental patients. And only by this magnitude of expenditure could programs be sufficiently extended outside the mental hospitals into the community. Toward these ends, the Commission outlined two major new roles for the federal government. It proposed substantial financial participation in the care of patients who heretofore had been considered the responsibility of the states. And it recommended, with far-reaching policy implications, that the federal government establish and maintain standards for the quality of care of the mentally ill.

President John F. Kennedy's "Message on Mental Illness and Mental Retardation," submitted to Congress on February 5, 1963, marked the beginning of an important new stage in the development of mental health services. President Kennedy called for a new approach to mental illness and mental retardation, an approach "designed, in large measure, to use Federal resources to stimulate State, local, and private action" (Kennedy, 1963). Relying heavily on new knowledge and new drugs to facilitate treatment in the community, the President asked Congress to authorize grants to the states for construction of "comprehensive community mental health centers," short-term grants for their initial staffing, and a relatively small sum for planning grants. These proposed comprehensive community mental health centers were to focus on both treatment and prevention. They were to provide a continuum of treatment, from diagnosis, to cure, to rehabilitation, without need to transfer patients to different institutions located in different communities.

On October 31, 1963, President Kennedy signed into law the Mental Retardation Facilities and Community Mental Health Centers Construction Act which promised to alter dramatically both the pattern of services available and the responsibility for providing them. The Act authorized $150 million for grants to states over a three-year period to pay one-third to two-thirds of the costs of constructing community mental health centers. Existing mental health services were to be augmented (some enthusiasts would have said replaced), by a network of comprehensive community mental health centers offering a range of coordinated services. Under the original regulations governing the construction of the centers (U. S. Federal Register, 1964), the *essential elements* of a comprehensive mental health center's program were inpatient, outpatient, emergency, and partial hospitalization services in addition to consultation and education services for the community. Each center was to serve a population of not less than 75,000 nor more than 200,000 and be readily accessible to the community to be served, "taking into account both political and geographic boundaries." Although grants for initial staffing of the centers were not authorized, two years later Congress passed additional legislation providing for initial staffing grants for three years and continuation funds in the necessary amounts for the succeeding four years.

Clearly, a substantial reorientation of mental health efforts was envisioned; a major emphasis on community services was to be brought about by federal government intervention with massive amounts of money. And while not expressly requiring it, the new program implicitly assumed a significantly expanded role for local governments.

By the end of fiscal year 1971, federal construction grants had amounted to $202 million. Under the matching formulas employed, this meant that a total of about $673 million had been expended on new or expanded facilities since the passage of the 1963 Act. Federal staffing grants had amounted to $274.2 million, and 452 comprehensive community mental health centers had been funded. With staffs totalling some 27,000 and providing direct services to some 512,000 patients (Taube, 1971), the 300 federally funded centers in operation at that time were playing a major role in the delivery of mental health services in a relatively very short time after the 1963 Act.

There is no doubt that there has been movement in the direction envisioned by the federal programs of the last three decades. In 1955, 77 percent of patient care episodes in mental health facilities were accounted for by inpatient services. In 1969, 54 percent of the total episodes were outpatient or day treatment episodes and only 46 percent were inpatient (Taube, 1972). The average daily resident population of state and county mental hospitals continued to decline, dropping to an estimated 317,163 for the period July 1, 1970, to June 30, 1971. Accompanying the decline in inpatient population, there has been a continued increase in the number of net releases from the hospitals, the number more than tripling since 1955, from 126,498 to 418,750 in 1971. At the same time the number of admissions to these hospitals has been increasing as has the ratio of full time staff to resident patients and the expenditures per patient under care per day (Bethel and Pedick, 1972).

Despite the changes that have occurred during recent years, however, there remains a significant gap between current reality and the goals sought by the proponents of intensified public efforts on behalf of mental health. While the 1971 level of public expenditures, an estimated $4.3 billion, represents a steep rise from the estimated $1.8 billion of 1962, because of inflation the increase in constant dollars is a good deal less than two-fold. And as a percent of national income, public expenditures for mental health have increased approximately one-fourth in nine years—from slightly less than four-tenths of one percent to five-tenths of one percent.

Well over half the public expenditures on mental health programs in 1970 still went to mental hospitals. The number of outpatient clinics had continued to rise, reaching 2088 in 1969, but most had long waiting lists and nearly half of all clinics were in cities in the Northeast. Moreover, an NIMH survey indicated that as of January, 1970, the number of forty-hour-equivalent psychiatrists in free standing outpatient clinics averaged just over one per clinc (Jones, 1970). As for federally funded community mental health centers, 452 by 1971 is an impressive number in so short a time, but it is a far cry from the number necessary to serve the entire population. Indeed, as of 1972, NIMH estimated that approximately 1000 more would be required. Further, it seems clear that the existing centers are finding it difficult to provide the range of community services for which they were designed. As of 1970, for example, consultation and education services accounted for a relatively small percent of total center services. While there was wide variation among individual centers, this *essential element* of a comprehensive mental health center's program accounted for, on the average, only 6.6 percent of total staff time, little more than general administration (Taube, 1970). A major focus of the centers as originally envisioned was to be prevention, but a far greater concentration on consultation and education services would appear to be necessary before the existing centers can have a significant impact in that regard.

The extent of governmental efforts on behalf of mental health services in the 1970's is a far cry from what it was a hundred years ago. Indeed, the last quarter of a century has been a period of startling advance. Yet, in view of the magnitude and costliness of the problem, current efforts to combat mental illness are puny at best. But the seriousness of a social problem is rarely, if ever, the sole determinant of what is done to cope with it. What should be or needs to be done may be professionally ascertainable, what *is* done is usually a pragmatic determination. And in the case of public programs, it is the determination of bureaucratic and political pragmatism. Moreover, mental health programs compete with many other worthy programs, each with its own constituency and supportive bureaucracy, complicated by dependence on three interacting levels of government—federal, state, and local. How scarce tax dollars are distributed among these competing activities is determined by the interaction of many groups of officials responding to a variety of practical considerations from differing political perspectives.

Shared Responsibilities in the Federal System

The delivery of mental health services provides a good example of the extent to which traditional patterns of governmental responsibility have been altered in recent decades and the extent to which public programs involve all levels of government. In this and other areas, federal government initiative and financial capacity have been increasingly brought to bear on what once were viewed as primarily, if not exclusively, state functions.

The framers of the United States Constitution created a federal system, dividing powers between national and state governments. The document restricted both levels of government and specifically listed the powers of the national government. By implication, later made explicit by the Tenth Amendment, state powers were general and residual. But some of the specifically listed powers of the national government were considerably less than precise in their implications. In the face of the proclamation that the Constitution and national legislation in pursuance thereof were to be the supreme law of the land, such clauses as those giving Congress the right to make all laws "necessary and proper" for carrying out the listed powers left rather unclear precisely what powers were reserved to the states. While some functions were assumed to be within the sphere of the national government and others were viewed as responsibilities of the states, the Constitution as written left open the possibility of considerable alterations in the allocation of responsibility in response to changing practical considerations.

Most of the change in the division of responsibility between national and state governments has been in the direction of broadening the federal role. Professor William Riker (1964) has compared the degree of involvement of the national and state governments in the performance of a number of functions at four periods in the nation's history—1790, 1850, 1910, 1964. He concluded that, in general, there had been a progressive rise in the participation of the national government and that the increase had taken place at the expense of the states. The growing role of the federal government in respect to functions once viewed as primarily state responsibilities can be shown in another way as well. In 1902, national government grants to state and local governments amounted to about $7 million, less than one percent of state-local expenditures. By 1932, federal aid to the states had grown to more than $200 million, and in 1969 it was in excess of $19 billion, over 16 percent of the direct general expenditures of state and local governments. Grants for health programs alone amounted to $3.2 billion, some 37 percent of state and local expenditures in this area.

The activities receiving federal grant-in-aid funds are quite varied. Hospital construction, public-health services, highway construction, old-age assistance, aid to dependent children, agricultural extension work, public housing, urban renewal—these are only a few of the more prominent. Nor is the federal role limited to providing money. Some early federal grants of land and money were made with no conditions attached, other than the requirement that they be used for the purpose specified. However, beginning with the Weeks Act of 1911 which provided funds for forest-fire prevention, grants have ordinarily been made subject to additional conditions of two types. First, aid is conditioned upon the states meeting federally prescribed standards and submitting to federal supervision. Second, there is usually a matching requirement. The state or local government receiving the grant must contribute from its own funds some prescribed proportion of the total cost of the project or function.

The existence of extensive grant-in-aid programs and their conditional nature enables the federal government to exercise a substantial amount of control over state and local activities. Theoretically, of course, a state is free to avoid federal standards and supervision by declining federal grant money. As a practical matter, however, there is ordinarily no real option. In the first place the state's residents pay their share of federal taxes with the result that if they do not meet the requirements for federal aid their money will be spent in states that do. Moreover, the costs of governmental services together with the fiscal realities of state and local governments make it all but impossible to decline available funds.

Many view the expanding activities and increasing supervisory role of the federal government with alarm, seeing it as a steady and rapid movement away from federalism in the direction of a unitary system. A 1963 survey, for example, indicated that a substantial majority of state and local government officials who expressed an opinion, believed that the American governmental system was becoming too centralized. As shown in Table 9-I, the proportion of respondents who expressed concern varied by categories of officials, but large-city mayors and city managers in the 50,000 to 250,000 population class were the only groups in which a majority took the opposite position.

In reality, of course, despite the significantly expanded role of the federal government, the federal system is far from dead. Indeed, one effect of increased national government activities, especially during recent years, has been to further complicate the allocation of power and responsibility by increasing the ability of local governments to act independently of their states and encouraging them to do so.

In theory, the federal system comprises two levels of independent governmental authority. Although their responsibilities may overlap, the national government and the states are distinct and independent, neither level deriving its authority from the other.

TABLE 9-I
VIEWS OF STATE AND LOCAL GOVERNMENT OFFICIALS ON
CENTRALIZATION OF GOVERNMENT

	Question: Do you believe that government in the U. S. is becoming too centralized:		
	Yes	*No*	*No Answer*
State government			
Governors	4	3	2
Attorneys general	6	1	2
Budget officers	4	3	8
Legislative leaders	19	5	4
County government (by population)			
Below 10,000	2	2	1
10,000-50,000	10	1	3
50,000-250,000	15	4	1
250,000 and over	21	11	8
Mayors (by population of city)			
Below 10,000	1	1	1
10,000-50,000	13	6	4
50,000-250,000	8	4	2
250,000 and over	3	4	1
City managers (by population of city)			
Below 10,000	30	20	12
10,000-50,000	39	20	10
50,000-250,000	4	9	5
250,000 and over	3	2	1
School board officials	23	22	16
TOTALS	204	118	81

Source: Adapted from Subcommittee on Intergovernmental Relations of the Committee on Government Operations, U. S. Senate: *The Federal System as Seen by State and Local Officials.* Washington, U. S. Government Printing Office, 1963, p. 183.

Local governments, on the other hand, are legally creatures of the state and have no independent status under the federal constitution. In fact, however, local governments have long enjoyed considerable independence although the degree varies widely both within and among the states. Federal programs such as urban renewal and public housing that make grant-in-aid funds available directly to local governments stimulate greater local independence in at least two major ways. The receipt of such federal funds reduces the localities' financial dependence upon state government. Further, prospects for obtaining federal funds increase the political leverage of local governments for the removal of state restrictions that interfere with meeting the conditions of the grant program.

As a consequence of these and other factors, governmental power and responsibility is currently shared by three distinct and significantly independent levels of government. A leading text on state and local government describes the resulting patterns of influence or control as follows (LeBlanc and Allensworth, 1971) :

1. Power in or dominance by the national government
2. Power in or dominance by the state government
3. Power in or dominance by the local government
4. Some combination of the above, to include:
   a. Both national and state governments exercising power
   b. Both national and local governments exercising power
   c. Both state and local governments exercising power
   d. All three levels exercising power

Examples of each pattern are apparent but it is important to recognize that this description of power allocations is further complicated in several important ways. In the first place, when two or more levels of government exercise power in a particular functional area, they may administer programs jointly or separately. The provision of mental health services provides examples of both. While the Community Mental Health Centers Program involves the joint participation of federal, state, and local governments, state mental hospitals and Veterans Administration neuropsychiatric hospitals are programmatically distinct and separate. Whenever two or more levels of government are responsible for a single function, their relationship will involve both cooperation and competition; but clearly the problem of coordination as well as the means for coping with it will vary depending on whether the function is performed jointly or separately.

A second complication results from the complexity of the functions themselves. A particular activity may accurately be described as involving the exercise of power by all three levels of government, when in actuality it involves a number of related programs that are themselves examples of different kinds of power allocations. The provision of mental health services, for example, may be viewed as a functional area involving the exercise of power by all three levels of government. The operation of mental hospitals, however, despite the role of the VA and the existence of some county mental hospitals, is a function controlled principally by State governments. In assessing the pattern of influence or control that prevails, much depends on how the function is conceptualized. The ways in which those responsible for performing a particular function conceptualize their activity may affect significantly the degree of cooperation or competition with similar or related governmental programs.

Still another complication of the patterns of influence and control results from the nature of local government. To say that a particular functional area such as mental health services is wholly or partly a local responsibility is to say that a number of distinct and independent authorities with varying powers and overlapping judisdictions may be involved. The pattern of local government in the United States is, to put it mildly, exceedingly complex. And that pattern has significant implications for the development and administration of mental health programs.

Fragmentation of Local Government

According to the 1967 Census of Governments, there were in that year 81,248 local governments (U.S. Bureau of the Census, 1968). Included in the total were 18,048 municipalities, 3,049 counties, 17,105 townships (includes New England town governments), 21,782 independent school districts, and 21,264 special districts. The average number was over 1,600 per state, but there was wide variation from one part of the country to another, a variation not correlated with population size. Illinois, with 6,453 local governments, stood in stark contrast to Hawaii, with only 19. Texas, with approximately the same number of inhabitants as Illinois, had 3,446 local governments; and New Hampshire, with roughly the same population as Hawaii, had 515.

These units of local government fall into two broad types; general-purpose and special purpose. General-purpose governments are those responsible for the normal range of functions generally associated with local government such as law enforcement, fire, water, welfare and health. Counties, townships, and municipalities are in this category. School districts and special districts are special-purpose governments; they are given responsibility for one or a small number of locally performed public functions.

Counties (parishes in Louisiana and boroughs in Alaska) cover most of the United States. Only Connecticut, Rhode Island, and limited areas in other states (such as the independent cities of Virginia) are not served by county governments, though the extent and significance of the services performed varies from one area to another. Technically, county governments are unincorporated political subdivisions of states. Where strong systems of lower-level government (townships, towns, or cities) exist within the boundaries of counties, the county government may perform only a few functions. Nonetheless, they have been and continue to be important units in rural areas and frequently have key responsibilities in the area of public health. While they are relatively weak or non-existent in the New England states, counties exercise important functions in the Midwest, West, and South. In recent years, a number of counties have adapted to expanding populations and changing social and political patterns by reorganizing their governmental and administrative structures and adding urban-type activities. It is now not uncommon to find county governments in urban areas operating *city-type* programs such as planning, urban renewal, public housing, air pollution and model cities. Some counties have adopted home-rule charters permitting them to function more independently of state government and make it somewhat difficult to distinguish them from municipal corporations.

The term *township* as used by the Census of Governments includes the New England Town (including *plantations* in Maine and *locations* in New Hampshire), towns in New York and Wisconsin, and civil townships elsewhere.* In New England, the

---

*Two distinctions should be kept in mind. First, *towns* in areas other than New England, New York, and Wisconsin are incorporated and classified as municipalities. Second, civil townships, with governmental organization and functions, must be differentiated from *congressional* or *survey* townships, which are six miles square and used for land description and location, but not governing purposes.

town corresponds generally to township and county governments elsewhere in that it is unincorporated, serves both rural and urban areas, and virtually blankets the state. Apart from incorporated municipalities, it is the most important unit of local government and plays a significant role in the delivery of health and mental health services. New York and Wisconsin towns, like townships elsewhere, are unincorporated subdivisions of the county, usually covering all or most of the area within any county, where they are found.

Existing primarily in the Northeast and Midwest (they are nonexistent in the South and are found only in Washington in the West), civil townships typically contain a small population; only five percent had 10,000 or more inhabitants as of 1967. As might be expected from their typically rural character, township functions are often quite restricted. However, in some areas of the country, notably Pennsylvania and New Jersey, township governments, like New England towns, are often very similar to smaller incorporated municipalities, performing such urban functions as planning, zoning, and subdivision regulation, and operating as the principal local general-purpose government.

Municipalities differ from counties and townships in that the form was developed primarily for urban government and they are governmental, or municipal, corporations. They operate under charters granted by the state either by special act of the state legislature or under the terms of general statutes governing standards and procedures for incorporation. Home rule charters are now commonly allowed and municipalities exercise considerable discretion and independence in developing and carrying out local powers. In every state the larger municipalities are legally designated *cities;* in some states, all municipalities are so designated although they may be distinguished by size. Many states, however, apply a different designation, such as village, town, or borough, to their smaller municipalities which usually have less extensive powers.

By far the most numerous kind of special-purpose government is the independent school district. Of the 23,390 school systems in the nation in 1967, almost 22,000 were operated by independent school governments. In only four states—Hawaii, Maryland, North Carolina, and Virginia—were all school systems operated as part of general purpose governments. These school districts are of significance to the development of mental health programs in at least two ways. Since no other local activity even approaches the dollar volume committed to public education, the manner in which these funds are controlled and expended affects what is available for other local programs and services. Moreover, in many areas school districts bear primary responsibility for public health services offered to children and in some places this includes mental health services as well.

Other special districts are as varied and numerous as the considerations that bring them into existence. They include such functions as local sewage disposal, mosquito abatement, water supply, soil conservation and flood control, as well as those with multiple functions and extensive regional responsibilities such as the Port of New York Authority.* A significant number of special district governments, however, bear responsibility for programs or services closely related to mental health concerns. These include 234 health districts, 537 hospital districts, 613 parks and recreation districts, and 1,565 housing and urban renewal districts. Although almost 30 percent of the special districts are in three states—Illinois, California, and Pennsylvania—this form of government is common throughout the country. Thirty states contain 200 or more such units and only two, Virginia and Hawaii, have less than fifty.

When this pattern of local government is related to contemporary patterns of living, the potential complications for the formation of public policy and the delivery of mental health services become readily apparent. As of 1970, the United States population was 73.5 percent urban. More significantly, 68.6 percent of all Americans lived in 243 metropolitan areas, technically termed "Standard Metropolitan Statistical Area" (SMSA's). As defined by the Census Bureau, an SMSA consists of one or more counties which contain a central city or twin cities with a population of at least 50,000. But it may, and usually does, also include numerous other incorporated municipalities as well as

---

*As of 1967 only 453 special districts had multiple responsibilities. The remaining 20,811 were single purpose governments.

special districts and unincorporated rural lands served by county and township governments. Thus, the general concept of an SMSA is an integrated economic and social unit, but not an integrated governmental unit. As of 1967,* there were nearly 21,000 local governments in 227 metropolitan areas, an average of 91 per area. Although the total number and the number of each type varied widely from one area to another, multiple local governments, in most instances a veritable host of local governments, are the rule in contemporary metropolitan America.

To be sure, generalization is difficult because metropolitan areas differ greatly both in population size and in the number of governments. And in a few areas, such as Tucson, Albuquerque, Austin, and El Paso, a large proportion of the people live within the central city; but generally, the metropolitan population is widely dispersed among a number of independent jurisdictions. Indeed, as of 1970, the central cities contained only 45.8 percent of the metropolitan population; over half were suburbanites. And in some metropolitan areas, notably Boston, Washington, and Pittsburgh, population decentralization is so great that three-fourths of the area's people live outside the central city.

The division of governmental authority that results is startling. Not only are nearly all functions of local government within the metropolitan area performed by agencies and officials on a local rather than a metropolitan-wide basis, but there is considerable overlap of governmental authority as well. Less than one-fourth of the school districts in SMSA's have boundaries that correspond to those of a general purpose government, and over three-fourths of special districts are also noncoterminous with other local government areas. As a result, local government in metropolitan areas is all too often characterized by an inefficient duplication of efforts, an insufficient coordination of related activities, and an inequitable apportionment of responsibility for area-wide problems.

To many, the obvious solution to this *balkanized* pattern of government in metropolitan America is some sort of urban con-

---

*The census of governments is taken every five years, three years before and two years after the decennial census of population. 1967 figures are, therefore, the latest available at this writing.

solidation. But whatever the type of consolidation proposed, it is fraught with practical difficulties. Extending the jurisdiction of the central city is both politically and legally difficult. The typical metropolitan pattern is that of a central city surrounded by a number of incorporated suburbs or even two or three central cities each with its bedroom satellites. In most states, annexation of incorporated areas requires popular approval by referendum in each affected jurisdiction; an approval very difficult to obtain since there are almost always some significant local interests furthered by independence. And in view of the increased representation in state legislatures for suburban areas resulting from the Supreme Court's one-man one-vote reapportionment decisions, it is highly unlikely that state laws will be changed to make annexations easier for the central cities.

City-county consolidation is both difficult to achieve and of limited usefulness. Quite apart from the political obstacles that must be overcome, a merger of city and county governments does not necessarily affect the status of other municipalities contained within the county's boundaries nor does it automatically eliminate the numerous special purpose governments or the factors responsible for their existence. Moreover, over one hundred metropolitan areas encompass two or more counties, over fifty spread over three or more, and thirty extend across state lines. Obviously, the probability of multi-county areas increases with the size of the SMSA, and in 1970, metropolitan areas with 500,-000 or more residents accounted for over half the United States population.

Annexation and city-county consolidations have, of course, been employed with considerable success in a number of instances in the past and will, no doubt, prove a viable means for rationalizing metropolitan government in some areas in the future. And there are, of course, other approaches to metropolitan-wide organization. These include the metropolitan federation approach of Miami-Dade County, Florida; the service contract approach long associated with the Los Angeles, California area; the more recently emerging land development and regulation contracts; metropolitan-wide special districts; and various bodies such as metropolitan planning commissions and councils of govern-

ments which, though typically lacking enforcement and implementation authority, often play significant advisory and coordinative roles. These and other approaches will be employed, with
varying degrees of success in various places, to bring about greater
governmental integration in metropolitan areas. But the chances
of major structural alterations and dramatic rationalizations of
the pattern of metropolitan government in the immediate future
seem very slim.

In addition to a host of self-interest considerations that militate against change (on the part of the various publics concerned,
and on the part of elected officials and the various bureaucracies),
opposition to governmental centralization has deep roots in the
American intellectual and political tradition. The almost mysti-
cal infatuation with the concept of "local community" is reflected
in a number of contemporary federal government programs,
among them the Community Mental Health Centers Program.
And there is considerable evidence to suggest the absence, in
most metropolitan areas at least, of a sense of community
broad enough to support any significant change in government
structure.*

The American population is an urban population residing
overwhelmingly in large metropolitan areas. But while metropolitan areas may be socially and economically integrated, govern-
mentally they are not; and at least for the immediate future, they
promise to remain that way. Thus, the three-tiered system of
governmental power and responsibility includes an immensely
complex third tier.

---

*See Advisory Commission on Intergovernmental Relations: *Metropolitan Social
and Economic Disparities: Implications for Intergovernmental Relations in Central
Cities and Suburbs.* Washington. U. S. Government Printing Office, 1965; Banfield,
Edward C.: The politics of metropolitan area organization. *Midwest Journal of
Political Science, 1:*77-91, 1957; Dye, Thomas R.; Liebman, Charles S.; Williams,
Oliver P., and Herman, Harold: Differentiation and cooperation in a metropolitan
area. In Danielson, Michael N. (Ed.) : *Metropolitan Politics.* Boston, Little, Brown,
1966, pp. 261-271; Dencan, Beverley: Variables in urban morphology. In Burgess,
Ernest W. and Bogue, Donald H. (Eds.): *Contributions to Urban Sociology.*
Chicago, University of Chicago Press, 1964, pp. 17-30; Wood, Robert C.: *Suburbia,
Its People and Their Politics.* Boston, Houghton Mifflin, 1958; and Connery,
Robert H. et al.: *The Politics of Mental Health.* New York, Columbia University
Press, 1968, esp. chapters XII and XIII.

Most Americans find themselves served by, and paying taxes to the federal government, the state government, and a number of independent local governments. More importantly, they are served by a number of independent governments that vary significantly in legal authority, fiscal capacity, structure, and constituencies served. Each factor has an important bearing on the policy-making process. Whether a particular policy determination *can* be made is obviously dependent upon a government's legal authority and fiscal capacity. Whether a particular policy determination *will* be made and how it will be executed is largely dependent on access patterns—which interests exercise effective influence in what direction.

Who will have effective access to the decision-makers, which values will be reflected in the decision-making process and whose views will prevail in the determination and execution of policy are largely determined by governmental form and structure and by the nature and size of the relevant constituency. All of these factors affect the development and administration of mental health programs.

Separation of Powers and the Decisional Process

In a book published a decade ago, Professor E. E. Schattsneider (1960) observed that the outcome of all conflict is determined by the scope of its contagion. The number of people involved in any conflict determines what happens; every change in the number of participants affects the result. It follows that the most important strategy in politics is concerned with the scope of conflict. Probably no governmental system in the world provides a better illustration of the accuracy of Schattsneider's observation than does the federal system of contemporary America.

At each level of government the resolution of a particular political struggle is potentially different because the participating publics are different. And each level of government is characterized by an organizational complexity sufficient to produce outcomes that vary according to which part of the institutional apparatus assumes primary responsibility for decision-making. To change the level of government at which a decision is made, or to shift the forum for decision-making at a particular level, is to alter the probabilities as to what precisely will be decided. This results in large part from the simple fact that the varying institutional forms reflect and favor different political alignments.

What will happen in respect to mental health policy in the future, just as what has happened in the past, will be greatly affected by where the decisions are made. Whether present programs will be expanded or contracted, whether certain types of services will be emphasized at the expense of others, how ongoing mental health programs will fare in the annual appropriations competition, depend in good measure on what parts of the governmental apparatus are involved.

At the national level, significant policy determinations involve the interaction of an executive department and both houses of Congress, each designed to be responsive to different combinations of interests and therefore to varying political considerations. The varied representation systems reflected by the House of Representatives, the Senate, and the Presidency as well as the internal organization of these different parts of the policy-making apparatus assure that decision-making will occur within significantly varying political contexts.

The fact that the 435 seats in the House of Representatives are apportioned among the states according to population whereas each state elects two senators makes for significant variations in the manner in which different population groups are represented in the two bodies. Representatives are elected from geographic districts including some 475,000 people while the senatorial district is the entire state. Consequently, save for those few states (five as of the 92d Congress) entitled to only one seat in the House, representatives are responsible to smaller, and usually more homogeneous, groupings of people than are senators. The potential effect of this difference on their political outlook can be illustrated by current demographic patterns.

As of 1970, over half the population lived in 65 metropolitan areas containing 500,000 or more people. Thirty-two states had at least one such area within its boundaries; thus, 64 of the 100 senators had such an area within their districts. Since, on the average, less than half the population of metropolitan areas lives in the central city, it is apparent that a senator's district typically includes significant numbers of rural/small town, suburban, and big-city residents, while the representative's much smaller district is considerably less likely to approximate national living patterns. Moreover, socioeconomic, racial, and ethnic groupings tend to be reflected in residential patterns and, therefore, in urban/suburban/rural divisions.

Consequently, there is a considerably greater likelihood of socioeconomic, racial, and ethnic homogeneity and thus a greater unity of political outlook within a representative's district than in a senator's district. Thus, despite the fact that representation is proportionate to population in the House and disproportionate in the Senate, a far greater percentage of senators than representatives are responsible to constituencies approximating national population patterns and issue orientations.

On the other hand, the district system and greater size of the House of Representatives offer a greater opportunity for direct representation of diverse population and interest groupings through *their own* spokesmen. And to these differences must be added the varied terms served by senators and representatives. A senator's six year term almost inevitably produces a degree of independence enjoyed by few representatives who must face the electorate every two years.

The workings of the electoral college system ensure that the selection of the chief executive will reflect still another alignment of people and interests. It is commonplace to observe that both Democratic and Republican presidential candidates are normally somewhat to the left of the ideological center of their parties. This results from the fact that a state's electoral votes are cast in a block for the candidate receiving the greatest number of poplular votes in that state, thus exaggerating the importance of the large, *close* states and the political interests concentrated there. The large states are, for the most part, heavily urbanized and industrial with concentrations of organized labor, minorities, and the social and economic problems that give rise to demands for governmental intervention commonly regarded as politically *left*. This is not to say that such interests dominate presidential politics to the exclusion of all others, but the coalition politics necessary to win the Presidency differ from the constituency patterns reflected in the House of Representatives and the Senate.

To the extent that decision-making reflects constituency reality, the decisions of the House, the Senate, and the President will vary significantly, reflecting different pressures and considerations. However, the impact of constituency on the decisional process is a complicated matter, involving far more than the nature of the districts represented and the electoral considerations of particular officials. Both the internal organization and the decisional process itself also significantly affect access patterns, playing a major role in determining who exercises effective influence toward what ends.

The internal organization and decision-making processes of the Congress and the Presidency are, of course, quite complex. However, a summary of some major differences between the two branches suggests their critical role in policy determination.

While there are important differences in the organization, rules and procedures (both formal and informal) of the two houses of Congress, several generalizations about congressional decision-making are possible.* First, each house of Congress is a highly decentralized body in which power is widely dispersed. Committees are almost entirely autonomous and, in the case of some committees, notably Appropriations, subcommittees are also relatively autonomous. As a consequence, the actions taken by the committees are most commonly the actions taken by the parent body.

Second, while political party affiliation is a highly important organizing and coordinating force, reciprocity is also a major factor. As Lewis Froman (1967) puts it: "Committees, and committee members, tend not to interfere with the work of other committees. . . . There is a strong tendency for members to accept the work and expertise of the other committees. In return, of course, they expect little interference in their own work."

Third, legislative decision-making is serial; a number of successive approvals is necessary. While a single negative action may be sufficient to defeat a bill, agreements must be cumulative. Forming a winning coalition, then, requires putting together a

*The following discussion of Congress draws heavily on Froman (1967).

majority at a number of different decision-points involving different people in different situations at different points in time.

Fourth, the legislative process is lengthy and time-consuming
with many opportunities for delay. And delay ordinarily works to
the advantage of the opposition by prolonging the period of time
over which the proponents must maintain an intensity of support
sufficient to sustain a particular measure at each of the numerous
decision-points. The points at which delay and defeat may occur
in the House of Representatives are shown in Table 9-II. A similar
table, with some modifications, notably the omission of those
points involving the Rules Committee and the addition of the
filibuster, could be constructed for the Senate. And it is impor-

TABLE 9-II

POINTS AT WHICH DELAY OF DEFEAT MAY OCCUR IN THE HOUSE

Delay	Defeat
Committee inaction in refering to a subcommittee	Committee inaction
	Negative vote in committee
Subcommittee inaction (prolonged hearings; refusal to report	Subcommittee inaction
	Negative vote in subcommittee
Committee inaction (prolonged hearings; refusal to report	Rules Committee inaction
Rules Committee inaction (refusal to schedule hearings; prolonged hearings; refusal to report	Negative vote in Rules Committee
	Defeat of rule on the floor
Slowness in scheduling the bill	Motion to strike enacting clause
Floor action (demanding full requirements of the rules) reading of the journal repeated quorum calls refusing unanimous consent to dispense with further proceedings under the call of the roll prolonging debate various points of order	Motion to recommit
	Final passage

Source: Froman, Lewis A., Jr.: *The Congressional Process: Strategies, Rules, and Procedures*. Boston, Little Brown, 1967, p. 18.

tant to recognize that when a measure survives all these decision-points and is passed by both houses, differences between House and Senate versions will often require negotiation and compromise in a conference committee and then favorable action in each house on the conference report. Thus, two additional decision-points with opportunities for delay and defeat are added. And the appropriation of monies to implement an authorization involves still another journey through the legislative process.

These aspects of the congressional decision-making process have a significant bearing on who exercises power in the legislature and what interests are most likely to be favored. It is evident that the fate of a measure lies largely in the hands of the relatively small group of legislators who deal with it in committee or subcommittee.

Power in the committee structure is largely a matter of seniority (Goodwin, 1959). The seniority rule has much to do with the appointment of members to committees and determines the designation of the chairmen. The ranking majority member of each committee, in terms of seniority on the committee, is the chairman. Seniority results from consistent reelection, consistent reelection is most likely to occur in those areas that are *safe* for one or the other party, and those areas are likely to be the more homogeneous districts. This has important effects on the distribution of power. Not only are committee chairmen older members, but Democratic chairmen are disproportionately from the South and Republican chairmen disproportionately Midwestern. More importantly, the kinds of districts that produce committee chairmen are ordinarily those least approximating a microcosm of the nation as a whole.

The powers possessed by committee chairmen give them a position of importance in the policy-making process not enjoyed by other members. Froman (1967) summarizes this position as follows:

> Almost all bills are referred to committee. Whether a bill is considered, whether hearings are held, and whether the bill is reported, then, is up to each individual committee. To a large extent it also hinges on the actions or inactions of committee chairmen. Committee chairmen, among other things, set meeting times, determine the committee agenda, preside over meetings, decide whether there will be

subcommittees, and who will be on the subcommittees, hire the staff, recommend conference committee members to the presiding officer, who in most cases routinely accepts the recommendation, and manage bills on the floor (or designate subcommittee chairmen or others to do so).

The purposes for which these powers are used vary considerably and there are important constraints that can be applied by the committee members, by the party organization, and by the parent body. Both House and Senate have procedures whereby the chairman and even the committee can be by-passed, procedures that are used successfully on occasion. But the considerations underlying the general practice of reciprocity as well as the potential for future retaliation on the part of the chairman are powerful deterrents to circumventing the normal legislative process. A major consequence of the seniority rule, then, is to distribute extraordinary power in the policy-making process to members who on some issues, reflect a minority position even within their own party caucus.

It is this bias in favor of minority interests that is the most striking, and from a policy perspective, the most salient feature of the legislative process. The decentralization of power within Congress, the distribution of power within the decentralized structure, the serial nature of decision-making, and the complexity of the rules and procedures all work in the direction of inhibiting positive action that is opposed by significant minorities. Even a small minority, if strategically placed and intensely opposed, can play a potentially dominant role.

These factors, together with the workings of the seniority system, the procedures for assigning members to committees (especially the *exclusive* committees in the House, i.e., Appropriations, Ways and Means, and Rules);* and the correlation be-

---

*Under House rules, members assigned to exclusive committees may not hold another committee assignment. Assignment to one of these committees carries great prestige and power and few members are appointed to them until after they have served several terms and are fully acceptable to the leadership. In the Senate the most sought after, and most carefully considered committee assignments are Foreign Relations, Appropriations, and Finance.

For discussions of assignments to committees, see Clark, Joseph S.: *The Senate Establishment.* New York, Hill & Wang, 1963; and Masters, Nicholas A: House Committee Assignments. *American Political Science Review, 55:* 345-359, 1961.

tween seniority and the ability to manipulate the rules and structure of the organization work to the advantage of those favoring the *status quo*. Particularly with economic regulation and social-welfare policies such as mental health programs, the proponents of liberal legislation requiring expanded governmental activity face an arduous task indeed. They must build support (or at least assent) at a number of key points in a process with a natural bias in the opposite direction.

But to equate national policy-making with the congressional process is to mistake the nature of contemporary American government. In part because of the nature of the office itself, in part because of the ever expanding demands on government in an increasingly complex world, the modern President has assumed the dominant role in the policy-making process.* This is, of course, no new or sudden development. Although the Constitution vested "all legislative powers" in Congress, by giving the President the veto power and primary responsibility for the conduct of foreign affairs, the founding fathers assured that the presidential role would include more than merely the "faithful execution of the laws." With a few notable exceptions, Presidents back to and including George Washington have taken expansionist views of their functions. And the modern view of presidential responsibility dates at least from President Theodore Roosevelt.

After leaving the Presidency, Theodore Roosevelt (1916) set forth the following views on presidential responsibility:

> My view was that every executive officer, and above all, every executive officer in high position, was a steward of the people bound actively and affirmatively to do all he could for the people, and not to content himself with the negative merit of keeping his talents undamaged in a napkin. I declined to adopt the view that what was imperatively necessary for the Nation could not be done by the President unless he could find some specific authorization to do it. My belief was that it was not only his right but his duty to do anything

---

*For one treatment of this development, see Corwin, Edward S.: *The President: Office and Powers 1787-1957*. New York, New York University Press, 1957, especially chap. VII and "Resume." For an evaluation of the role of Congress *vis-a-vis* the President from a different perspective as well as an evaluation of the contemporary Congress and its prospects for the future, see Saloma, John S. III: *Congress and the New Politics*. Boston, Little Brown, 1969.

that the needs of the Nation demanded unless such action was for-
bidden by the Constitution or by the laws. Under this interpretation
of executive power I did and caused to be done many things not previously done by the President and the heads of departments. I did not
usurp power, but I did greatly broaden the use of executive power.
In other words, I acted for the public welfare, I acted for the common well-being of all our people, whenever and in whatever manner
was necessary, unless prevented by direct constitutional or legislative
prohibition. I did not care a rap for the mere form or show of power;
I cared immensely for the use that could be made of the substance.

To the extent that Roosevelt's "Stewardship Theory" contemplated the assumption by the President of major responsibility
for legislative initiative and the direction of national policy, it
has proved prophetic of subsequent developments.

The current allocation of roles between the President and
Congress has been summarized as follows (Saloma, 1969):

1. The President, as chief legislator, normally takes the initiative in the legislative process. He develops, through the executive
budget and the central clearance of agency requests for legislation, a coordinated agenda for congressional action. The expertise of the executive bureaucracy is used to develop legislative
proposals, and he works through the legislative leaders to enact
the priority items of his program.

2. The Congress, exercising its legislative powers, reviews the
requests of the Executive—accepting, amending, or rejecting. It
retains *secondary initiative* in the legislative process, i.e., while
leaving to the President the responsibility for the preliminary
work of screening and coordinating agency requests, Congress retains the right to *second-guess* his determination of national
priorities.

3. With the increase of delegated *(executive)* legislation, Congress has extended its control or review function. While permitting the Executive wide discretion in complicated areas of
public policy by specifying its intent in broad legislation, Congress increases its own role in the oversight of administration.

In at least two major ways, then, the Executive plays a major
role in the policy-making process—by a significant participation in
the legislative process itself and by administrative rule-making
which is often of great policy importance. In both respects, the

organization and decision processes characterizing the Executive are significantly different from those of Congress and have important implications for the play of interests and the kinds of determinations made.

Normally, Executive participation in the legislative process occurs, at least initially, through the participation of the various agencies responsible for particular areas of public policy. Whether acting in response to directives from above or on their own initiative, the bureaucracies directly involved in the execution of policy are responsible for the development of much of the proposed legislation eventually acted upon by Congress. Moreover, although subject to numerous constraints and many stages of review, these same officials play a crucial role in the development of the President's budget, with all of its significance for what will eventually be done.

Whether one chooses to point to the professional expertise and commitment resulting from an intensive involvement in a particular area of activity or to the personal ambitions served by the expansion of an agency's domain, clearly the perception of *the public interest* guiding the development of legislative proposals and budgetary requests from the executive agencies will ordinarily be quite different from that of popularly elected legislators. At the very least, there is likely to be a considerably greater conviction on the part of the executive agency of the overriding importance of its particular area of responsibility. Consequently, there is a somewhat greater probability of a coincidence of views between the relevant administrative agency and those interests seeking expanded governmental activity.

There are, however, other participants who play crucial roles in the decision-making process. Through its dominant position in the budgetary process and its legislative clearance operations, the Office of Management and Budget (formerly the Bureau of the Budget) operates as a powerful aid to the President in controlling and coordinating agency activities.

The budget, according to President Kennedy's first Director of the Bureau of the Budget, is

a major means for unifying and setting forth an over-all executive program. . . . (It) reflects (the President's) judgment of the relative priority of different federal activities. Thus, the President's budget necessarily reflects his policy judgments and the Congress in acting on the President's budget necessarily reviews these policy judgments as to the relative importance of alternative uses of national resources. . .

The essential idea of the budget process is to permit a systematic consideration of our Government's program requirements in the light of available resources; to identify marginal choices and the judgment factors that bear on them; to balance competing requirements against each other; and finally, to enable the President to decide upon priorities and present them to the Congress in the form of a coherent work program and financial plan. (Bell, 1961) .

The dominant function of the Office of Management and Budget (OMB), is to help the President carry out his purposes (Wildavsky, 1964). The OMB occupies a key position in the development of the executive budget through (1) its participation in establishing the tentative assumptions that will guide the preparation of the budget; (2) its communication of guidelines to agencies along with the annual call for budgetary estimates; and (3) its intensive review, followed frequently by revisions, of agency estimates when received. Since the budgetary process determines to a great extent what activities the federal government shall undertake, and to what extent it shall undertake them, the OMB is a most powerful participant in the policy-making process.

The Office of Management and Budget participates in the legislative process in still another important way. It reviews the hundreds of legislative proposals generated by federal departments, bureaus, and independent agencies and assesses their acceptability as component parts of the presidential program. Richard E. Neustadt (1954) has described legislative clearance as "by far the oldest, best intrenched, most thoroughly institutionalized of the President's coordinative instruments—always excepting the budget itself." Although no longer possessing the veritable monopoly claim on clearance decisions held by the Bureau of the Budget in the 1950's, OMB continues to play an important role at three successive stages in the legislative process.

First, once agency initiated bills have run the gamut of clearance channels in the sponsoring bureau and in the departmental hierarchy above, they must clear OMB before submission to Congress. Second, once bills are introduced in Congress, regardless of their sources, the committees considering them ordinarily solicit views from interested agencies. Official agency responses, in whatever form and to whomever addressed, first channel through OMB for coordination and advice on each bill's relation to the President's program. And third, when legislation comes from Congress to the President for signature or veto, OMB obtains, coordinates, and summarizes agency opinions, preparing a presidential dossier complete with covering recommendation.

There are, of course, means by which OMB restraints on agency perspectives can be minimized or averted. Revisions of budgetary estimates typically involve a process of negotiation and bargaining between OMB and the agencies, and agency personnel are not unskilled in that process. Not only may decisions be appealed to the President, but an agency may have powerful allies in Congress, as has long been the case with the National Institutes of Health.

In regard to legislative proposals, the trend in recent years has been for Presidents frequently to short-circuit normal clearance channels to put a personal stamp on high priority legislation, with a consequent increase in the influence of the White House staff. Moreover, White House deadlines for policy proposals, particularly in respect to new programs deemed politically crucial, can work to allow more discretion to individual agencies. Robert S. Gilmour (1971) reports that "an experienced observer" in HEW noted that deadlines have "more than once facilitated a shortcut in the clearance process." He went on to suggest:

> As a department strategy for approval of its bills, specific departments have dragged their feet until the eleventh hour. Thus when the draft went in from the line departments to the OMB there was virtually no time for Budget clearance, much less for a thoughtful and coherent response from other concerned departments. In the face of a firm White House deadline, the initiating department's proposal would earn the official blessing of the President as a reward for tardiness.

And finally, just as in the case of budgetary requests, agency relationships with strategically placed congressmen can be employed to *get around* the confines of clearance procedures.

In short, executive participation in the legislative process is, to a very significant degree, participation by line agency personnel directly involved in a particular functional area. And the nature of the decisional process, though subjecting the agencies to significant restraints, assures that the perspective of the relevant bureaucracy will greatly influence the legislative and budgetary proposals that are produced. Thus, the federal health bureaucracy's views of programmatic needs and the skill and intensity with which it pushes those views play a major role in the development of national health policies. A case in point is the Community Mental Health Centers Act of 1963, which was largely the product of professionals within the National Institute of Mental Health (Connery, 1968).

Administrative rule-making provides still another avenue for significant participation by the executive in the policy-making process. And, once again, the bureaucratic perspective can play an all-important role. Largely as a result of the complexity of the social and economic problems toward which public programs are directed, Congress must ordinarily be content with enacting legislation that sets policy objectives and prescribes general standards while delegating to the President and his subordinates in the executive branch the job of filling in the details. As a result, an enormous quantity of executive *legislation,* or administrative rules and regulations, is issued. Much of this quasi-legislative output governs simply the form and procedure of government action, but a large proportion is actually definition, elaboration, or amplification of the substantive provisions of federal statutes. The policy importance of this executive decision-making and of the views held by the administrative officials involved is apparent in the very earliest stages of the federal Community Mental Health Centers Program.

The Community Mental Health Centers Act authorized grants for the construction of public and other nonprofit community mental health centers, which were defined in the legislation as facilities "providing services for the prevention or diagnosis of mental illness, or care and treatment of mentally ill patients, or rehabilitation of such persons, which services are provided principally for persons residing in a particular community or communities in or near which the facility is situated." What would be the primary emphasis of the centers was not spelled out; the key conjunction in the Act's definition of community mental health center was *or,* not *and.* Precisely what sorts of services a facility would have to provide and in what mix in order to qualify for federal funds was left undetermined. This was to be prescribed in regulations developed and issued by the Secretary of Health, Education, and Welfare after consultation with the Federal Hospital Council and the National Advisory Mental Health Council.

The regulations issued provided that the facilities funded would be those providing, either alone or in conjunction with other closely related facilities, at least the *essential elements* of comprehensive mental health services. Those *essential elements* were defined as (1) inpatient services, (2) outpatient services, (3) partial hospitalization services—including at least day care service, (4) emergency services provided 24 hours per day, and (5) consultation and education services available to community agencies and professional personnel. Not surprisingly, the regulations in this regard and in others as well reflected the community orientation of the National Institute of Mental Health, a perspective not universal among mental health professionals. A significant movement in a particular policy direction, no doubt contemplated by the legislation, but not precisely prescribed, was ensured by administrative determination.

Through the process of legislative initiation and through the issuance of rules and regulations governing the execution of the laws, then, the executive plays a crucial role in the policy-making process. And in both cases, the nature of the decision-making process ensures that the kinds of policies made will reflect to a significant degree the programmatic dispositions of the professional administrators. In many instances, this will mean a favorable climate for proposals seeking to expand governmental activities, particularly when the nature of the expansion sought involves the enlargement of current programs.

On the other hand, the importance of the bureaucratic perspective in executive decision-making increases the odds against certain kinds of change. New policy directions, whether expansionist or restrictive, that threaten an ongoing program are likely to meet stiff resistance and skillful opposition from those responsible for its administration.

It is clear that attempts to substantially alter the nature of governmental activity in a particular functional area must survive a veritable obstacle course of potentially adverse reactions, both in the legislature and in the executive. In an area such as mental health, the nature of the problem as well as the need for new approaches is likely to call for frequent programmatic changes that, at least in appearance, may pose a threat to the interests of a number of related bureaucracies. How this facet of the decisional process is dealt with will be a major determinant of what can and will be done.

State Decision-Making

Much of what has been said above about the policy implications of varied decision-making contexts at the national level might be repeated for state and local government. But there are important differences. And since state and local governments continue to bear primary responsibility for the delivery of mental health services, decision-making at this level is vitally important to the development and administration of mental health programs. Although there are significant differences from one state to another and details will vary depending on which of the fifty states one is considering, some generalizations about the context of decision-making and its policy implications are possible.*

As with the national government, state governments are

*There are a number of good basic texts on state and local government. Especially recommended are Dye, Thomas R.: *Politics in States and Communities.* Englewood Cliffs, Prentice-Hall, 1969; Jacob, Herbert, and Vines, Kenneth N. (Eds.) : *Politics in the American States, A Comparative Analysis,* 2nd ed. Boston, Little Brown, 1971; and LeBlanc, Hugh L., and Allensworth, D. Trudeau: *The Politics of States and Urban Communities.* New York, Harper & Row, 1971. An extensive analysis of the linkages between socioeconomic environment, the character of state political systems, and public policies in education, health and welfare, highways, taxation, and public regulation is provided by Dye, Thomas R.: *Politics, Economics, and the Public: Policy Outcomes in the American States.* Chicago, Rand McNally, 1965.

characterized by separately organized executive and legislative branches in which popularly elected officials are representative of significantly different constituencies. All states save Nebraska have bicameral legislatures; and although since the Supreme Court's 1964 reapportionment decisions both houses may be apportioned on the basis of population, variations between the two bodies in the number of seats and the consequent size of districts may produce very significant differences in their constituency patterns.

More importantly, legislators represent territorially defined districts each comprising only a small segment of the state while governors are elected by the people of the state as a whole. Just as with the President and Congress, then, each legislator represents a more homogeneous constituency than does the governor. Since the legislator's constituents share a local environment they are more likely to have roughly similar opinions on policy matters. As a result, constituency influences on legislators are relatively clear, unmixed, and unambiguous whereas the governor must please a wider, more heterogeneous constituency. As Thomas R. Dye (1969) puts it, "No single local interest can dominate (the governor's) judgment; he can balance one interest against another; he is free to represent widely shared interests throughout the state; and he is free to direct himself to statewide problems."

The significance of the executive in the policy-making process is even more pronounced at the state level than at the national. Most state legislatures function as *arbiters* of public policy rather than as *initiators,* responding to the stimulus provided by the governor, the bureaucrat, and the interest group. As with Congress, however, the rules and procedures by which state legislatures operate make the passage of bills tedious and difficult, lending themselves easily to those who would delay or block legislation.

Committees play an important role in the process and provide an important opportunity for obstruction by less than a majority of legislators. But for many reasons, such as the abbreviated length of legislative sessions, lack of staff, and a high rate of legislative turnover, committees in state legislatures are not nearly so powerful as committees in Congress. Nor is the seniority system as prevalent as it is in Congress, with the result that committee assignments, even the selection of chairmen, are more likely to be controlled by the legislative leadership, frequently in consultation with the governor. The criteria commonly used in picking chairmen and the members of major committees include competence, experience in the subject matter, the maintenance of geographical balance, and an effort to respect the desires of members.

Given the typically large turnover of committee membership in each session in state legislatures—unlike Congress—expert knowledge comes less from committee experience than from the custom of putting on a committee legislators with specific occupational or professional experience. This frequently turns the committee into an arena for competing interest groups, each with direct representation on the committee. Once again, the likelihood of the committee becoming a tightly run citadel of power is reduced.

The committee system in the state legislature, then, does not usually offer the legislator a power base independent of party or factional control. As a result, party considerations and each legislator's personal convictions and perceptions of constituency interest play a more important role in the decison-making process. Although these influences may conflict, they are often difficult to distinguish. Where the constituencies of a state are divided along social and economic lines and where the party division coincides with these district divisions, loyalty to party and support for constituency interests are likely to push in the same direction. Indeed, a number of studies suggest that this division of constituencies is the major basis of party cohesion and influence in the legislature (Becker, 1962; Dye, 1969; Flinn, 1964; Grumm, 1963; LeBlanc, 1969; and MacRae, 1952).

Moreover, while most legislators appear to believe that a representative should be guided not by "local purposes" or "local prejudices," but by "his unbiased opinion, his mature judgment, his enlightened conscience (Walke, 1962)," a real conflict between district demands and personal judgment occurs rarely. Legislators are, after all, products of their constituency and share its goals and values. In most instances they have roots deep in the constituency and the party with which they identify is also a creature of the constituency. Hugh L. LeBlanc (1969) sums up the interrelationship of party and constituency influences and personal convictions as follows:

> Constituency influences on legislative voting are sometimes difficult to disentangle from party influences and the dictates of the legislator's own conscience or convictions. Often the several influences reinforce one another. Thus an individual of liberal convictions is politically involved in the Democratic party for that reason and, as the Democratic party's candidate for senator, is victorious at the polls in a constituency conventionally associated with Democratic party success—perhaps a racially mixed, low-income, urban constituency, heavily populated with industrial workers. In voting to increase workmen's compensation payments, the senator could be said to vote his convictions, his party's program, and his constituency.

As a consequence, the responses of state legislatures to the policy initiatives of governor, bureaucrat, and interest groups are likely to be significantly influenced by the parochial concerns of their members. State legislatures represent locally organized interests that are manifested in local, not statewide constituencies. And those constituencies are typically much smaller, and therefore likely to be even more homogeneous, than those of the national House of Representatives. As a consequence, although it may be difficult to distinguish a district's interest from the state's interest on many issues, local considerations will have a major impact on how a legislator views the state's interest and, therefore, on how the legislature performs its *arbiter* functions.

In an area such as mental health services, new or expanded programs or alterations in existing ones can have a direct and obvious impact on local interests in a number of ways—perhaps most obviously by establishing new facilities and payrolls or by contracting or eliminating existing ones. When that is the case, the nature of state legislatures assures that parochial considerations that have little or nothing to do with professional judgments of program merit are likely to play a major role in determining what happens.

The governor is the central political figure in state government. The functions he performs are often described, like those of the President, by referring to the various *hats* he wears—as party chief, legislative leader, head of the administrative establishment, leader of his party, ceremonial head of the state government and leader of public opinion. Viewing the governor as the political leader of the state charged with developing a successful program, his activities may be divided into three broad areas. As described by Coleman Ransome (1956), these are policy formulation, management, and public relations. The three are, of course, interrelated; but the distinction is useful for analytic purposes and the governor's success in each area as well as his own political inclinations will significantly affect public policy determinations.

Policy formulation activities include efforts to influence the legislature, lead his administration, and exert policy control over his political party or, in some cases, party factions—in short, developing his program, enacting it into law, and funding it. The management function, though difficult to distinguish, is more directed toward the successful execution of his program, once enacted. As summarized by Hugh L. LeBlanc and D. Trudeau Allensworth (1971),

> The primary effort of governors in management is not in overseeing day-to-day operations; they have neither the time nor the authority, given the dispersal of power in the typical state administrative establishment. Rather, it is a broad effort at coordination which requires bargaining, persuasion, and compromise to insure that the gubernatorial program is put into operation with a minimum of conflict or resistance on the part of the administrative agencies.

Public relations activities are designed to ensure a favorable view of the governor and his program throughout the state, building the public support necessary to success in the other areas.

Public demands for governmental responses to the problems of an urban-industrial society and the inability of deliberative assemblies to answer effectively the calls for prompt and decisive action combine to create a popular expectation of positive policy leadership on the part of the governor. This, together with the nature of their constituencies, assures that governors, even those committed to a *caretaker* role, will put forward some kind of legislative program and will play, at least to some extent, the role of the *initiator* of public policy decisions. Because the executive has become the initiator of public policies, the governor's office, like the Presidency, has become the best instrument for pursuing new or different approaches to public problems. The legislature, at both the state and national levels, has become increasingly the critic or check upon executive power, the primary instrument of those pursuing a defensive strategy. But the formal powers of the governor, though varying widely from state to state, are considerably less than those of the President.

Joseph A. Schlesinger (1971) has assessed the relative position of the governors in the 50 states. By assigning ratings of one to five to the strength of a governor's tenure potential and his appointive, budgetary, and veto powers, Schlesinger constructed the index of gubernatiorial authority shown in Table 9-III. The maximum possible rating is 20, found only in New York, Illinois, and Hawaii. The lowest rating is 7, found in Texas. The median is 15.

TABLE 9-III
A COMBINED INDEX OF THE FORMAL POWERS OF THE GOVERNORS

	Tenure Potential	Appointive Powers	Budget Powers	Veto Powers	Total Index
New York	5	5	5	5	20
Illinois	5	5	5	5	20
Hawaii	5	5	5	5	20
California	5	4	5	5	19
Michigan	5	4	5	5	19
Minnesota	5	4	5	5	19
New Jersey	4	5	5	5	19
Pennylvania	4	5	5	5	19
Maryland	4	5	5	5	19
Utah	5	3	5	5	18
Washington	5	3	5	5	18
Ohio	4	4	5	5	18
Massachusetts	5	5	5	3	18
Wyoming	5	2	5	5	17
Missouri	4	3	5	5	17
Alaska	4	3	5	5	17
Tennessee	3	5	5	5	17
Idaho	5	4	5	3	17

TABLE 9-III (Continued)

	Tenure Potential	Appointive Powers	Budget Powers	Veto Powers	Total Index
North Dakota	5	1	5	5	16
Kentucky	3	4	5	4	16
Virginia	3	5	5	3	16
Montana	5	3	5	3	16
Nebraska	4	3	4	5	16
Connecticut	5	4	4	3	16
Delaware	4	1	5	5	15
Oklahoma	4	1	5	5	15
Alabama	3	3	5	4	15
Wisconsin	5	2	5	3	15
Colorado	5	1	4	5	15
Louisiana	4	2	4	5	15
Georgia	3	1	5	5	14
Oregon	4	2	5	3	14
Nevada	5	2	5	2	14
Arizona	2	1	5	5	13
South Dakota	1	4	5	3	13
Maine	4	2	5	2	13
Vermont	2	4	5	2	13
Kansas	2	2	4	5	13
Arkansas	2	4	3	4	13
Iowa	2	3	5	2	12
New Hampshire	2	2	5	2	11
Rhode Island	2	3	4	2	11
New Mexico	1	1	5	3	10
North Carolina	3	2	4	1	10
Mississippi	3	1	1	5	10
Indiana	3	5	1	1	10
Florida	3	2	1	3	9
South Carolina	3	1	1	3	8
West Virginia	3	3	1	1	8
Texas	2	1	1	3	7

Source: Schlesinger, Joseph A.: The Politics of the Executive. In Jacob, Herbert and Vines, Kenneth N. (Eds.): *Politics in the American States: A Comparative Analysis*, 2nd Ed. Boston, Little Brown, 1971, p. 232.

An examination of the general ratings reveals that there is a relationship between the size of a state and the formal powers of its governor. Texas is the only populous state where the governor's formal strength is low. The urban industrial giants—New York, Illinois, California, Pennsylvania, and New Jersey—all rate near the top, while those at the bottom of the rankings tend to be the smaller, rural, agricultural states.

One can conclude that size, urbanization, and industrialization increase the complexity of state administration and the need for explicit means of control by the governor. As Schlesinger points out, however, this does not necessarily mean that within their states the governors of Mississippi and North Dakota have less influence than the governors of New York and Illinois. It means only that the governors of New York and Illinois need more formal powers in order to control the large complex bureaucracies in those states and to cope with other competing powers such as the mayor of a large city. Within their own states, governors with less formal powers are still central figures in their state's political system, perhaps attaining a degree of influence by dispensing minor jobs, contracts, and patronage that rivals or exceeds the power of governors in the urban industrial states.

The formal powers of the governor are, in fact, not necessarily related to the governor's influence, either in his policy formulation or his management activities. As Thomas R. Dye (1969) puts it,

> The governor's real power rests upon his abilities at persuasion. His power depends upon his ability to persuade administrators over whom he has little authority, legislators who are jealous of their own powers, party leaders who are selected by local constituents, federal officials over whom the governor has little authority, and a public that thinks he has more authority than he really has.

Some governors, of course, possess great persuasive abilities and combine these with their formal powers to exercise very effective political leadership. Nonetheless, the fact is that decision-making has not been effectively centralized in most state governments, and this has significant implications for the policy-making process at the state level.

Even a strong governor is seldom the master of his administrative house. As a consequence, the bureaucracies are likely to be even more influential in the budgetary process and in administrative rule-making at the state than at the national level. Moreover, the incentives to adopt a protectionist stance are greater. Due to the federal government's virtual monopoly of the personal and corporate income tax, state governments are dependent on considerably less flexible revenue sources. This financial constraint increases the threat to existing programs posed by new or expanded activities in other fields and increases bureaucratic resistance to anything new that appears to compete for already scarce resources.

This may explain why, despite great increases in state and local expenditures over the past 20 years, there has been such remarkable consistency in the manner in which the funds have been allocated. As shown in Table 9-IV, the five most costly activities of state and local governments in 1950 continued to occupy their same relative position in 1969. While there have undoubtedly been changes in state and local programs in at least some of these policy areas, as well as in the quantity and quality of services, the same basic patterns emerge today that were present 20 years ago. This would strongly suggest that the success of efforts

9-IV

DIRECT GENERAL EXPENDITURE OF STATE AND LOCAL GOVERNMENTS:
1950 TO 1969
(Prior to 1960, excludes Alaska and Hawaii)

Item	1950	1955	1960	1965	1966	1967	1968	1969
Total mil. dol.	22,787	33,724	51,876	74,546	82,843	93,350	102,411	116,728
Percent of Total								
Education	31.5	35.3	36.1	38.3	40.2	40.6	40.2	40.5
Highways	16.7	19.1	18.2	16.4	15.4	14.9	14.1	13.2
Public Welfare	13.0	9.4	8.5	8.5	8.2	8.8	9.6	10.4
Health & Hospitals	7.7	7.5	7.5	7.2	7.1	7.1	7.4	7.3
Police Protection & Correction	3.4	3.6	3.6	4.7	4.6	4.5	4.6	4.5
Natural Resources	2.9	2.4	2.3	2.3	2.5	2.5	2.4	2.2
Sanitation & Sewerage	3.7	3.4	3.3	3.2	1.2	2.7	2.6	2.5
Housing and Urban Renewal	2.0	1.5	1.7	1.7	1.7	1.6	1.6	1.6
Interest on General Debt	2.0	2.5	3.2	3.3	3.2	3.2	3.2	3.2
All Other	17.3	15.3	15.8	14.4	14.0	14.0	14.3	14.6

Source: U. S. Bureau of the Census, *Statistical Abstract of the United States 1971.* Washington: U. S. Government Printing Office, 1971, p. 404.

on behalf of mental health, for example, is dependent upon assuaging the fears and enlisting the support of the existing state and local health and mental health bureaucracies.

Local Decision-Making

Still another complication of the governmental/political context within which public policy is developed and administered in the United States is provided by the decision-making process at the local level. In addition to the intricacies presented by multiple and overlapping jursidictions, local decision-making is further complicated by differences in government form and variations in the structure of community power. Both affect the kind of policy determinations likely to be made.

There are three forms of government* used in municipalities in the United States: mayor-council, council-manager, and commission. The mayor-council form is prevalent in both the largest and smallest cities and is the most widely used. Under this plan, a mayor is elected at large by the city's voters and serves as chief executive while the city council is independently elected and has general policy responsibility for the municipality. At least in theory, this form corresponds to the separation of powers model employed at the national and state levels. There are, however, two variations, one of which departs significantly from the pattern of executive-legislative relationships common at the other levels. The strong mayor system is characterized by (1) a concentration of executive and administrative authority in the mayor's office; (2) an executive budget prepared under the direction of the mayor; (3) restriction of the council to broad policy-making responsibilities; and (4) the veto power. Under the weak mayor plan, the executive authority is restricted and shared with the council. This gives the city, at least in some instances, what is effectively a plural executive.

Council-manager government is gaining adherents and is most popular among middle-sized cities, those ranging in population from 25,000 to 500,000. First adopted in this country by Staunton, Virginia, in 1908, this form stresses the principles of econ-

---

*The summary of forms or local government which follows relies heavily on Le-Blanc and Allensworth (1971).

omy, efficiency, and professional administration. It is based on the same concepts that have guided the structuring of the private business corporation. The voters (stockholders) elect the city council (board of directors). It is responsible for policy-making and for hiring and holding accountable the city manager (president) who is responsible for executing policy and running the city (company).

The commission form is used in less than 10 percent of American cities and is seldom employed by the largest or smallest cities. Adopted first by Galveston, Texas, and originally highly regarded by reformers, the commission plan rapidly fell into disfavor and was largely displaced by the council-manager form. There is no separation of powers under the commission system; the commissioners constitute both a policy-making board and a plural, or collegial, executive with each commissioner assuming administrative authority over specific major departments or functions.

The typical county has essentially a commission form of government, with the members of the governing body elected by districts, by political subdivisions of the county, or at large. The governing body, variously called board of commissioners, board of supervisors, commissioners court, county court, and the like, normally has both policy-making and administrative powers, although it shares the latter with other elected county officials (for example, sheriff, treasurer, county clerk, and coroner). Some counties in urban areas have, in recent years, switched to county-manager and county-executive systems. The former closely resembles the city-manager form and the latter approximates the mayor-council plan.

In New England towns, the town meeting, at least in theory, is still the legislative body, with a board of selectmen chosen by the qualified citizens serving as the executive agency. In some places, especially Massachusetts, the *representative* town meeting has been adopted, with representatives of the voters, numbering perhaps a hundred or so, attending legislative sessions, expressing their views, and electing officers, but not voting on policy matters. Increasingly, towns are hiring managers to supervise the administrative activities of government.

Townships vest policy-making authority in a board of trustees, supervisors, or commissioners and divide executive authority among several officers. Special districts and school districts have governing boards selected by popular election or by officials (often the governing bodies) of the general-purpose local governments in the area served. These boards are typically responsible for hiring and holding accountable a professional administrator or school superintendent.

These varied forms of decision-making have important effects on the content and direction of public policy. At the local level, as elsewhere, citizens differ on what they consider important, on what government should do, on what policies should be adopted. And local governmental structure and organizational form are directly related to specific types of public policy and political groups and interests (Kessel, 1962; Schnore and Alford, 1963; Sherbenov, 1961).

The council-manager form of municipal government, for example, is frequently the choice of communities in which the upper-middle class comprise a substantial proportion of the residents whereas lower and working class jurisdictions are unlikely to adopt this system. Similarly, special district governments seem to encourage access patterns not necessarily found in general-purpose governments (Scott and Corzine, 1966). And the independence of school districts from general-purpose governments has often assured that interest groups (the professional educators and their lay allies such as the PTA), would control educational programs.

In short, the form of local government is likely both to reflect and to affect the power structure of the local community and has a direct bearing on policy decisions. Local governments are the primary determinants of where populations will live, what kinds of services will be available, and the way in which land will be used. Moreover, local governments spend more than state governments and collect almost as much in tax revenues. And largely as a result of federal initiatives during the last two decades, local government has become an increasingly important participant in the provision of mental health services.

CONCLUSION

The provision of mental health services involves the complicated interrelationship of a host of public and private organizations and agencies. Public programs involve three distinct and immensely complicated levels of government, each with multiple decision-making processes that tend to provide varied patterns of access favoring differing social groupings and political interests. Moreover, mental health programs are closely related to and often require close cooperation with other governmental programs that involve a similarly complicated web of interrelationships.

Understanding the intricate governmental/political context within which the mental health administrator must work is, to put it mildly, no easy task. Yet understand it he must, if the administrator is to be able to operate within it successfully. And successful administration requires the securing of adequate budgetary support, the coordination of related activities, and sometimes the initiation of programmatic change; all are essentially political tasks.

The concluding paragraph of *The Politics of Mental Health* observed in 1968 that the successful unfolding of the Community Mental Health Center Program was dependent upon reconciling the conflict between programmatic ideals and practical problems of implementation and that "such reconciliation can occur only when professional zeal is adequately tempered by political adaptability and administrative flexibility (Connery, 1968)." It might just as well have said that in mental health administration, real professional zeal is evidenced by political adaptability and administrative flexibility.

REFERENCES

Becker, Robert W., *et al.*: Correlates of legislative voting: Michigan House of Representatives, 1954-61. *Midwest Journal of Political Science, 6*:384-396, 1962.

Bell, David E.: *Organizing for National Security, The Budget and the Policy Process.* Hearings before the Subcommittee on National Policy Machinery, Part 8. Washington, 1134-1135, 1961.

Bethel, Helen and Pedick, Richard W.: *Provisional Patient Movement and*

Administrative Data, State and County Mental Hospital Inpatient Services, July 1, 1970–June 30, 1971. Statistical Note 60. Washington, National Institute of Mental Health, 1972.

Connery, Robert H., et al.: *The Politics of Mental Health*. New York, Columbia University Press, 1968.

Dye, Thomas R.: *Politics in States and Communities*. Englewood Cliffs, Prentice-Hall, 1969.

Dye, Thomas R.: A comparison of constituency influences in the upper and lower chambers of the state legislature. *Western Political Quartely, 14:* 473-480, 1971.

Felix, Robert H.: A comprehensive mental health program. In National Conference on Social Welfare: *Mental Health and Social Welfare*. New York, Columbia University Press, 1961.

Flinn, Thomas A.: Party responsibility in the states: Some causal factors. *American Political Science Review, 58:*60-71, 1964.

Froman, Lewis A., Jr.: *The Congressional Process: Strategies, Rules, and Procedures*. Boston, Little Brown, 1967.

Gilmour, Robert S.: Central legislative clearance: A revised perspective. *Public Administration Review, 31:*150-158, 1971.

Goodwin, George, Jr.: The seniority system in Congress. *American Political Science Review, 53:*412-437, 1959.

Grumm, John G.: A factor analysis of legislative voting. *Midwest Journal of Political Science, 7:*336-356, 1963.

Jacob, Herbert and Vines, Kenneth N. (Eds.) : *Politics in the American States, A Comparative Analysis*, 2nd Ed. Boston, Little Brown, 1971.

Jones, Ronald R.: *Staff and Manhours in Mental Health Facilities in the United States: 1970*. Statistical Note 51. Washington, National Institute of Mental Health, 1970.

Joint Commission on Mental Illness and Health: *Action for Mental Health*. New York, Basic Books, 1961.

Kennedy, J. F.: Speech to the Congress, *U. S. Congressional Record*, 88th Congress, 1st Session, 1963, CIX, Part 2, 1744-49, and as H. R. Document 58.

Kessel, John H.: Governmental structure and political environment. *American Political Science Review, 58:*615-620, 1962.

LeBlanc, Hugh L.: Voting in state senates: Party and constituency influences. *Midwest Journal of Political Science, 13:*33-57, 1969.

LeBlanc, Hugh L. and Allensworth, D. Trudeau: *The Politics of States and Urban Communities*. New York, Harper and Row, 1971.

MacRae, Duncan: The relations between roll call votes and constituencies in the Massachusetts House of Representatives. *American Political Science Review, 46:*1046-1055, 1952.

Neustadt, Richard E.: Presidency and legislation: The growth of central clearance. *American Political Science Review, 48:*642, 1954.

Ransome, Coleman B., Jr.: *The Office of Governor in the United States,* Part III. Alabama, University of Alabama Press, 1956.

Riker, William H.: *Federalism.* Boston, Little Brown, 1964.

Roosevelt, Theodore: *An Autobiography.* New York, Macmillan, 1916.

Saloma, John S.: *Congress and the New Politics.* Boston, Little Brown, 1969.

Schattsneider, E. E.: *The Semi-Sovereign People.* New York, Holt, Rinehart and Winston, 1960.

Schlesinger, Joseph A.: The politics of the executive. In Jacob, Herbert and Vines, Kenneth N. (Eds.) : *Politics in the American States, A Comparative Analysis,* 2nd ed. Boston, Little Brown, 1971.

Schnore, Leo F. and Alford, Robert R.: Forms of government and socioeconomic characteristics of suburbs. *Administrative Science Quarterly, 8:* 1-17, 1963.

Scott, Stanley and Corzine, John: Special districts in the San Francisco bay area. In Danielson, Michael N. (Ed.) : *Metropolitan* Politics. Boston, Little Brown, 1966.

Sherbenov, Edgar L.: Class, participation, and the council-manager plan. *Public Administration Review, 21:*131-135, 1961.

Taube, Carl A.: *Caseload of Federally Funded Mental Health Centers, 1969.* Statistical Note 38. Washington, National Institute of Mental Health, 1971.

Taube, Carl A.: *Distribution of Patient Care Episodes in Mental Health Facilities, 1969.* Statistical Note 58. Washington, National Institute of Mental Health, 1972.

Walke, John C., *et al.: The Legislative System.* New York, John Wiley and Sons, 1962.

Wildavsky, Aaron: *The Politics of the Budgetary Process.* Boston, Little Brown, 1964.

U. S. Bureau of the Census: 1967 Census of Governments, Volume 1. *Governmental Organization.* Washington, United States Government Printing Office, 1968.

U. S. Federal Register: 54.201-215. pp. 5951-56, 1964.

CHAPTER 10

CHANGE AND INNOVATION

HOWARD R. DAVIS

To THE ADMINISTRATOR, change is a constant companion. Continual adjustments must be managed in response to shifts in social and political circumstances, availability of funding, broad trends in mental health services, the needs of key personnel, and more. The parade of pressures to change seems never-ending. Less recognizable as change events are the day-to-day crises that require new ways of coping. Administrators may become virtual experts in the process: rearranging resources, reckoning with power patterns, involving exactly the right personnel, even making *end runs* to ensure effective and efficient change.

Sooner or later, however, every administrator, no matter how skillful he is in playing it by ear, finds himself in the midst of change that has not gone so well. People expected to use a new approach may be complying on the surface only. Change may have caused unnecessary loss or hardship to employees. Power factions may be distorting the needed change to fit their own special values. Fiscal resources required to sustain the change may be short-lived, with consequent reversion to the former pattern. The administrator, in stepping back and looking at change that has occurred, may see things being done differently but without manifestly better results. Resistance to change may set in because it always seems to be added to old ways rather than replacing them.

Bennis (1965), Rogers and Shoemaker (1971), and Fairweather (1972) point out that changes perceived as threatening to employees—from the most powerful to the least—are apt to be

289

ambushed. It would be less of a problem if this sort of resistance were out in the open where negotiation could occur. But counter-movements to change characteristically are subterranean. One of the outcomes of unmanaged change is that its unworkability usually evokes another unmanaged effort to launch a replacement or modification. Not only is effectiveness reduced during the duration of the first change, but it begins an unnecessary escalation of changes.

So unmanaged change can be costly! Practical approaches toward the management of planned change clearly are needed (Morgan, 1972). Institutions no longer have the choice of planning for a period of stability or non-change. Any plan must assume dramatic unforeseen change. Either we manage change or change will manage us.

The Increasing Tempo of Change

Within the field of mental health, it might seem that the major trends have come along slowly enough: moral treatment, custodialism, psychoanalysis, community mental health. But closer examination reveals that innovation, if not other varieties of change, has become a way of life within mental health organizations. Glasscote and Gudeman (1969) report that 96 percent of 320 respondents in community mental health centers indicated that recent changes had taken place. Roberts and Larsen (1971) contacted a sample of mental hospitals and were flooded with some 350 reports of innovations from all of the institutions. Larsen (1972) recently has contributed pertinent information on the progress of her study on innovation in community mental health centers. She has received reports on 500 innovations from 307 federally-funded centers. That early result already represents over 90 percent of the centers contacted. The number of proposals dealing with innovative mental health service delivery techniques submitted to the National Institute of Mental Health has increased by a factor of four in the past few years.

The current rapid rate of change is generalizable to our society as a whole. In a recent 36-month period, 66 major corporations out of 100 surveyed announced significant organizational changes. A major restructuring about every two years is probably average for most medium and large operations (Morgan, 1972). Increased tempo is reflected in reduced time span between introduction and saturation of certain devices, such as appliances. For the vacuum cleaner, the electric range, and the refrigerator, all produced before 1920, the span was about 34 years. Yet for a group introduced between 1939 and 1959, including the electric frying pan, television, and the washer-dryer combination, the time span was only eight years.

Another phenomenon that has implications for change is the increasing diversification of services. In seeming defiance of a technological world that would impose sameness on people, their demand for individualized products and services is growing. The consequence is that providers must shift rapidly as they go about their work; the same factors that determine the effectiveness of major innovations and change determine the effectiveness of shifts in responses. No longer can a mental health worker be effective by specializing in, say, one form of psychotherapy for all clients. Either the client has to shift from one worker to another or the worker shifts from client to client. Early results of an unpublished study conducted at the Hennepin County Mental Health Center in Minneapolis illustrate the point. When client and mental health workers together negotiate the goals of treatment based upon the client's perception of the prevailing problem, the result over time is a vast array of highly differentiated problems calling for highly diversified service responses. Most problems cluster around the broad topics of work experience and interpersonal relationships; older classifications of personality breakdown symptoms seem simple in comparison.

Again, the trend toward diversification of demand is not unique to mental health. Toffler (1970) has called attention to the case of Ford's Mustang: there are 145 different combinations of bodies, engines, and transmissions. But added to this are all the different colors and accessory options. This means that Ford, apparently in response to a judged public demand, produces 25 million different combinations just on one new family sports car!

The Inevitability of Change

Probably people have always tried to stem the tide of change but history suggests that change cannot be stopped in the broad sense, even if it were desirable to do so. French and Belgian peasants threw their wooden shoes (sabots, hence the word saboteur) into the textile machinery that threatened the handicraft way of life, but obviously to little avail. It has become an immutable fact that the steam drill, sooner or later, will always replace John Henry.

Some Impellers of Change

At least two reasons can be cited for the ever-increasing rate of change:

(1) Change begets change. The swift emergence of new knowledge and technology forces response. NIMH alone has sponsored some 7,000 researches in mental health; even more significant is the increase from 38 in the year 1948 to 1,700 in 1972. *Psychological Abstracts* has accommodated, since 1967, 120,000 entries (American Psychological Association, 1972). Even assuming a flat, non-accelerating rate, it can be inferred that 2,000 articles with new information of some sort are abstracted each month. Beyond the mental health field, the same growth in the availability of knowledge is evident: In the last 15 years, while our Gross National Product doubled, research and development soared 400 percent in the United States. When confronted with knowledge, people fundamentally have only two choices: assimilate it and change, or turn away. Perhaps this is why the rate of reading scientific journals is so appallingly low (Glaser and Ross, 1971; Garvey and Griffith, 1965): It's better not to know.

(2) A primary human need for stimulation may be manifested in the need for change. This need for stimulation has been documented for at least 50 years (Thomas, 1923). More recently, Maslow (1954) cast a new light on the motive for change as a form of self-actualization. Self-actualization is the desire that comes with ideal human development. Individuals seek first to fulfill their basic needs for physical comfort, for love, for security, for achievement, and then for self-actualization. Since it is easier

in society today to satisfy these fundamental needs there may be growing motivation and opportunity for self-actualization through change. Jenning (1970) gives a new term to the change-driven person—"Mobicentric." The mobicentric person spurns stability of the usual sort. He moves about, seeking change. As reported by Jenning, investigations in industry have indicated that mobicentricity and effectiveness go hand-in-hand.

Morgan (1972) has said that the people who will populate the successful organization of the future are those who look at change as a creative, thought-provoking, dynamic way of life. We might even go further: at one point in our evolution, survival was a function of physical strength. The machine helped take care of that. At a later point, survival had become a function of the mind. Computers are helping to take care of that. In the near future, survival may be a function of our capacity to deal with change. Nothing is yet here to take care of that. This is particularly true of extra-organizational change—change that occurs in the society at large, beyond the environs of the organization in which one is involved. Though this change may have a major impact on the ethos of an organization, it is very difficult to anticipate.

At the same time, it is important to recognize that the forces of change do appear over and over again throughout history. For example, the influence of the prevailing values of both public and special interest groups is a powerful determinant of change. Another critical factor is the ability to sustain change through the resources of manpower and funding. The obligation to change, or the need for action as sensed by the public, frequently has directed the course of development. But the motivations for change are not always those we would expect to be out front; subtle, never-discussed motivations are often the power behind change. Equally subtle are resistances to new movements; sometimes they are open and attacking but more often they are reflected in disinterest and neglect (Gardner, 1964). As in all human activity, the yield of payoff of the change determines whether it will survive. Again, the rewards often are not those that might be expected. Manifestly ineffective programs commonly survive because they quietly meet the needs of key persons. In some instances, we have seen that the total constellation of circumstances lies in wait for a convincing pattern of action, of information to be offered. Appropriate timing is almost without exception another influencer of change.

Though broad change in the development of mental health services and other areas does not lend itself to precise management, limited forecasting is feasible that does allow some planning. And in instances, of course, opportunities do occur for modification of the influential factors at hand.

There are some guesses one could make about events in the future that may modify the factors influencing broad change. For example, the quality of information available is likely to improve. It may provide mental health services with something better to deliver. Still more efficient and effective chemical control of extreme and debilitating emotional reactions to stress may be on the way. Methods likely will be found to exploit learning principles toward more rapid and precise extinction of maladaptive emotions and behavior and the reinforcement of more adaptive ones. Modest, but promising progress probably will be made toward knowledge on how mental health workers can collaborate with others in changing social and environmental conditions deleterious to mental health. New information on the process of delivering mental health services also will be made available: in collaboration with other human service agencies, in systems application to the development of services, and on administrative techniques. Information probably will, as in the past, offer the greatest opportunity for change. But by itself it will bring only modest modification. The yield of mental health services will become increasingly evident through the use of more appropriate methods of program evaluation. Values within the mental health profession may progress toward the human development concept, but prevailing values elsewhere are apt to move much more slowly in this direction. The ability to sustain improved changes seems likely to be increased through more vigorous activity and support in the form of staff development programs. But new funding mechanisms have the greatest impact on the direction of change. Where money goes, program is likely to follow. Funding for medically-oriented services and for public mental hospitals seems secure in the immediate future; the most exciting changes are likely to be in concepts of funding for community-oriented programs, particularly indirect services.

These are, of course, only examples. Forecasting, even utilizing such techniques as Delphic predictions and scenario-writing, is a game anyone can play. Despite the predictably wide margin of error, is is a useful pastime contributing to improved management of organizational change; for sound planning and management of intraorganizational change requires cognizance of supra-organizational trends. Sooner or later, all but the most minor innovations and changes will be influenced by the flux of the broader scene.

There are some general barriers, stimulants, and resources for intraorganizational change in mental health services of which the mental health executive should be aware. A number of these are not specific to the field of mental health alone, but would apply to many of the human services. Some natural barriers to the adoption of change are:

(1) There seldom is a profit motive for being an innovator in mental health services.

(2) There is no core of specifically-trained change consultants in mental health comparable to those in other fields. Agriculture, of course, has had extension agents for many years. Social and Rehabilitation Services and the U.S. Office of Education now have specialists in Regional and State offices, respectively. They not only consult on specific changes but work with administrators toward broader utilization of change technology.

(3) Innovations in mental health services are less clear-cut in their advantage over the existing methods they would replace than is true in some other fields.

(4) Innovative mental health services—unlike many practice modifications—are influenced by complex variables inherent in the formal structure of the system in which the services are delivered.

(5) So far, there is no systematic way of getting findings from

more fundamental researches into service settings. Consequently, many of the changes in mental health are ad hoc solutions to problems rather than the implementation of scientifically validated information.

On the other hand, there are multiple forces that stimulate change in the delivery of mental health services that include: (a) cultural change, itself, such as human liberation; (b) State and federal legislation; (c) regulations and requirements of community boards and State mental health programs; (d) court decisions; (e) State, regional, or national accrediting agencies; (f) research and experimentation; (g) study committees appointed for special purposes; (h) financial grants for special purposes; (i) crises; (j) dissatisfaction of citizens; (k) creative practitioners and administrators who redefine problems, perceive new problems, and create new ways of dealing with them.

Various national resources may provide a base for building programs that can foster broad adoptions of new services delivery ideas and practice:

(1) The National Clearinghouse for Mental Health Information continually expands and refines its services. For instance, it is now possible to obtain print-outs of literature abstracts on virtually any topic in mental health. A new NIMH publication, *Information Sources and How to Use Them* (NIMH, 1971), details how to contact whom for what information from a comprehensive variety of sources.

(2) The Joint Commission on Accreditation of Hospitals has, for some time, stimulated and guided change through offering standards. Of course, standards can discourage change as well.

(3) The American Institutes for Research, in collaboration with the National Council of Community Mental Health Centers and NIMH, is developing and testing a system of exchange of problems and innovative solutions among community mental health centers. If it proves effective and feasible, such a system may continue as an ongoing service.

(4) Experimental projects in health services delivery are in some instances stimulating change in mental health services toward integration with general health services delivery.

(5) New federal funding programs for services to special at-risk groups are making new program changes possible; for example, children's mental health services, new services for alcoholism and drug abuse; etc.

(6) The NIMH program on mental health services research and development is specifically designed to stimulate improvement of services through the use of new knowledge.

(7) In addition to a number of professional journals giving special coverage to innovations in mental health services, publications specifically designed to facilitate the continual improvement of services are issued from time to time by the Federal Government. For instance, the NIMH publication, *Innovations,* presents summaries as well as more comprehensive descriptions of new service techniques. A new series, *Planning for Creative Change in Mental Health Services* (NIMH, 1971-72) is designed to help in the implementation of new techniques. The Joint Information Service, representing collaborate efforts between the American Psychiatric Association, the National Association of Mental Health, and NIMH, frequently publishes books reviewing selective aspects of services delivery.

(8) Technical assistance consultants in Regional Offices often assist with the implementation of new services techniques. In some states, such as New York, staff consultants carry major responsibility for assisting with change.

The Use of Planned Change Techniques

The availability of information about a different way of approaching a problem does not necessarily lead to use of that information. That holds true for information on organizational change! As with all change, there are some disinclinations to utilize information about the administration of change. In discussions with numerous mental health service administrators certain reactions seem to repeat. While administrators do indeed recognize that the key to their effectiveness is the success with which necessary change is ushered in, several likely resistances to the practice of full-scale change management can be sensed:

(1) *The use of power is an easier way to bring about change.*

Actually, if the change at hand is non-elective, if it is resistance-proof, then the use of power to bring about change probably is a defensible choice. However, reaching that decision should be part of the planned change process. In organizations there is a *normative sanction* for *orders from above*. People expect orders as a condition of employment. The tedious manipulation of each factor in influencing change not only might be counterproductive in some instances, but discomforting to staff. So use of authority should not always be avoided. It is difficult to think of situations, however, when at least the prior involvement of the staff to be affected by the change would be inappropriate. Katz and Georgopoulas (1971) imply that even though concern for the views of staff need not be overemphasized, maintaining respect for democratic principles and processes increases the probability of success. Rogers and Shoemaker (1971) report that changes brought about by the authoritative approach are more likely to be discontinued than are those from a participative approach.

The skill comes in knowing when to use authority and when to proceed more slowly with planned participative techniques. The Deputy Commissioner of the Department of Mental Hygiene in an Eastern State had struggled for some time with the problem of excessive numbers of elderly people unnecessarily admitted to State mental hospitals. He assessed all relevant elements in the situation and decided, in this instance, to bring about the change by fiat. He dispatched a memo banning the use of State mental hospitals as repositories for aged persons not actually in need of treatment for mental illness. That was in 1968. The document still is commonly referred to in that State as *the June memo on aging*. But it did the job.

The same Deputy Commissioner was faced with the need to promote decentralization among the State hospitals. This time, on assessing the relevant variables, he decided the participative approach would work better. It did, but he had to expose himself to long hours of meetings to consider motivation, resistances, abilities, values and the like, and to work them through. That experience later was recounted to a superintendent of a Midwestern hospital. He felt it would be a waste of time to go through the laborious participative change process. He told of calling in his department heads at two o'clock one afternoon and ordering decentralization to begin the subsequent morning. The superintendent reported that there had been no problem at all in implementing the plan. Alas, less than a year later he was no longer in his position. A controversy reportedly had arisen over employees' perception of his continual authoritarian manner. Perhaps the moral is that authority may be used inappropriately as the sole instrument of change, one time, two times, or more. But its failure may become apparent only in the accumulation of incidents.

Power through the use of money is another way to bring about change. Roberts and Larsen (1971) found that among 350 commonly used innovations reported in hospitals, 40.5 percent had been supported through Federal funds. In the course of conducting experiments on promoting the adoption of change, Glaser and Ross (1971) and Fairweather (1972) found that one of the first questions asked was "Will NIMH fund the program?" It seems quite obvious that the promotion of change is rendered considerably easier if the ability to pay for the change is provided!

As it has been put by others, the big dollar is an ineluctable carrot; the administrator may be pressured by its availability to implement the stipulated changes in pursuit of the money. The trouble is that when the funds to stimulate innovation expire, the innovation may follow suit. For instance, among mental health demonstration projects supported through NIMH, over half expired upon termination of federal funds. (That was prior to the incorporation of organizational change factors in the planning, review, and conduct of project grants.) Rein and Miller (1966) go so far as to suggest that externally-funded demonstration projects may diminish an organization's own investment in problem-solving and growth.

While the use of power through authority and/or money is a tempting way to initiate change quickly, too-ready use may thwart enduring change.

(2) Another resistance to the use of planned change processes

is expressed as *Good ideas will be employed on the basis of their own merits.*

Some administrators have stated that if an idea is good enough it will be adopted; if it is not, it will be turned down as it should be. The assumption is that while good ideas may need some help along the way to implementation, generally they will clear their own paths. But it is a false assumption that the world will beat a path to the door of a man who builds a better mousetrap. Furst and Sherman (1969) cite the case of the *truly better mousetrap,* used as an illustration at the Harvard and Stanford graduate schools of business administration. The problem was that the mousetrap worked perfectly, too good to be thrown away. What the manufacturers ignored was the prevailing *value* in middle-class America to dispose of mousetraps. The functional worth of the idea was not the sole determinant of its adoption.

Another danger in assuming that a worthy idea does not need to be carried along by planned change is that subtle, unspoken resistances can drain off the effectiveness of the change even if it does reach apparent stabilization. Despite the placid countenances that are often maintained, below the surface many organizations are hard jungles. For example, NIMH consultants visited mental health facilities with grants to research innovative service programs. Sanguine pictures of peace and harmony were perceived. But when neutral and confidential independent investigators visited the same group of facilities, a quite different overall picture emerged (Glaser and Taylor, 1969; Weiss, 1972). Repeated instances were described in which innovations were sabotaged, where intense rivalries waged, where destruction-with-a-smile was the rule. Often the directors and administrators of the facilities genuinely had no awareness of what was going on at staff levels.

The point is that if the change process is not considered carefully, particularly from the people standpoint, full success may not be achieved, and the reasons never known.

(3) *The deliberate manipulation of change is too Orwellian.*

At a high-level conference on the subject of science and social change, one eminent person registered his strong rejection to the very word, as well as the concept of, change. The subject of the day was switched accordingly! Though the expression and action were extreme, the notion is by no means unique. The prerogative of self-determination is fiercely guarded, no matter how much of an illusion it may be. Even people with the title *change consultant* may come to hold a negative valence. As Floyd Mann, Director of the University of Michigan's Center for Research on the Utilization of Scientific Knowledge, warned during a symposium on change in August of 1969, "If the change agent does not tread carefully, he will find himself in Siberia."

The fact is that the manipulation of organizational change, like the modification of individual behavior, is not nearly so predictable in efficacy as most of us might fear—or wish! Nevertheless, the administration of change calls for scrupulous and sincere regard for the rights and feelings of those involved in the change. Perhaps Rule and Regulation No. 1 in the practice of change should be to respect the dignity of persons in the organization by frank openness in all activities. In addition to the moral reasons for observing dignity, there is the matter of the changer's own durability!

(4) *Taking time to administer planned change can be a dodge from action.*

Thorstein Veblen, over 70 years ago, used the term *conspicuous consumption* to describe activity that displays preparation for action—studies, training, even planning—which in fact drains off the drive for action. Some people have suggested that Presidential commissions at times have served that function. Caplan and Caplan (1969) describes classical instances of this phenomenon in mental health during the days when moral treatment was giving way to custodialism.

Larsen and Roberts (1971) provide data that may be helpful in estimating appropriate planning time for the introduction of change: 20 percent of the innovations that occurred within a six-month period were preceded by one month's planning; another 20 percent required over seven months. But when to admit *conspicuous consumption* and give up is hard to judge. Operation Decimal, the conversion of Britain's monetary system, has been under *planning* for some time. It was proposed by an Oxford scholar, Robert Wood, in a paper he published in 1655!

So it perhaps is true that planning for change may be an unnecessary stall. But good administration should discern accurately whether or not protracted planning is necessary. In many instances, of course, the manager of change must hustle into action in order to make effective use of the fleeting timely moment. It goes without elaborating that undue time taken in change is ipso facto poor administration of change.

The Value of Managed Organizational Change

The management of organizational change is hard. There are no quick tricks. It is the long-cut route to goal achievement. It makes work. On the other hand, if the *management* of change is a struggle, so is natural change, without management. The chances are that when great effort is called for in the management of change, failure to invest that effort will result in a less effective end point reached and excessive expense.

Change management is a young, still not fully developed field, but one which is growing at great speed. Over a 15-year period citations on the topic of innovation grew from an estimated 450 to over 10,000.

An occupational specialty pertaining to the management of change is just beginning to emerge though it has been discussed in the literature for a number of years. The titles used for it vary and suggest different concepts. Among the earliest was *social engineer* (Watson, 1964; Guetzkow, 1959). Lippitt (1965) suggested *linking agent.* Schwartz (1966) called for a *popularizer* and suggested the name *knowledge linker.* A frequently used name is that of *change agent* (Rogers, 1962). Mackie and Christensen (1967) used *research translator* and also *learning engineer.* Archibald (1968) favors *applied behavioral scientist* while Riley, Hooker, Massar (1968) and Engstrom (1969) prefer *research utilization specialist* (RUS). Glaser (1970) suggested *knowledge utilization specialist* (KUS).

Fairweather (1972) found in his experiment on social innovation that active use of a change consultant was associated with successful change in mental hospitals. He points out that this is not proof of the worth of the change consultant; it may be that the hospitals with a greater potential for change also tended to seek consultation more readily.

Perhaps the most important question about the management of change is "Does it work?" The evidence suggests that it does. But similar to the utility of psychotherapy as a general concept, the efficacy of change management is a very difficult matter to prove. Its worth may not lie in the simple criterion of the achieved change rate. Sometimes the outcome of employing change techniques may be just the opposite, averting change. A good change administrator does not necessarily go all out for change. One may well agree with George Bernard Shaw who said, "If it is not necessary to change, then it is necessary not to change." So the *rate of advisable non-change* also could become a criterion measure of the worth of change practices. Further, perhaps the best payoff of planned change is not the eventuality of change itself but greater organizational effectiveness. Judging that is not simple.

References to the effectiveness of change techniques in the literature pertain mostly to changes in what we might describe as *values,* specifically, management styles. Bennis (1965) reports several early efforts to evaluate the use of change agent skills. He refers to the work of Blake, Mouton, Barnes, and Greiner, reported in 1964, which evaluated their participative management efforts in a large petro-chemical plant. Not only did they find significant changes in the values, morale, and interpersonal behavior of employees, but significant improvements in productivity, reduced turnover, and absenteeism, in addition to a significant improvement in attitudes and subjective feelings. Argyris (1965) has described his efforts to change management styles through "laboratory training," one approach to planned change. The executives involved did indeed perform more effectively when they were working with associates who had been in the group, but not with others. That suggested that what had been acquired was relationship change rather than the adoption of new ideas about management techniques.

Morgan (1972) describes the efforts of executive Arthur H.

Kuriloff of Texas Instruments who had too many defective products coming off the assembly line. The change he decided to promote was the delegation of authority down the ranks. Time clocks disappeared. The workers on the assembly line, who formerly had learned to perform small tasks, were reorganized into teams of seven, each team responsible for producing a complete instrument, with distribution of tasks left to mutual agreement. Man-hour productivity increased by 30 percent while reports of customers of defective instruments had decreased by 70 percent. Absenteeism fell to half the local average.

It would be invalid to hold these testimonies up as evidence of the efficacy of planned change. But they do feature the most salient aspect of change management: consideration of the dignity and worth of people who are affected by the change.

Another approach to the question is represented by the work of Fairweather (1972). After extensive traditional dissemination of the results of his work on the lodge innovation—a system of self-help through work programs for chronically ill mental patients—Fairweather could locate only one mental hospital in the Nation that had adopted his program. Even that adoption had been supported by a Hospital Improvement Project grant. But after employing his approach to change, described in the next section as "Experimental Social Innovation," he could report that 25 hospitals were in the process of adopting the program without special funding.

Still not proof of the worth of planned change, data from the evaluation of the NIMH applied research grants offer encouraging evidence. Projects included in the study had the purpose of producing new information on the delivery of mental health services that should be utilizable throughout the mental health field. In 1968, six months after termination of the project grant, 41 percent of the innovations had been adopted at the facilities where they had been developed. But for only 11 percent could other users of the innovative idea be identified. Efforts were then implemented to encourage investigators to incorporate in their projects techniques to facilitate change and to provide technical assistance on change when requested. By 1971, the percentage of facilities where the innovative programs had endured had risen from 41 percent to 77 percent; the percentage of completed projects for which other users could be identified had risen from 11 percent to 54 percent.

Studies are now under way that should provide more specific information on the worth of organizational change practices. The Utah State Division of Mental Health is testing the value of a change consultant who will serve all State and community mental health facilities. In addition to working with those organizations on all phases of change from the assessment of needs through evaluation of the payoff, people from outside the State will be helped to adopt innovations developed in Utah. The American Institutes for Research, in collaboration with the National Council of Community Mental Health Centers, is exploring the contributions center directors or staff themselves can make as change consultants. Following an orientation program at Palo Alto, selected center representatives, functioning as administrators of change, will experiment with the adoption of innovations in their own organizations. But they also will help others in the process of adopting innovative ideas with which they may be particularly familiar. A major study to specifically evaluate the worth of planned change techniques is being carried out by the Human Interaction Research Institute of Los Angeles. A special design will be employed to determine where change is more successful, by several criteria, when techniques of administration of change are fully applied.

As the Democratic Ethic, the recognition of the human rights of employees in the organization, gains recognition, so will the value of planned change. For the essence of planned change is the consideration* of those individuals affected by it. By the value, the worth of planned change is inherent.

---

*A sense of responsibility for meeting the human rights of all of the members of an organization is one that is growing in the corporate conscience (Shepard, 1965; Katz and Gorgopoulas, 1971). The responsibility is to provide not only humane working conditions but opportunities for self-actualization. This position, referred to as the Democratic Ethic, is supplanting the Protestant Ethic, as defined by Max Weber, as surely as it supplanted the Soul Ethic of an earlier day (Furst and Sherman, 1969).

MODELS AND APPROACHES

The vast literature on innovation and organizational change*
is as flimsy as it is substantial, as impressionistic as it is experimental, as narrow, as encompassing, and as academic as it is practical. Some, but not great, progress has been made since Bennis
(1965) said this:

> Unfortunately, no viable theory of social change has been established.
> Indeed it is a curious fact about present theories that they are
> strangely silent on matters of *directing* and *implementing* change.
> What I particularly object to . . . is that they tend to explain the
> dynamic interactions of a system without providing one clue to the
> identification of strategic leverages for alteration. They are suitable
> for *observers* of social change, not for practitioners. They are theories
> of change, and not of *changing*.

McClelland (1968) provides an insightful overview of existing change models. He says that it is premature to do more than
wish for a general model, let alone a general theory of changing.
McClelland goes on to point out that researchers in the field have
developed a variety of sub-system models, each of which deals
with some aspect of the change process or with a specific setting.
They vary widely in comprehensiveness, complexity, and elegance.

Bennis (1965, 1966) reviews approaches to change according
to two dimensions: The first pertains to *strategies* based on sundry assumptions about change. Examples of the strategies are: *exposition and propagation*, which assumes that those who have
knowledge should be listened to and followed; *elite corps*, a strategy stemming from the view that knowledge plus important roles
are necessary for change, as when a scientist goes into government; *human relations training*, which holds that those already
in power positions should be helped to assimilate behavioral
science concepts into their leadership.

The second dimension addresses *types* of change according to
the relationship between the changer and the organizational system. For instance, planned change entails equal power and mutual

*The term organizational change is taken to mean the adoption of a *different*
response to ensure the well-being of the organization. Well-being pertains to attainment of the mission of the organization. *Innovation* is a subset of change referring to the process of implementing *new* practices or devices.

goal-setting; emulative change occurs through identification with power figures by subordinates; and *coercive change* is characterized by non-mutual goal-setting and the one-sided deliberateness of an imbalanced power ratio.

Leavitt (1965) sees three different dimensions of change models:

Structural approaches—Systems of communication, systems of authority, and systems of work flow. Decentralization is a change that is often approached structurally.

Technological approaches—Direct problem-solving inventions like work-measurement techniques. Computerization of management systems would represent an example.

Actors (people) approaches—Concerned chiefly with people and their psychological reactions to their experiences. Sensitivity training represents a favorite *people approach.*

In the structural and technological approaches, people are expected to perform appropriately to accommodate new organizational charts, functional statements, new management information systems, and hardware devices. People are not left out of consideration, but they are treated as manipulable entities. The emphasis is on internal responsiveness to duty, orderliness, and hierarchial coordination. People are to fill specified roles, to serve as nodes in communication networks and respond accordingly. Structural approaches are common to the military in the purer sense. In technological approaches the regard for people is typified by Taylor's concept of *scientific management,* introduced formally in 1911. Its technique was work measurement.

The literature on these approaches has dwindled in recent years. But both *social engineering* (modifying the behavior of people and systems to improve past performance) and *scientific management* (manipulating eye-hand and muscle coordination against time) have had a profound effect on such large classifications of organizations as government and industry, respectively. The literature and rhetoric are now more humanistic; assumptions and policies, however, still retain the strong flavor of both approaches.

People approaches try to change organizations by first changing the behavior of its members. By contrast, structural and technological approaches focus chiefly on problem-solving mechanisms, sliding past the processes by which new problem-solving means are generated and adopted into the organization. Two people approaches have prevailed:

(1) MANIPULATION. Dale Carnegie approaches, usually scoffed at by social scientists, have nevertheless been effectively employed. Festinger (1957) suggests that the Carnegie model is not foolish at all. The formula is simple: One does not assault with logic and criticism and advice. A offers B support, approval, a permissive atmosphere; having engendered a close relationship, A then asks B to change in the way A wishes, holding the change as the price of continuing the relationship.

Other manipulative approaches connect group needs through discussion and then redirect them toward the desired change. A classical example is the work of Lewin (1952) in convincing housewives, through persuasive involvement, to purchase and consume more varieties of meat. Still others sought change through catharsis. Morale and attitude surveys, fed back to power groups for planning subsequent changes, also came to the front. All of the manipulative *people approaches* have one feature in common: the power balance remains unmolested.

(2) POWER-EQUALIZATION. Client-centered therapy (Rogers, 1942) may have been one of the prime movers in this approach to people change. The techniques are unique and explicitly aimed at allocating equal power to the changes. One changes the world by changing people; and further, it is held that one changes people either by helping them change themselves or by some collaborative effort between changee and changer.

Three prominent routes have been followed in the power-equalization approach:

(a) *Participative management* is typified by McGregor's (1960) *Theory X-Theory Y* proposals. Theory X is the traditional authoritarian assumption in organizational life. Theory Y is a participatory approach that shifts some of the total power of superiors dealing with impotent subordinates to those subordinates. The contrast is between external control of human beings (Theory X) and self-control and self-direction (Theory Y). The well-known

Scanlon Plan—a union-management cooperative plan—is a mechanism for implementing Theory Y. It consists of bonuses to all members of the firm in proportion to their base rates and company efficiency, and of a system of work-improvement committees that cross organizational levels.

Blake and Mouton (1961) reify the concept in their managerial grid. Espousing neither *task management*—viewing employees as rented services—nor *country club management*—viewing employees as people whose morale must be kept up at all costs—they seek to bring the organization into a state of balance, termed *team management*. The managerial grid is widely used in industry change activities.

(b) *Sensitivity training* was invented out of Gestalt tradition by Lewin in the late 1940's (National Training Laboratories, 1953). Among the outstanding contributors have been Lippitt, Bradford, Bennis, and Marrow. The T (for training)—group long has been the mechanism of choice in power equalization. What brings change about is felt to be the beliefs and skills of people.

At first human relations training was offered to supervisors and foremen. Then it became a favorite approach in working with executives, often away from home with anonymous others. More recently, sensitivity training has been carried on within the work setting and with colleagues. There it has proved to be a much more daring approach.

Argyris (1965) used T-group methods to bring human fulfillment closer to the issue of organizational efficiency. The achievement of becoming oneself, of authenticity, through the T-group is related to improvement in decisions and performance of tasks. Authenticity leads to personal competence which leads to facilitation and the spread of authenticity among others.

(c) *Organizational Development* is an "effort (1) planned, (2) organization-wide, (3) management from the top, to (4) increase organizational effectiveness and health through (5) planned interventions in the organization process, using behavioral science knowledge" (Beckhard, 1969). Or as Thomson (1971) more simply puts it, "OD is . . . a strategy of planned change directed toward making organizations more supportive of human growth and development." Both the philosophies and techniques of T-groups are evident in OD approaches. Many of its leaders are those who also led in the T-group movement. One difference is that OD efforts are—in the Argyris tradition—specifically related to the organization's mission.

OD differs from management development, which might better be termed *manager development*. That approach is concerned with upgrading the skills and abilities of managers to handle broader assignments. It involves career planning, job rotation, and management education. OD, on the other hand, is focused on improving the systems that make up the total organization. The emphasis is on training *of* groups in: intergroup relationships; examination of communication systems; organization structure and roles; and in improving the goal-setting process.

These people approaches can offer much help to the administrator of change as specialized techniques to use where appropriate. But as models of change they are a bit out of company in the hurly-burly, extremely variable and demanding circumstances of most operating organizations. Those settings hardly fit with the sanitary, cultural island atmosphere under which many of the people approaches have been spawned and developed.

A different model that has been hammered out within the real-life setting of mental hospitals is Fairweather's (1972) Experimental Social Innovation approach. Fairweather sees the process of innovation in three stages: (1) approach, (2) persuasion, and (3) implementation. Over a period of several years he experimented in controlled studies with various techniques in each stage. Not surprisingly, he found that personal contacts at each stage were far more effective than letters and even detailed manuals.

In the *approach* phase, a telephone call is made to the person considered most likely to be interested in the innovation. The identity of that person, naturally, will have been ascertained beforehand. Fairweather does not believe that the top-level staff necessarily represent the best starting point, as advocated by many in the change field. He found that less visible staff members often achieved more in the long run than persons with more power in the institution.

The *persuasion* phase is best carried out through a type of demonstration at the facility. The plan that has worked most effectively is to ask the organization to commit its own resources to putting on the demonstration. There are fewer willing to do that than there are who would welcome a no-commitment demonstration. But Fairweather found that this step is an excellent one to *weed out* those that have a low probability of staying with the change to its final stages. One of the critical determinants of the success of the innovative effort is the development of a cadre of advocates.

The *implementation* phase is carried out most effectively when the action consultant stays in the environment for a period. During that time help is provided to the innovator group in the form of consultation.

Requirements for a Working Model of Organizational Change

There are certain characteristics that a model of change should contain if it is to be of use in everyday organizational situations. These encompass the criteria proposed by Chin (1961). None of the models and approaches considered so far include all of these characteristics. The model to be outlined in the next section is an attempt to incorporate all of them. The degree to which it succeeds, however, is certainly open to debate.

1. The model, above all, should be practical. Change is not always a voluntary option. Demands for change not uncommonly come from higher levels and from compelling social and political sources. Lead time may be extremely short. A usable model occasionally must allow application with a small investment of resources. It must have some utility even if it is only used in part.

Maguire (1970) stated well what the everyday situation is like: He points out that the practitioner and administrator can find very little practical help in models as they are presented in the literature. For the most part, these models portray change as a novel event interposed between periods of organizational stability. The practitioner and administrator, on the other hand, do not have the luxury of viewing change as a novel event. They are daily involved in crisis decision-making that entails making the most of less-than-satisfactory circumstances. They must solve the plethora of immediate, non-postponable problems if they are to survive.

2. The parts of the model should be manipulable. Guidance on the theoretical phenomena to observe will help the administrator little. He should be able to do something about those factors that the model assumes influence change.

3. Economy of use should be a primary consideration. Though it is agreed that a small investment will usually yield a small achievement, there are many circumstances in which the administrator does not have the prerogative of hiring action consultants or people to run sensitivity groups.

4. Ease of communication is important. Not only should the model lend itself to brief discussion, it should be readily understood and easy to recall. Administrators are not likely to go back and read about change each time they employ the model.

5. The model should be comprehensive. In delineating the various phases in a change process, many models tend to focus on a segment of the change process without indicating which segment is being explicated. Or they imply that all segments are being explicated when, in point of fact, they are not (Maguire, 1970). Little is achieved in overstressing one aspect of change to the exclusion of others. Resistances may be handled with skill, but it will be a wasted effort if resources necessary to sustain the change are taken for granted.

6. Synergism—the force of factors working together—is important to consider. A general weakness of most models is that they seem to view, or at least report, changes as linear, rational processes. As McClelland (1968) says, most models seem to be predicated on the assumption that there is an orderly process from research to development to use, but the existence of such a process is largely a myth. The process of change might be visualized as a diagram from Lewinian field theory. Change is the resultant arrow created by multiple force vectors acting simultaneously. Dealing with too many variables simultaneously is like being a juggler with too many objects in the air. Yet, the change

process is facilitated by marshalling the interactive effects of the multiple determinants of change.

7. The model should lend itself to intervening in phases. This may appear to be in contradiction with what we just said about synergism. But all this means is that the change manager should be able to set up a plan of action depending upon where the organization is in the process at any given time. It does not matter if the intervention steps are carried out more or less sequentially, so long as continual attention is given to all factors at play.

8. Differential investment in working with the components of the model should be possible. A way to influence the effects of any change lies in applying the "Pareto Principle." Zilfredo Pareto (1848-1923) was an Italian sociologist and economist living in Switzerland who discovered and applied the idea that in most situations a few factors influence the outcome, while a great many others prove largely irrelevant and can have little effect on the situation no matter what one does about them. Pareto's statistical analysis revealed that 80 percent of the results come from 20 percent of the action.

9. The model should call attention to how the change process influences the rest of the system. The errors here result in so many instances of change becoming *additional* functions of an organization, requiring new resources. Change that takes the place of the old way always encounters the problem of molesting the rest of the system.

10. The model should be flexible and versatile enough to apply to different organizational systems.

11. The model should provide a basis for a subsequent evaluation of the effectiveness of change. One way this is achieved is to require a specific statement on the expected outcome of the change.

12. The model should recognize the humanness of the participants involved. This is more than human dignity; it implies that an organization is "behavioral, as are the people within it." Shepard (1965) puts it this way: "Organizations, like persons, can be viewed as organisms, whose parts are living and in com-

munication. Organizations can be understood as learning and adapting, as being and becoming. If one takes this view, then change is to be understood in terms of development and regression, of health and illness, of adaptive and maladaptive processes."

THE *A VICTORY* MODEL

The *A VICTORY* acronym comes from the first letters of the eight factors considered to be necessary for organizational change. The model is a behavioral one; it considers organizations to be living systems (Leavitt, 1965; Shepard, 1965).

The model suggested represents one attempt to provide something more than a review of observations about the phenomenon of change; it is a working guideline for use in the everyday administration of innovation and change in mental health facilities. But it would be a mistake to imply that it is anything more than a stage toward the development of a technology. The current state of knowledge on organizational change hardly warrants anything more. The bulk of the literature consists of observations about change made from the sidelines. Many of the studies that have involved the manipulation of variables have been carried out under relatively artificial conditions. So the potential user of the guidelines is urged to draw upon his own experiences and ingenuity in refining the suggested model.

On the other hand, the derivation of the model should allow at least moderate confidence in its use. Basic contributions came from the many persons involved with project grants on innovative mental health services over the past ten years. A synthesis of over 1,200 publications on knowledge utilization did, of course, strongly influence the direction and substance of the model. Some of the significant variables in change began to emerge from special projects on the adoption of new ideas (Glaser and Taylor, 1969; Roberts and Larsen, 1971; Fairweather, 1967). Certain of those variables were employed in controlled experiments bringing about change (Fairweather, 1972; Larsen, 1972; Glaser and Ross, 1971). Valuable counsel was given by specialists on change in academic settings, research institutes, and federal agencies. Components of the model have been employed in the NIMH mental health services research and development program over the past two years. Its soundness and practical value will continue to be assessed through studies of its application in the NIMH program and in special projects that were described earlier.

The factors that constitute the A VICTORY model can be illustrated by referring to a study on the adoption of innovation carried out by Glaser and Ross (1971). A chief purpose of their study was to investigate the factors that influenced the decision to adopt—or not to adopt—an innovative mental health service. The innovation was a *weekend hospital,* employing saturation group therapy, a marathon approach. The program was designed to help persons so precariously adjusted that they needed intensive help, yet who because of job or family responsibilities were quite unable to accept inpatient status. Such persons also lived too far from available partial hospitalization services requiring daily or nightly attendance. The weekend experiences extended from Friday evening through Sunday afternoon, and continued for a period of 16 weeks.

Before Glaser and Ross began their study on the nationwide adoption of the innovation, the program had been thoroughly evaluated in a controlled design by Dr. Frank Vernallis of Olive View, California, who had developed and demonstrated the program over a period of several years. Patients served in the program improved significantly more—both statistically and practically—than did control patients who were provided traditional outpatient treatment over the same time period.

An analysis of the responses of community mental health centers as potential users of the weekend program helps to illustrate the eight variables in the A VICTORY model:

ABILITY—Resources necessary to implement and sustain the change

For change to be carried out successfully, the resources necessary to achieve and sustain it must be available. For the individual, this capacity might be represented by intelligence, the biochemical condition of the nervous system at a given point in time, constitutional predisposition, and so forth. In organizational change, the most common resources required are (1) funds, (2) manpower and training, often specialized, and (3) physical facilities.

The adoption of the weekend hospital called for two kinds of resources; namely, staff competence in conducting marathon therapy and up to $9,000 for staff time and incidental costs for one group of patients. Glaser and Ross found that even such modest resource requirements as these constituted perhaps the greatest deterrent to the adoption of the program. Community mental health centers did not have the *ability* to implement the change.

Strangely, the literature on organizational change is almost silent on this critical determinant.

VALUES—Consistency of the change with the beliefs and styles of the organization

Probably no other single determinant of change is so important as this one. *Values* encompass the guiding principles that predetermine which direction will be taken when a choice point is reached. Though values are not sufficient to bring about change, they do constitute gatekeepers. Only change that is consistent with the beliefs and styles of a person or organization is likely to survive.

For the individual, *values* encompass self-expectancy and characteristic ways of handling stimuli. For the organization, *values* include its perceived mission and attitudes, characteristics such as management style and openness of communication, the personal characteristics of the top decision-makers, relationships with benefactors and the supporting community, and the personal attributes of the individuals participating in the change process.

One requirement of the weekend hospital innovation—that therapists be away from their families for 16 straight weekends—clearly clashed with the personal values of most potential participants. Further, the concept of marathon group therapy was allied with a school of thought different from that in which most of the mental health workers had been trained. Glaser and Ross also found that the agencies most resistant to adoption of the innovation were strongly centralized, unaware of the agency mission, engaged in staff/administration power struggles, and rigidly committed to orthodoxy.

INFORMATION—The pattern of action

It is apparent that all change requires some pattern of action. Even in relatively unstructured approaches, such as sensitivity training groups, the expected pattern of performance is demonstrated or shaped by the group, if not expressed verbally.

Patterns for individual behavior commonly are presented through processes of identification, modeling, and group approval or disapproval. However, occupational behavior may be channeled by explicit and detailed communication of patterns for action. An example is the process in a behavior modification endeavor.

For the mental health facility, patterns of action for change may be communicated as research findings, program descriptions in the literature, visits to the sites of innovations, and so forth. Qualities of the information—clarity, relevance, apparent advantages, etc.—and the method of communication determine whether it will be used in a change process.

Despite good traditional dissemination of project results on the weekend hospital, only about 5 percent of the potential users initially were familiar with it. Glaser and Ross found that supplanting journal publication with an attractive brochure carrying concrete examples and illustrations increased the proportion of potential users familiar with the project to 55 percent. Unfortunately, the excellence of the communication still did not lead to implementation of the information. Insofar as community mental health centers were concerned, the quality of the information presented problems: it was limited in terms of relevance, relative advantage, and credibility; the investigators further reported difficulties with regard to the complexity of the idea and the degree to which it would lend itself to a trial or partial use.

It is hardly surprising that research findings, even those dealing with innovative services as such, play a relatively minor role in change among mental health service programs. Research so often is designed to meet the sole criterion of scientific merit, and journal publication traditionally is looked on as a sufficient method of dissemination.

CIRCUMSTANCES—Relevant shaping situations in the environment

Environmental characteristics surrounding an organization exert a profound influence on the phenomenon of change. Perhaps by dint of their pervasiveness, environmental circumstances are taken for granted. They constitute the forest that may not be seen for the trees.

Learning theorists refer to this factor as *stimulus conditions* impinging on the individual. They help make one work at work and dance at a dance. Circumstances influencing organizational change, as in a community mental health center, may range from the rural nature of its setting to a public concern with crime in the catchment area.

The weekend hospital idea proved to be more relevant to the concerns of centers serving suburban neighborhoods. Those neighborhoods contained a high proportion of family units in which the roles of the potential patients in the family were more necessary to preserve than in other areas. Also, in catchment areas where poor transportation facilities made it impracticable to travel daily for partial hospitalization services, there was a greater likelihood that the weekend hospital would be valuable.

Considerations that may fall under certain of the other variables in this model also might be thought of as *circumstances*. For instance, the ability to furnish free bed space on Saturday and Sunday for the weekend hospital may be thought of as a circumstance rather than an *ability*. However, items under *circumstances* usually are considered not to be manipulable by the administrator. Their utility comes in predicting the nature of change that may be successful.

TIMING—Phases of events that may help or hinder change

Timing is one of the most critical and difficult determinants of change to manipulate. The keenest administrators of change are those who can predict when the best opportunity to bring about change will occur. But more than accurate anticipation is required. The marshalling of all influencers of change at the appropriate *move-out* time requires consummate skill.

The probability of individual change is greatest if it is planned to coincide with a peak drive stage. This also is true in organizations: crises, if they can be anticipated, represent fruitful occasions for change. Other events that present good timing opportunities are the start of a budget cycle, a change in top decision makers, and an overall reorganization of the facility.

At the time the weekend hospital idea was presented to community mental health centers, most were in no particular state of change that would make the adoption of the innovation timely. In fact, some centers indicated that they would have to wait for a new funding cycle to even consider adopting the weekend hospital.

OBLIGATION—The motivation of change

A fundamental tenet of behavior is that it is motivated. Even so-called autonomous behavior was originally a response to a state of motivation. It is safe to say that organizational change does not take place unless some need for the change is *felt* by persons who are in a position to influence that change. The problem is that the need is not always a front-stage one. In the administration of change, one might hope that the *obligation* to change always would be based upon an organization's need to achieve its goals. However, much organizational change probably stems from the back-stage needs of the participants.

Few of the centers approached about implementing a weekend hospital were aware of any pressure from patients for an alternative to the traditional hours of service. A few staff people felt there was a need for such service. Others seemed to reflect a need to be creative, to start something new. But beyond that, there was virtually no felt need to launch such a program as the weekend hospital.

Administrative change within a mental health organization usually does not involve the *selling* of a new idea, as was the focus in the Glaser and Ross study. But change that is based upon an ascertained need will come off more smoothly if the persons involved are helped to gain an *awareness* of that need. Helping people feel the need for change is hardly less important than determining that the need exists. Making the task all the more difficult is the fact that some of the individual motivations will be consistent with the change but will be different from the front-stage need of the organization. For instance, a staff member not otherwise greatly concerned with the need to provide patients with the opportunity for weekend service might be motivated by an opportunity to earn extra income for 16 weeks.

RESISTANCES—Inclinations to preclude the change

No matter how strongly the force vectors of all the other determinants point toward change, the desired change will not occur or will not be sustained if the resistance force is too great. Even if resistance is not the greater force, the smoothness and effectiveness of the change will be diminished in more or less direct proportion to the amount of resistance that does exist.

The tendency to resist change is one of the most obvious phenomena of individual behavior. Behavior that pays off even mildly is not abandoned readily. And situations that have been associated with anxiety are particularly avoided, even without the conscious decision to do so.

Some organizations that are at least surviving are reluctant to give up their existing behavior in favor of an innovation when its benefits have not been directly experienced. Paradoxically, it is often the less well-off organization that is most reluctant to change its behavior. The fear of collapse is so great that the organization does not dare risk backing off from what is keeping it safe for the moment.

Anxieties of individuals or groups within the organization can impair the change process in sundry ways. (One reason to regard resistances seriously is that they may indeed be realistic and give cause to reconsider the plan for change.) Resistances become particularly difficult to deal with when they are unspoken; more common than not. Most harmful of all are the resistances manifested only by disinterest. It is probable that more change comes a cropper because of disinterest than because of resistance expressed in direct confontation.

A special kind of resistance evoked by the weekend hospital proposal was related to *product loss*. Since new funds and personnel are not conjured up by a snap of the fingers, the resources had to be taken away from some other activity, at least until a new funding cycle. Most administrators are familiar with what happens when a new high priority topic is announced. Program heads begin to squirm in their seats because everyone realizes that the needed resources will have to come from somebody's program.

It is in the consideration of resistance that awareness of the total system becomes most pronounced. True change almost always causes some shifts in other parts of the system. An apparent exception to this is when the innovation is simply added to the program rather than replacing anything else. But even in such cases, the administrator should give high regard to monitoring possible consequences in other parts of the system.

YIELD—The rewards for changing

Despite the readiness of all the other factors to move toward change, it will not come about unless there is at least some implied promise of payoff. And the experience of reward in some form after the change will be what sustains it.

The problem with *yield* is that both for individual and group performance in organizations, reward is an elusive and complicated as it is powerful. In the idealized situation, there would be clear evidence that a change in staff activity, for example, solved a particular problem. This is difficult to achieve. But the closer the administrator can associate the felt *obligation* to change, *information* about how to meet the obligation, and the *yield* from implementing the information, the more successful the change will be. However, rarely do all of the people involved in the change process feel a common sense of need for that change. What will be perceived as rewarding will vary as much as will the sense of need. Job security may be the felt need. The consequent reward will be retention of the job. When that occurs, the behavior that intervenes will tend to be continued.

There were few rewards even implied for launching a weekend hospital. Certainly no power figures in the community mental health centers approached were sufficiently sold on the innovation to make the reward of job security a relevant one for staff members. There would be little yield in terms of creativity because no staff member could claim the innovation as his own. Because the idea already had been written about and published, the promise of adding to one's bibliography was not even there. A number of staff members who participated in a conference on the weekend hospital acknowledged that it could offer certain patients a more convenient service. Not surprisingly, that became the chief verbalized reason for showing interest in the idea. But the stated reason for not pushing its adoption was that the evaluation did not cogently promise sufficient reward in terms of patient improvement. The project, they felt, should be replicated to make sure that the results would hold true for subsequent groups of patients. Given sufficient grant funds, many of the staff members were willing to try out the program in modified form—an event that would have rendered them creators rather than users.

The reaction of the potential users in the Glaser and Ross study highlights a problem that may be rather special in the mental health services field. Graduate training, particularly for psychologists, ingrains the need to be a producer of knowledge rather than a user. This may be one reason why the development and demonstration of new methods in mental health services outrun the adoption of those methods. An implication of this that may be worth exploring is that in the mental health field, the opportunity to help change a change may be significant reward in itself.

A case example:

An illustration of how easy it is to propose change and how difficult that change may be to implement took place in the office of the Commissioner of Public Welfare in a Midwestern State.

Aftercare programs were of paramount interest at the time. The Commissioner was responsible for the county welfare departments, which in turn held legal responsibility for services to many patients discharged from State mental hospitals. His department also had authority for the State mental health program, including the hospitals. So he was the appropriate person to be approached about a minor change in the State-wide aftercare program.

The visitors, who included members of the Commissioner's own staff, as well as outside consultants, were reporting results from a major aftercare study. An important finding was that when patients were seen by the same worker both during hospitalization and after return to the community, the probability of readmission would be significantly lowered; that is, *statistically* significantly lowered. The seemingly minor change proposed to the Commissioner was a policy whereby county welfare workers would initiate relationships with patients several weeks before their anticipated discharge. There had been little doubt that the Commissioner would agree. He was known for progressive administration. Surely he would be grateful for this *simple* way to reduce readmission rates. But after listening to the news he merely lit his cigar and said nothing. So his visitors added that for aged patients included in the experimental group, their scores on the MMPI scale reflecting depression had dropped significantly—again, *statistically* significantly. Still the Commissioner seemed unimpressed—he had a few questions to ask. They were essentially as follows; though the order was a bit different:

"In your project, you used experienced MSW psychiatric social workers and public health nurses with master degrees. How do I know that our county welfare workers will be able to match the skills of your project workers? How will we pay for the training programs necessary to prepare the county workers to carry out the same aftercare services? Where do I find funds to pay for their travel expenses to the State hospitals? Who will carry out the work that they will be unable to accomplish while they are spending the required time at the hospital helping the patients prepare for discharge?"

(The Commissioner was asking about the *ability* to produce the resources needed for the change.)

"How will people in our hospital social service departments feel about county workers coming in and taking over a major portion of what they have seen as their roles? And how will the counties feel about extending the duties of their employees beyond the responsibilities which they normally carry?"
(He was concerned with violating the assumed *values* of the system.)

"Your findings sound almost too simple and pat. How do you know the results you've obtained did not stem from the high skills of the workers on the project; and how do you know that their small caseload of only about 6 patients at any given time wasn't the determining factor?"
(The soundness of the *information* was being appropriately questioned.)

"In your project, your workers had their offices in a city very close to the hospital and the locations of the patients after discharge were also fairly close. There aren't many parts of the State where things are that convenient. Will the plan still be feasible.?"
(The *circumstances,* the Commissioner was pointing out, would likely work against the success of the change.)

"The counties aren't going to volunteer to use their scarce resources for added service unless legislative and budget adjustments are made. The State Legislature just met. How will I bridge things throughout the rest of the biennium?"
(*Timing* had not been given consideration.)

"Readmission rates already are respectably low. Who is so critically concerned about the problem that the increased expenditures would be warranted? Of course, I'd like to see readmission made unnecessary even for one patient, but it would help if the Legislature, the Governor, or at least some groups were concerned enough to back this change."
(His point was that the *obligation* to change was not all that pressing.)

"The need for social workers in our hospitals would be considerably less. Some may lose their jobs. How will I handle their unhappiness? And the county workers are going to be raising cain

because of the hardships they will have to face, even if compensation is arranged. They'll have to stay away from their families during trips to the hospital, for instance."
(The Commissioner seemed to be reminding us that *resistances* had been overlooked.)

"Though your results are statistically significant, would the improvement in the readmission rate be sufficient even to be noticed? Will anyone feel a sense of betterment for having gone along with this proposal?"
(The reinforcing reward necessary to sustain successful change, the *yield*, admittedly was minimal.)

This true incident took place some 12 years ago. But with only a slight reordering and restructuring of the questions, it demonstrates the critical importance of precisely the same factors in extensive investigations carried out since.

Using the A VICTORY Model

The guidelines that follow are presented to help the administrator quickly review the factors to be considered when organizational change is contemplated. In most instances, major planning and action will not be carried out in detail. But in thinking about even the most minor or technical changes, referring to a checklist can help to avoid costly errors in the *people aspects* of the change. The guidelines are intended for use not only in bringing about desired change, but in averting change that would be deleterious to the organization.

The factors in the A VICTORY model are presented as though they are discrete linear steps toward a specific desired change as an end result. While this may be necessary for description, in actual use something much more fluid, interacting, and harmonious must take place. Perceptive and skillful administration is the key to successful innovation and change. Without the administrative touch, using a model is like playing a 1912 Wurlitzer automatic orchestra—the clarinet, marimba, tambourines, drums, and cymbals may all be there and play on cue, but something akin to cacophony comes out. Morgan (1972) puts it this way: "Managing change effectively often requires more than technique and strategy. It calls for a new kind of thinking about change—as an element in planning, as a factor in all decision-making, and as a pervading force in practically all other aspects of management."

The four steps in the use of the A VICTORY model are: (1) Analysis (2) Goal Definition (3) Action (4) Follow-through.

The extensive literature pertaining to analysis of and action on the eight A VICTORY factors has been condensed to a guideline format for Steps 1 and 3. However, the relatively barren literature on goal definition and follow-through does not warrant synthesis into documentable guidelines for Steps 2 and 3.

Elaboration of recommended techniques outlined in the guidelines, together with references to their sources in the literature, can be found in the series of publications *Planning for Creative Change in Mental Health Services* (NIMH, 1971; 1972a; 1972b; 1972c; 1972d).

(1) Analysis

Because types of change and the conditions under which they may be planned vary so greatly, the user's own judgment will have to be invoked to judge the probability that change can be administered as desired. For a fully adequate assessment, some items in the guidelines would require painstaking measurement. Argyris (1965), for example, details a procedure for analyzing and scoring individual and group behaviors within organizations which indicate the probability that change can occur.

Administrators who have had at least several months' experience with their organizations usually can estimate conditions with sufficient accuracy to reach educated conclusions. On the other hand, because some of the items require judgment about top-level management—of which the person administering the change may be a part—it is usual to enlist the help of at least one person from a different echelon in the organization or of a consultant who knows the organization well.

If one had the opportunity in practice to analyze and arrange the A VICTORY factors sequentially, the order would be as follows: OBLIGATION (determination of felt needs for change); INFORMATION (selection of knowledge or a pattern of action likely to lead to a reduction of the need); VALUES (determination of the consonance between the chosen pattern of action and the beliefs and styles of the organization); ABILITY (estimation of the resources necessary to carry out the action); CIRCUM-STANCES (assessment of aspects of the environment that pertain to the appropriateness of the intended action); TIMING (anticipation of events that may influence the success of change); RE-SISTANCES (reckoning with both rational and irrational objections to the proposed change); YIELD (establishing meaningful rewards for participation in the change).

OBLIGATION

Has the origin of any existing proposal for change been reviewed?

Are there informal clues indicating needs for change: mistakes, vague or conflicting goals, lack of communication, poor decision-making, complaints, rumors, low morale?

Has a formal attempt been made to evaluate the program? Have forecasts been made about new needs?

Have individual needs of staff or employees been considered, especially those that might represent secondary or back-stage motivations? If multiple needs exist throughout the system, has a priority ranking been made?

Following the determination of needs, have steps been taken to amplify awareness of those needs among staff and employees?

INFORMATION

Has vigorous effort been made to explore all sources of information toward finding the most suitable action to meet the obligation—work experiences, group discussions, literature retrieval, special publications? Does proposed information meet the CORRECT criteria—Credibility, Observability, Relevance, Relative advantage, Ease of understanding, Compatibility, and Timing?

Has special attention been given to methods of communicating the information to all relevant persons?

Have persons concerned been given an opportunity to challenge the selection of the information, to simplify it, to elaborate it?

VALUES

Has the organizational climate been assessed—open communication rather than one-way, supportive administration, mutual support among colleagues, participation in decision-making, high morale, adequate time for reflection and testing new ideas?

Are the organizational goals clear and written down?

It the organizational structure characterized by decentralized and distributed power?

It the organization large enough to accommodate the kind of change being considered?

Is the organization reasonably affluent, secure, and "in good" with its benefactors?

Is the community served by the facility a reasonably supportive and liberal one?

Are social and physical distances among staff and employees so great as to impede innovation?

Are social relationships of staff so closed as to render unlikely individual initiative of innovators?

Has the tenure of chief decision-makers been reasonably short?

Has the organization had a history of successful innovations?

Are staff members rewarded for performance rather than status?

It the top man at the organization a self-renewing, goal-oriented type of person himself?

With respect to the persons who may be involved with the change, are they either younger or older than most? Is their economic status reasonably adequate? Are they people with a personal sense of security in the facility? Are they the sort who attend meetings and mix with other professionals beyond the mental health facility in which they work? Are they bright, authentic, not afraid to be deviants from the total group? Has consideration been given to the danger that supporters of the change are motivated by their own dissidence, indifference to the organization, disaffection, or resentment?

ABILITY

Have the funds necessary to support the change been identified?

Have sources of the needed funds been identified?

Has a prediction been made regarding manpower required to carry out and sustain the change?

Will special orientation or training in the new patterns of action be necessary?

Has the need for additional facilities been determined—office space, meeting rooms, parking, etc.?

Has there been a review of the product-losses that would occur; that is, if resources have to be taken from another part of the system, have the consequences of that withdrawal been given consideration?

CIRCUMSTANCES

Have fixed organizational characteristics—openness, attitude of leadership, clarity of goals—been assessed from the standpoint of the probability that any change can take place? Have restrictions on the nature of the change been judged vis-a-vis the organizational values?

Have characteristics of the catchment area or region served been considered in relation to the proposed change?

Are there changing organizational situations that would bear upon the success of the change—new budget periods, change in leadership, new mission for the facility?

TIMING

Has the time for predicted major changes in the organizational milieu been estimated?

Has the possible advent of new community concerns, legislative interest, and economic circumstances in the community been assessed from the standpoint of timing?

Are there impending crises relative to the proposed change with which the initiation of change might be timed?

Has the phasing of events in the personal lives of staff and employees been considered—holidays, for instance?

Has continual sensing of staff readiness for change been employed?

RESISTANCES

Have plans been made to sense reactions to the proposed change?

Has the advisability of the proposed change been reconsidered in the light of any rational resistances that have been detected?

Has there been a sensitive exploration of the irrational resistances of staff—fear of loss of status or job security, misunderstanding, etc.?

Has thought been given to those who might be affected by the change, such as beneficiaries of the program, even though their support isn't necessary to bring about the change?

YIELD

Have reasons for expecting the change to pay off been communicated to persons concerned?

Have direct, tangible rewards been planned for persons instrumental to the change?

Have indirect rewards been considered, such as better working conditions, opportunity for professional advancement, and for self-actualization?

Has direct and personal support from the top of the organization been planned?

(2) Goal Definition

When the change is structural (e.g. "mental health staff will fill 24-hour duty rotations on emergency service instead of being on-call only") or technical (e.g. "group transactional analysis will be employed on the alcoholism service"), the *information*, or pattern of action, is often taken to represent the goal of the change. But when behavioral or people change is kept in focus along with structural or technological change, the definition of the goal should extend beyond a mere restatement of the pattern of action. Prescribing action to be taken is one thing, but defining the elements of the outcome state is quite another. As Maguire (1970) stresses, the task of defining meaningful goals and structuring operational objectives should be of the greatest concern to the administrator. But the political and other considerations involved in the task are immense.

It is because factors other than *information* strongly influence the outcome of the change process that Step 2, Goal Definition, follows rather than precedes the analysis of factors. So a second major task of the change administrator is to estimate the most realistic outcome that can be hoped for on the basis of estimating *resistance, values,* and the other factors.

The worth of defining the goal lies in its eventual use during the follow-through evaluation. Only if a goal has been clearly defined will the administrator be able to determine whether it is working out successfully and, accordingly, whether further modifications are indicated.

One device that can be helpful in defining the goal and increasing the benefits of the follow-through evaluation is the Goal Attainment Scale developed by Kiresuk (NIMH, 1972c). In brief, the Goal Attainment Scale may be used as follows: Assuming the change to be evaluated is the utilization of group transactional analysis with alcoholic patients, the goal might be divided into several aspects. With regard to the sobriety rate, one might predict that 60 percent of the patients participating in the groups would maintain sobriety to the six-month point. The aspect concerned with patient reaction might be expressed as the prediction that only 15 percent of the patients would drop out of the program prematurely. Staff reaction could be represented by a prediction that three out of four therapists will express comfort in using the technique. The best estimate of outcome for other aspects could be stated in the same manner. Then statements are made for each aspect about what would happen if the results were better or poorer than expected.

In the formal use of the scale, outcome statements that are sufficiently objective for consensual judgments to be made about them at a subsequent point in time are prepared along a five-point scale. A statistical manipulation then allows one to not only see whether the change is achieving the anticipated success, but which aspects of the outcome are relatively better than expected and which are worse. Such an evaluation provides for a more discriminating review and feedback for further modifications.

(3) Action

Predicting how the A VICTORY factors, as they stand, will influence the outcome of the change process is not enough, of course. The profit from administering planned change grows out of ensuring an optimum outcome to the change process.

The suggestions for action follow, in outline form, the same sequence of factors as in Step 1, Analysis.

OBLIGATION

Involve key participants in a re-evaluation of the need for change.

Hold group discussions with participants in the change about problems in present working conditions, etc., which might be influenced by a change.

Assign responsibility for specific outcome concerns.

Obtain the personal endorsement of a significant authority. This endorsement should be delivered personally and a followup visit should be promised and carried out after efforts have begun.

When appropriate, withdraw supports that have kept the old order intolerable.

Cite examples of other facilities that have already moved ahead to take care of the problem.

Encourage a public statement of concern about the problem by a respected pacesetter within the group.

Fight fire with fire, as it were; if true, indicate that a participative change at this time will preclude a coerced one later on.

If necessary, invoke the most common of all methods to stimulate motivation; namely, *normative sanction*. The ultimate motivation for participating in change is to fulfill one's commitment to the job.

INFORMATION

Encourage participation in the selection of the action pattern, the solution and the information about it. Encourage participants to challenge the information, to simplify it, to think of improvements.

Use available systems of retrieval, specialized journals, and digests.

Seek out expert consultants. If practicable, attend professional meetings and conferences in specific search of the needed information; take part in problem-solving exchange programs as they are developed.

Conduct discussion with key participants in change regarding treatment of the *information*—rendering it, prior to its communication to others, credible, observable, relevant to the *obligation* to change, manifestly superior in payoff to the present way of handling the problem, easily understood, and compatible with the agency's *value* systems.

Conduct a deliberate communication of the information or plan of action among all persons in groups concerned with the proposed change.

VALUES

Obtain consultation to help with objective review of the analysis already made of organizational values and characteristics, and also to help with feasible modifications.

Depending upon the change administrator's influence in the organization, in advance of specific attempts to bring about change, encourage top decision makers to:

> Advocate self-renewal of staff and employees.
>
> Let it be known that experimenting persons have the right to make mistakes.
>
> Create an atmosphere receptive to pilot experiments.
>
> Encourage attendance at workshops, etc.
>
> Arrange for rewards and recognition related to performance.
>
> Encourage staff to express views on administration and policy-making.

If there is top-level support for modifying the organization toward being more receptive to change in general, any of several techniques might be employed, usually through the assistance of a consultant:

Direct systemic alterations—bringing power systems (policy-making, administration, socialization) into alignment with product systems (direct service and care to patients, community work).

Tavistock group therapy—working through deeper interpersonal feelings about organizational social and working relationships.

Balancing the *managerial grid*—bringing about a *team* management system that is neither task-oriented (treating personnel as rented instruments) nor country club-oriented (treating personnel as though all stress were to be avoided).

Temporary systems—conducting a group session such as sensitivity training away from the work setting so that the usual barriers to close interpersonal relationships do not prevail; the purpose is to give staff self-understanding about their own roles in the organization.

Emerging needs monitoring—development of a standing group of personnel who carry the responsibility for continually advocating an orientation toward assessment of needs for change and stimulating their consideration.

In order to help adjust the fit of organizational values with a specific prospective change, the following might be employed:

Peer group discussion—participants in the change—without the presence of power figures from the organization—discuss their personal reactions to the change proposal and offer recommendations accordingly. (This approach also will be considered when dealing with *resistances* arising out of a clash between the *values* of the participants and requirements of the *information,* or action pattern; for instance, the values of professional mental health workers about new assignments of paraprofessional mental health workers within the organization.)

Mann systematic use of feedback—trial of the new approach followed by pre-arranged discussion sessions of relevant personnel about their experiences and appraisals of the trial vis-a-vis the organization.

Orientation sessions with benefactors and beneficiaries—early introduction to the planned change, when appropriate to pertinent representatives of the community, board, or other parts of the supra-system and with representatives of the client groups, including patients, their *significant others,* and consultees.

Team piloting and specific change—early formation of key participants within the organization who will carry primary responsibility for bringing the change into actuality.

Legitimization of the change—arranging for the manifest endorsement and commitment of respected authorities.

ABILITY

Prepare specific budget for start-up costs and continuing costs.

Arrange inclusion of requests for funds in the organization's next periodic budget proposal.

Propose sources of immediate funds and discuss product-losses that would be involved, and how they might be covered. (If you use resources from A to start B, what happens to cover the losses of A?)

Explore grant mechanisms for start-up costs, using state and regional consultation.

Prepare manual or provide written references for participants if the information or pattern of action to be followed is sufficiently unfamiliar or complex.

Obtain an *action consultant* if available—a person thoroughly familiar with the *information* or action pattern and who also is familiar with organizational problems and its employment.

Conduct a formal training program from the use of the *information*— conference, demonstration, study group, anticipatory rehearsal (dry run through the new practices followed by discussion).

Estimate specific facilities required and propose ways of arranging for them.

CIRCUMSTANCES

Review of earlier analysis—through group discussion or consultation, review of organizational characteristics in situations in a community conceivably influencing the proposed change.

Examine *circumstances* out of which the *information* grew—investigation, by visit if possible, of the attributes of the situation where a new action pattern was developed and tested. (Rarely are these adequately described in communications about new service methods.)

Assess the interaction of all factors influencing the change—consideration of how all of the A VICTORY factors might be brought into interaction more conducive to fulfilling the desired change.

TIMING

Review *timing* of *circumstances*—anticipation of changes and events that might influence the process of change.

Coordinate staff readiness with timing of circumstances.

Prepare for mustering of resources and support at move-out time.

RESISTANCES

Appraise resistances deemed to be rational—final consideration of whether the change should be modified or even abandoned.

Decide on advisability of fait accompli approach—bringing about change quickly and without working through resistances if the change is imperative and indeed non-negotiable; it may be preferable not to evoke expressions of resistances about which nothing can be done.

Employ rational persuasion—intensification and broadening of communication approaches.

Use selective individual counseling—personal discussions with individuals who seem to have unique problems in reaction to the change.

Resolve complex resistances through group dynamics—utilization of some of the same techniques suggested for changing organizational values, such as Tavistock Therapy, T-groups, discussion at retreats, etc.

Use listening as a deliberate approach—allowing persons to express their resistances through the rare experience of being listened to.

Use advisory groups—involvement of representatives of participating factions.

Approach the change implementation slowly—introduction of elements of the change a few at a time, beginning, if possible, with the least disturbing.

Settle on partial change, if necessary and if better-than-nothing.

YIELD

Provide information on adequacy of proposed pattern of action as a solution to the problem, by:

Special presentations, especially by a person who has employed the pattern.

Demonstration of the pattern and its yield, if practicable.

Visit to a site where pattern has been employed.

Reward participants with timely feedback, attention, and interest.

Provide and *carry out* plan for specifically deserved rewards—pay incentive, new titles, professional opportunities, group recognition.

(4) Follow-through

There are two compelling reasons for planning careful follow-through. The first is to prevent the occurrence of an almost invariable phenomenon about change; namely, regression back to practices it was intended to supplant. Jenkins (1962) points out that whenever planned change occurs, care must be taken to ensure that the new condition is stabilized; otherwise the resistant forces tend to push back toward the former condition. Innovations require time to prove their worth and early disappointments are apt to snowball into counterproductive pressures. So during the follow-through months, the continuing task of the administrator is to reassess, and modify if necessary, the conditions that are influencing the progress of change.

The second reason the follow-through step is necessary is that some determination must be made about the effectiveness of the change. If it is working well, this fact can be fed back as reinforcement that will speed the stabilization of the change. If the outcome is deficient, steps should be taken to correct them before they become fatal. And, of course, if the results of the change are all significantly below what was anticipated, a major overhaul is indicated.

One of the reasons that change is so frequently resisted is that after making the investment, there is little evidence that things are any better as a consequence. Understandably, repeated failure to demonstrate improvement extinguishes positive attitudes about change. So evaluation becomes a key element in the follow-through stage.

Gardner (1964) has identified continual evaluation and further improvement as the essence of self-renewal. The adoption of a recommended innovation should not be a finished act; it should be only the beginning of a continuing process that may lead to something much better than the original design.

The key to effective evaluation is goal definition. Without a clearly defined goal, sensible evaluation becomes almost impossible. The more precise and systematic the goal, the simpler the evaluation. For example, if the Goal Attainment Scale is used as the basis for defining the goal and predicting the outcome, then evaluation is simply a matter of an objective assessment of the status of progress at any point in time. The evaluation results will be more cogent if the ratings have been made by group examination or through the use of outside observers.

At this point, the cycle is repeated for continued organizational improvement and renewal, with an accompanying increment in the organization's capacity (Havelock, 1970). Campbell (1969) underscored the point that in many ways the first cycle in the administration of systematic change is much like an experiment, with smoother operations and greater payoffs likely with subsequent cycles and refinements. Each cycle should require a lesser investment of time and effort, allowing attention to other problems in the effective delivery of services.

CONCLUSION

Administrators of mental health programs find themselves continually dealing with innovation and change. Beyond specific major changes are the countless everyday minor changes made necessary by shifting pressures and needs. Success of the mental health program, to a significant extent, depends upon how skillfully the administrator manages the change process within his organization.

Increasing tempo of change can be predicted. There seems to be a growing tendency for individuals to become *mobicentric*—desirous of change, of moving on—as they achieve self-actualization. Another clear contributor to change in the mental health field is the swiftly mounting body of knowledge. Legislation, court decisions, crises, and new appreciation of human rights all militate toward change. Backing-up the natural stimulators are such facilitators as new developments in information retrieval and change techniques.

Full use of change technology currently available appears to be delayed because of prevailing assumptions about planned change. Some administrators feel that the use of power in the form of either authority or money is easier than employing the more tedious change management techniques. That assumption is sometimes valid, but simplistic adherence to it has proved to be false economy. Others feel that if an innovation is sufficiently worthy it naturally will be adopted through its own merits. But the hidden jungle of conflicting personal motives, characteristic of many organizations, can subvert the most promising innovations.

When it comes to planned change management, a legitimate question asked by executives is "Does it work?" A cogent blanket answer is not easy to produce. But there is indeed sound evidence that the use of planned change in certain circumstances yields results. Management styles, for example, have been shown to be

responsive to planned change approaches. The adoption of research results in mental health services has been found to have
increased dramatically with the use of techniques to promote their
utilization in program change.

Among models of change, the two most familiar are concerned
with structural approaches (e.g. decentralization) and technological approaches (e.g. computerization of management information systems). But they tend to disregard people. Recently,
humanistic models have been awarded increasing attention. The
people approaches involve either manipulation or equalization of
power. The brighter focus now is on the latter, featuring such
techniques as participative management, sensitivity training, and
Organizational Development. A further model developed recently, Experimental Social Innovation, combines aspects of the
structural, technological, and people approaches.

A new working model of change has been derived through a
comprehensive assessment of the state of knowledge on innovation and change, plus special researches on the process. Toward
meeting ideal standards for change models, it has been designed
to be practical, manipulable, economical, flexible, evaluative, and
consistent with the humanistic view of organizations as living
systems. The model is termed *A VICTORY,* an acronym formed
from the first letters of the factors influencing organizational
change: *Ability* (fiscal, manpower, and physical resources required) ; *Values* (consonance between the organization's characteristics and the nature of proposed change) ; *Information* (pattern for action and its characteristics and communication) ; *Circumstances* (environmental features or events relevant to the
change); *Timing* (critical phases of events relevant to the change);
Obligation (awareness of the need to change, including both
front-stage and back-stage motivations) ; *Resistances* (inhibitors
of the change, both rational and irrational) ; *Yield* (felt benefits
from participating in the change). Use of the model proceeds
through four steps: (1) analysis of the status of each factor; (2)
goal definition based upon the analysis; (3) action steps to modify conditions within the factors; and (4) follow-through, including evaluation and recycling toward maximizing benefits of the
change.

REFERENCES

American Psychological Association: *APA Monitor, 3*(8): 5, 1972.

Archibald, Kathleen: *The Utilization of Social Research and Policy Analysis.* Doctoral dissertation, Washington University. University Microfilms No. 68-10, 771, Ann Arbor, 1968.

Argyris, Chris: *Organization and Innovation.* Homewood, Dorsey, 1965.

Beckard, Richard: *Organizational Development: Strategies and Models.* Reading, Addison-Wesley, 1969.

Bennis, Warren G.: Theory and method in applying behavioral science to planned organizational change. *J Appl Behav Sci, I,* October-November-December, 1965.

Bennis, Warren G.: *Changing Organizations.* New York, McGraw-Hill, 1966.

Blake, R.R. and Mouton, J.S.: *The Managerial Grid. Houston, Gulf,* 1961.

Campbell, Donald T.: Reforms as experiments. *Am Psycholog, 24:* 409-429, 1969.

Caplan, Ruth and Caplan, Gerald: *Psychiatry and the Community in Nineteenth Century America.* New York, Basic Books, 1969.

Chin, R.: The utility of systems models and development models for practitioners. In Bennis, W.G.; Benne, K.D., and Chin, R. (Eds.): *The Planning of Change.* New York, Holt, Rinehart & Winston, 1961.

Engstrom, George A.: Where we stand on research utilization. *Rehabilitation Record,* November-December, 28-32, 1969.

Fairweather, George W.: *Methods for Experimental Social Innovation.* New York, Wiley, 1967.

Fairweather, George W.: *The Challenge to Survival.* Final report, NIMH Grants #R12 MH09251 and R12 MH17888. Michigan State University, E. Lansing, 1972.

Festinger, L.: *A Theory of Cognitive Dissonance.* Evanston, Row & Peterson, 1957.

Furst, Sidney and Sherman, Nathan: *The Strategy of Change for Buisness Success.* New York, Clarkson N. Potter, 1969.

Gardner, John W.: *Self-Renewal: The Individual and the Innovative Society.* New York, Harper & Row, 1964.

Garvey, W.D. and Griffith, B.C.: Scientific communication: The dissemination system in psychology and a theoretical framework for planning innovations. *Am Psychol, 20(2):157-164,* 1965.

Glaser, Edward M.: *Facilitating the Utilization of Validated Knowledge.* Paper presented at meeting of American Orthopsychiatric Association, San Francisco, March, 1970.

Glaser, E.M. and Ross, H.L.: *Increasing the Utilization of Applied Research Results.* Final report to National Institute of Mental Health, Grant # R12 MH09250-02. Los Angeles, Human Interaction Research Institute, 1971.

Glaser, E.M. and Taylor, S.: *Factors Influencing the Success of Applied Re-*

search. Final report to National Institute of Mental Health, contract 43-67-1365. Washington, 1969.

Glasscote, Raymond M. and Gudeman, Jon E.: *The Staff of the Mental Heatlh Center*. Washington, Joint Information Service, 1969.

Guetzkow, Harold: Conversion barriers in using the social sciences. *Administrative Science Quarterly, 4(1)*:68-81, June, 1959.

Havelock, Ronald G.: *A Guide to Innovation in Education*. Center for Research on the Utilization of Scientific Knowledge, Institute for Social Research, University of Michigan, 1970.

Jenkins, David H.: Force field analysis applied to a school situation. In Bennis, W.G.; Benne, K.D., and Chin, R. (Eds.) : *The Planning of Change: Readings in the Applied Behavioral Sciences*. New York, Holt, Rinehart & Winston, 1962.

Jenning, Eugene: Mobicentric man. *Psychology Today*, July, 1970.

Katz, Daniel and Georgopoulas, Basil S.: Organizations in a changing world. *J Appl Behav Sci*, 7:342-370, 1971.

Larsen, Judith: Innovation in community mental health centers. Personal communication on NIMH research project progress, 1972.

Larsen, Judith and Roberts, A.O.H.: *Effective Use of Mental Health Research Information*. Final report to National Institute of Mental Health, Grant # 1 R01 MH15445. Palo Alto, American Institutes for Research, 1971.

Leavitt, Harold J.: Applied organizational change in industry: Structural, technological and humanistic approaches. In March, James G. (Ed.) : *Handbook of Organizations*. Chicago, Rand McNally, 1965.

Lewin, K.: Group decisions and social change. In Swanson, C.E.; Newcomb, T.M., and Hartley, E.L. (Eds.) : *Readings in Social Psychology*, 2nd ed. New York, Holt, 1952.

Lippitt, Ronald: Roles and processes in curriculum development and change. In Leeper, R.R. (Ed.): *Strategy for Curriculum Change*. Washington, Association for Supervision and Curriculum Development, 1965.

Mackie, R.R. and Christensen, P.R.: *Translation and Application of Psychological Research*. Technical report 716-1. Goleta, Calif., Santa Barbara Research Park, Human Factors Research, Inc., 1967.

Maguire, Louis M.: *Observations and Analysis of the Literature on Change*. Philadelphia, Research for Better Schools, Inc., 1970.

Maslow, A.H.: *Motivation and Personality*. New York, Harper & Row, 1954.

McClelland, W.A.: *The Process of Effecting Change*. Paper presented to the Division of Military Psychology, American Psychological Association, San Francisco, September, 1968.

McGregor, D.: *The Human Side of Enterprise*. New York, McGraw-Hill, 1960.

Morgan, John S.: *Managing Change*. New York, McGraw-Hill, 1972.

National Institute of Mental Health: *Planning for Creative Change in Mental Health Services: Information Sources and How to Use Them.*

Publication No. (HSM) 71-9058, U.S. Government Printing Office, Washington, 1971.

National Institute of Mental Health: *Planning for Creative Change in Mental Health Service: A Distillation of Principles on Research Utilization, Vol. I.* Publication No. (HSM) 71-9060. U.S. Government Printing Office, Washington, 1972a.

National Institute of Mental Health: *Planning for Creative Change in Mental Health Services: A Distillation of Principles on Research Utilization, Vol. II, Bibliography.* Publication No. (HSM) 71-9061. U.S. Government Printing Office, Washington, 1972b.

National Institute of Mental Health: *Planning for Creative Change in Mental Health Services: Use of Program Evaluation.* Publication No. (HSM) 71-9057. U.S. Government Printing Office, Washington, 1972c.

National Institute of Mental Health: *Planning for Creative Change in Mental Health Services: Manual on Research Utilization.* Publication No. (HSM) 71-9059. U.S. Government Printing Office, Washington, 1972d.

Rein, M. and Miller, S.M.: Social action on the installment plan. *Transaction, 3(2):*31-38, 1966.

Riley, P.; Hooker, S.; and Massar, N.: Introducing RUS: a link between clinical and research teams. *Rehabilitation Record,* 22-24. November-December, 1968.

Roberts, A.O.H. and Larsen, J.K.: *Effective Use of Mental Health Research Information.* Final report to National Institute of Mental Health, Grant # 1 R01 MH15445. American Institutes for Research, Palo Alto, 1971.

Rogers, C.R.: *Client Centered Therapy.* Boston, Houghton Mifflin, 1942.

Rogers, Everett M.: *Diffusion of Innovations.* New York, Free Press, 1962.

Rogers, E.M. and Shoemaker, F.F.: *Communication of Innovations: A Cross-Cultural Approach.* New York, Free Press, 1971.

Schwartz, David C.: On the growing popularization of social science: The expanding publics and problems of social science utilization. *Am Behav Sci, 9(10):*47-50, 1966.

Shepard, Herbert A.: Changing interpersonal and intergroup relationships in organizations. In March, James C. (Ed.) : *Handbook of Organizations.* Chicago, Rand McNally, 1965.

Thomas, William I.: *The Unadjusted Girl.* New York, Little-Brown, 1923.

Thomason, Harvey A.: The psychologist as a change agent. *Can Psychol, 12:* 506-512, October, 1971.

Toffler, Alvin: *Future Shock.* New York, Random House, 1970.

Watson, Goodwin: Utopia and rebellion: The new college experiment. In Miles, M.B. (Ed.): *Innovation in Education.* New York, Teachers College, Columbia University, 1964.

Weiss, Carol H.: *Evaluation Research,* Englewood Cliffs, Prentice-Hall, 1972.

CHAPTER 11

PROGRAM EVALUATION

PAUL BINNER

PART I: THE ROLE OF EVALUATION

Introduction

A S MENTAL HEALTH programs, especially in institutions, have evolved from a basically custodial to a treatment orientation during the decade of the 1960's, the meaning of program evaluation has changed as well. In a custodial setting, much of the emphasis on evaluation is related to program standards. For instance, did the institution provide adequate food, clothing, and shelter for the patients? This might be evaluated by the incidence of disease or death in the population, per capita expenditures for food, or the number of square feet of living space for each patient. The efficiency of the program might be judged by its per diem expenditures. Since patient movement was not the major focus, it could be evaluated adequately by monitoring the average length of stay or the percentage of patients discharged each year. The volume of work in the program could be monitored by counting the number of admissions and the year end census. In general, evaluation could focus *within* the program under consideration, i.e. intra-institutional behavior. There was little expectation that much improvement in the patients would be accomplished, so there was no great interest in measuring such changes.

With the evolution of the treatment orientation, evaluation has begun to pay much more attention to what is accomplished for patients. This has meant more than merely counting discharges, since discharge rather than custody is now the expected outcome of institutional care. In general, this has meant increasing concern for how well the patient manages his life after he has been discharged. Moreover, with the greater variety of treatment approaches, there has been a greater need to evaluate the relative effectiveness of alternative methods in order to choose among them wisely.

In this sense, the successful changes in the mental health field over the past decade have made our previous evaluation programs obsolete and have required the development of more adequate information and techniques for evaluating mental health services. These changes call for information on important aspects of a patient's community functioning in relation to his family, his friends, and his work; information that can assess changes in the mental health of an entire community; and information that assesses the economics of a program, such as cost-benefit or cost-effectiveness analyses.

It is in the light of this changing emphasis on program evaluation (Roberts, Greenfield, and Miller, 1968; Dent, 1966; Suchman, 1967; Schulberg, Sheldon and Baker, 1969) that the modern mental health executive seeks to meet his responsibilities. In doing so, however, he is often confronted with a contradictory picture. On the one hand, the resources allocated to program evaluation are seldom a large part of his budget. In this respect, it is a relatively small and unimportant part of his responsibilities. In many organizations, resources specifically allocated for program evaluation may be nonexistent in a formal sense, with these duties performed by staff with other primary responsibilities, such as discipline chiefs or department heads, if they are performed at all. Mental health has not been noted for the lavishness of its expenditures for research and evaluation. In 1967, the field spent less than 2 percent of its resources for research and development. Only 36 percent of the psychiatric hospitals spent anything at all on research and development and even this group spent less than 5 percent of its resources (Resources for biomedical research and education, 1970). There were only six psychiatric hospitals in the entire country that spent as much as one million dollars a year on research and development in 1967. While current information is not yet available, the situation is not likely to be much different. In community mental health centers, evaluation is an optional rather than a required function and only 2.2 percent of staff time is allotted to it.

Perhaps, because the need for services is so pressing, it seems necessary to administer and justify programs without providing any formal or systematic evaluation of their accomplishments. Perhaps, too, there is a reluctance to even attempt evaluations because the requirements in terms of manpower, equipment, and design sophistication seem too formidable. As a result, many mental health programs feel that evaluation is simply beyond their means. Many organizations do not even have the facilities to efficiently collect and retrieve the kinds of information needed to monitor and evaluate a program, although most generate a great deal of the necessary data during the normal course of their work. The unwillingness of most funding sources to pay for the development of more adequate evaluation systems has made it easy for this situation to persist.

Even when funds and other resources are available, however, it is not easy to find people qualified to staff program evaluation positions. It is highly unlikely that enough people could be found if all or even most of our mental health organizations suddenly became able to staff such positions. But if the resources and staff were to become available, the problems would not be solved because of the reluctance on the part of mental health professionals to be judged by the measures currently available.

In contrast to these realities of the current organizational scene, the administrator is aware that evaluation is one of his primary functions. If he only plans and implements new programs or continues old programs, he is doing only part of his basic job. Without evaluation, he might better be described as operating his organization, i.e., keeping it alive and in motion rather than managing it toward some specified goals.

Undoubtedly, there are many difficulties in providing a reasonable evaluation of our programs. However, we have delayed longer than is necessary. A careful review of what is meant by evaluation and how a framework for evaluation might be developed will demonstrate that further delay is not warranted.

The Meaning of Evaluation

What is meant by program evaluation is critical for determining what is done to evaluate a program. A variety of questions, such as, "What is being done by this program?" "How much is being done?" "How much is being accomplished?" or "Are the accomplishments of the program worthwhile?" may all be asked within the general context of program evaluation. Rather than being concerned with which of these questions constitutes *real* evaluation and which something else, it is probably more profitable to think of them as different levels of evaluation and to examine each one briefly to see what information it may legitimately give us about a program and what it does not tell us.

Levels of Evaluation

Asking "What is being done by this program?" simply calls for some basic descriptive statements such as what services are being provided (outpatient, inpatient, partial hospitalization, consultation, education, etc.) or what people are being served (adults, children, all residents of a given area, all individuals on welfare, etc.). While the information is descriptive, it becomes evaluative if it is compared to the requirements or purpose of the organization. For instance, the question of the range of services offered is essential for an organization to qualify as a federally funded comprehensive center. If the required services are not offered, the organization would not qualify for this support. Similarly, if the purpose of an organization is to serve certain age groups, neighborhoods, or economic groups, it is relevant to ask whether or not its services are reaching these groups. Without an affirmative answer to this level of questioning, any additional evaluations of the program may be beside the point. By the same token, simply knowing a program is delivering the required services or is reaching the intended population does not answer the additional questions raised.

Once it is known that a program is *on target,* the next question might be, "How much service is being provided?" This might be answered by the number of hours of service rendered, the number of clients served, or the number of units of service rendered. Again, this information is descriptive until it is compared against some standard or expectation. For instance, if an organization is expected to render services 24 hours a day, but it is only open 40 hours a week and a telephone recording answers the rest of the time, the discrepancy between expectation and performance would likely result in a negative evaluation.

Similarly, the number of clients served is a neutral descriptive statistic until it is compared to the number served in previous years, the number anticipated, or the number served by similar organizations. The number of service units rendered may be used in similar comparisons, with the added complication of establishing what these units of service should be. These might be inpatient or outpatient days, consultation visits, students taught, talks given in the community, hours of individual or group therapy, prescriptions written, phone calls, or any number of other activities. All these data may be included among the variety of answers possible to the question of "How much is being done by the program?"

"How much is being accomplished by the program?" raises the evaluation effort to the next level of complexity. This question differs from the previous one on services provided in that it focuses on accomplishments or end products rather than service units. An answer might be as simple as counting the number of patients discharged, or made more complex by trying to take into account such factors as their condition at discharge, their level of adjustment in the community, the number of days spent in the community, or the degree of independence from some form of institutional or social support a given population achieves over a given time period. It is when trying to answer this question on accomplishments that the required data generally exceeds the information available within an organization. Consequently, most organizations can only begin to answer the question with the usual information available at discharge.

Asking "Are the accomplishments of the organization worthwhile?" directly introduces the issue of values. An organization may be giving the expected service to the right population at the anticipated volume but at a price that appears incompatible with its resources. This requires a judgment on the relative value of the accomplishments and their costs. How much is it worth to reunite families, reduce institutional care and relieve human suffering? Comparisons of these kinds of accomplishments with program costs are obviously impressionistic and highly subjective. However, while it is difficult to decide how much a given amount of suffering relieved is worth in an absolute sense, if relieved suffering could be quantified, it would at least be possible to examine its relationship to the cost of achieving that result. This kind of cost-effectiveness relationship could be monitored over a period of years to determine whether a program is giving a greater or lesser return for the resources invested in it. If the program's achievements can be translated directly into dollar values, it would then be possible to answer this question within a cost-benefit framework. Some beginnings have been made in this type of study (Conley, Conwell and Arrill, 1967; Fein, 1958; Fox, 1968; McCaffree, 1966; Binner and Halpern, 1971).

Program and Procedure Evaluation

Program evaluation has sometimes been given a limited meaning by identifying it with a kind of classical experimental design. In this type of design, some groups receive the treatment under study and some may receive other treatment or none at all. The treatment is then evaluated on the basis of the results of the various groups under study. Because of the system of comparison and controls, it is fairly safe to conclude on the basis of this design whether or not the treatment had any effect.

The program director is seldom in a position where he can compare the results of matched programs and populations. In a sense, he is not in a position to evaluate his program so much as he is to evaluate the attainment of the program's mission or goals. These are two different questions. For instance, it is possible that his program is quite effective but his goals are not being attained. It is also possible that his program is really ineffective, but that his goals are being reached. Perhaps a few examples will clarify this point.

Suppose that a mental health program is providing highly effective psychotherapy to the clients it serves. Assume also that the psychotherapy delivered is individualized and time consuming for both patient and therapist. Consequently, such a program is serving only a relatively small number of clients. If the aim of the program is to meet the mental health needs of a larger population, it may be unable to do so because of its individual psychotherapy orientation and the excessive resources necessary to serve a much larger number of clients. Consequently, while the program might be quite effective in treating those clients seen, it would not reach its goal of providing mental health services for the entire population to be served. Under these circumstances, the program director would be faced with the possibility of abandoning a highly effective program for another that will allow him to reach greater numbers at an acceptable level of effectiveness, or of finding ways to acquire greater resources to do the job.

In another instance, a program may be launched to reduce unemployment in the population of patients served. In due time it may be noted that unemployment has gone down. However, it may be that the program had little or nothing to do with this reduction, if there has been a marked upturn in the economy during the same time.

In both instances, some change is called for in the programs. In the first case, the program was effective but was still not attaining its goal. Some change would have to be made to reach the goal. In the second, the program may have contributed little or nothing to reach its goal, but other forces had operated in a way to attain it. Discontinuation of the program may be indicated, not because it failed but because it is no longer necessary. If it had been ineffective and unemployment had not been reduced because of other factors, it might have been justifiable to proceed with the program in modified form in order to continue efforts to reduce the unemployment rate.

The point is that simply evaluating the procedure would have missed the mark. Programs are created in order to reach certain goals. Ordinarily, they include a variety of procedures and the mere knowledge that a procedure is effective or ineffective does not reveal whether or not progress toward the goal is being accomplished. The administrator is basically charged with making progress toward this goal. If he conceives of his task as administering a collection of procedures, he may think primarily of evaluating the procedures rather than looking at his organization's progress toward its goals. Thus, the evaluation of a program does not measure the program so much as it measures the approach to the goal.

The evaluation of a procedure, on the other hand, may be accomplished by assessing its ability to produce a desired outcome. Ordinarily, the focus is on demonstrating that the procedure produced certain results, whereas program evaluation may only demonstrate movement toward a goal and does not necessarily demonstrate the program's role in reaching that goal. This could only be demonstrated by treating the entire program as though it were a variable and subjecting it to controlled manipulation, such as matched comparison groups, one of which received the program and one that did not.

It is clear, therefore, that program evaluation and procedure evaluation do not refer to the same evaluative model. The program evaluation model is concerned primarily with progress toward a goal and requires a clear enough conception of the goals to provide milestones that indicate relative distances from it. The procedure evaluation model is primarily concerned with establishing cause and effect relationships between procedures and their outcomes. As such, the two answer related but different questions and the answer to one does not necessarily provide the answer to the other. This distinction both frees the administrator from research design requirements that are usually impossible to fulfill in operating a day-to-day program and cautions against unwarranted causal assumptions about the results.

The Context of Evaluation

The suggestion that program evaluation be done in terms of goal attainment without any firm conclusion as to the program's precise causal role may be a disappointment to the administrator who hopes that some certainty can be attained as to the value of the program. The hard reality is, however, that all programs operate in a context of constantly changing forces that make their

350 The Administration of Mental Health Services

specific contributions exceedingly difficult to untangle. Even the most careful design can render an answer that is good for only a brief period of time and a specific set of circumstances. This means that even the most sophisticated evaluation must be considered within the total context of the information available.

These limitations may raise a question as to the value of even doing any program evaluation. While stress was placed in the last section on how the administrator must be very cautious as to what causal inferences are drawn from the program, the intent was not to discourage the answering of any questions or drawing any inferences.

There are several ways in which program evaluation can be useful. Evaluation can be helpful for gaining program support. The attainment of program goals by a new program can be part of the justification for continuing or expanding it. Evaluation can be helpful for identifying potentially valuable procedures. If several sub-programs are similar except for a new procedure used in one, and if evaluation reveals a higher level of goal attainment in that sub-program, there would be reason to examine the role of the new procedure more carefully. The preliminary evidence uncovered could help to justify the additional expenditures for the controlled studies needed. Evaluation can also be helpful for changing programs and goals. If evaluation continually reveals a failure to reach goals, either the goals or the program or both need modification. Evaluation can be helpful in finding the most productive deployment of resources.

Even when all programs are effective, the chances are that some will be more so than others. Knowing this can help the administrator obtain the maximum movement toward program goals with the amount of resources available. In all this the key word is *helpful.* Program evaluation can help an administrator with the variety of decisions he is called on to make. Certainly, if the evaluation has any meaning at all, he should be influenced by it. However, if he is fully discharging his responsibilities, he should not be dominated by it.

For instance, one program may be quite effective, but the goal it addresses now has lower priority than one related to a less effective program. It may be very sound administration to eliminate or reduce the more effective program in favor of the less effective one. In another instance, a program may be quite ineffective, but could continue because there is no better alternative. Continuing this program as is could be justified if it provides the experience needed to develop a better alternative. Evaluation will help identify the ineffective program, but it may not help improve it.

Considering evaluation in this light may help reduce the fear that evaluative information must, by definition, be used mechanically to determine the fate of programs. Even the most sophisticated management information systems in the most advanced business structures are not used in this fashion. The danger exists mainly if those using the information do not see the situation in a broad enough context. This may happen at any level of management in any organization, but it is clearly a function of the individuals involved and not determined by the evaluative information available.

A reciprocal danger is that other considerations will always be used to counter whatever evaluative information is available and that evaluation will never be allowed to influence a decision in a direction that might be unpleasant to someone. If this is allowed to happen, there is no sense in going through the trouble and expense of obtaining evaluative information. Moreover, if the evaluative information is never allowed to influence important decisions, almost inevitably the data collected to evaluate programs will deteriorate in quality. This will necessarily result in less credence being given to information, with the resultant further deterioration in quality. However, if the administrator uses the information to help make important decisions, the same cycle should work to constantly strengthen the quality of the information and increase the reliance that can be placed on it.

The Role of the Evaluator

By now it should be clear that evaluation cannot be expected to provide totally unambiguous information with which the administrator can automatically arrive at sound decisions. Programs are ordinarily too complex to provide unambiguous information and the context of decisions is too complex to allow easy choices. In such a difficult decision matrix, what should be the role of the evaluator?

Traditionally, the evaluator has been seen as the impartial analyst who develops an objective assessment of the program. In most instances, however, it seems unlikely that he can function as an impartial technician or scientist. The view that he can do so is nurtured by the myth that this is the way a true scientist operates. However, scientists do not ordinarily take a neutral stance toward the subject of their investigations. More often they have a pet theory or hunch they would like to confirm. The fact that they may report findings that are contrary to their beliefs attests to their strength of character and commitment to the scientific ideal. However, it does not contradict the general observation that theoreticians of differing persuasion tend to find results consistent with their positions and contradictory to opposing positions. This is not to suggest they are dishonest in doing so. This tendency relates more to the forces that determine where the scientist will look, how long he will look, and when he thinks he has found a satisfactory answer. The scientist who doesn't care what answer he gets or doesn't suspect there is something beyond the obvious results he is getting, will not persevere in order to attempt to prove his point. Scientists keep themselves honest by submitting their methods and results to the scrutiny of their colleagues. Over time, this system tends to discard incorrect or limited answers in favor of the more adequate ones. While the history of theories persisting after they had been demonstrated to have serious flaws attests to the imperfection of the system (Kuhn, 1970), the long range movement seems to be in the direction of generating better and better answers.

The administrator must, therefore, assume that the evaluator is less than totally objective about all or part of the program. If the organization has sub-programs, ideally each sub-program large enough to support the expense should have its own capacity for analysis. The same would be true of levels within the entire system. Again, the mechanism for keeping the analysis and counter-analysis honest would be the sharing of all assumptions and data so that each evaluator can judge the work of the other. The objective of the system is to find the best answer, not to surprise or deceive the opposition. In this sense, it is an open advocacy system modeled on scientific discourse rather than a closed one in which evidence is concealed from the opposition until presented before the jury, as is sometimes done in a court of law. An open system would make evidence inadmissible until the opposing analyst had been given sufficient time to examine it. If the program is only large enough to support a single evaluator, the administrator and other program people will have to play the role of counter-advocate.

The system works as a series of checks and balances. Analyses at different levels of the organization or system are no more redundant than having a lawyer for both the defense and the prosecution at a trial or having both candidates for an office discuss the issues with the voters. The crucial gain for the administrator in an advocacy system is that he does not become the captive of his own analysts. He hears the best possible case developed for both sides of an issue and decides on the basis of this evidence. Almost inevitably, this leads to a fuller consideration of the facts. The less the administrator knows about the technical content of the programs for which he is responsible, the more important this becomes.

One important spinoff from such a system should be that the administrator has a far better understanding of his programs than he would have if they were not critically and systematically analyzed. The utility of good program evaluation should go well beyond stop or go decisions in programs but should offer the kind of information helpful for better managing the daily operation.

Further, the administrator and the staff who will review the evaluation, will each find themselves forced to clarify their own thinking. Evaluation ordinarily calls for a clarification of terms than can result in the highly beneficial development of a common language. Often the lack of this common understanding results in the disregard of information because it does not relate to the point that the recipient has in mind. Indeed, until the participants in an evaluation can agree on what they want the program to accomplish and how they will know when it has been accomplished, evaluation cannot take place. Elementary as it may seem, many attempts at evaluation fail to ever achieve this basic level of agreement because they are not performed in this mutual advocacy framework.

Viewing evaluation and the role of the evaluator within the advocacy framework helps to dispel some of the mythical qualities the administrator may be tempted to look for in an evaluator. The evaluator need not be the wholly impartial individual who will apply his objective techniques and thereby produce unsullied truth. He may even be drawn from within the program he is to evaluate, if he has the needed technical skills. Such skills would include a knowledge of the type of program to be evaluated, its manner of operation, and its goals. Also needed would be technical skills in the design of data collection instruments and data collection strategies such as sampling and surveying; knowledge of data analysis; and, if large amounts of data are to be analyzed, data processing techniques; program knowledge to help relate any findings to their broadest bases; and knowledge of writing and other communication skills, to facilitate the interpretation and presentation of findings in the clearest possible way. It is not likely that one individual will embody all of these skills, and if possible, the administrator should think of evaluation team specialists highly versed in the various technical skills required.

The evaluator who is a program expert most closely fits the model of the program advocate described, while experts in the other technical skills might more closely approximate impartiality. Although technical experts could help evaluate different programs more easily than program experts, it would be a mistake to assume that any of these technical experts could be completely unbiased. If they are at all human, they will carry with them some subjective preference for one kind of program or another. If they really don't care one way or another, the administrator should be wary as they will probably do a totally superficial and uninspired job of analysis. The power of the system lies in the clarifying action of the advocacy and counter advocacy of the program evaluators. It assumes the respective advocates have normal human biases and it tries to take advantage of these characteristics rather than denying or suppressing them.

Where the administrator can find qualified evaluators varies widely. Certainly, the traditional mental health professions of psychiatry, psychology, social work, and nursing constitute a major source. Their mix of technical skills, however, will depend as much on the individuals as on their professional training. Others may be found in the related fields of sociology, public health, epidemiology, statistics, and computer sciences. With the increasing stress on economic aspects of evaluation, specialists with a background in economics, accounting, or business management may be very helpful. Individuals skilled in operations research and systems analysis would also be useful; they often have engineering backgrounds that provide the logical and mathematical tools of problem analysis.

The right mix of people and skills for a particular job of evaluation depends on the questions to be studied. Clearly, a wider variety of skills and knowledge are called for than could commonly be found in a single individual. The basic requirements are for a knowledge of data collection and analysis techniques together with sufficient program knowledge to identify relevant information. Other skills should be added as resources when the scope of the questions call for them.

PART II: THE NEED FOR A FRAMEWORK

Even with agreement that the evaluation of a program consists of assessing movement toward its various goals, a great deal more structure must be introduced before the process of evaluation can actually proceed. To bring some coherence to the essentially infinite number of facts and observations that may be considered in evaluating a program, requires a framework for both the questions to be asked and the data to be considered. The framework for the questions may be seen as a kind of contract between the funding source (or sources) and the organization. The framework for the data to be considered provides a logical organization within which observation of the program may be arranged. Without a specification of these constraints, which essentially spell out what the program will try to do and how to tell if it has done so, any attempt to evaluate will be a futile exercise. Without guidelines, evaluation will be either a random search for possibly relevant facts or an arbitrary measuring that may have little or no relevance to program objectives.

The Need for a Contract

The need for a contract is so fundamental that it is ordinarily not even given explicit consideration. By a *contract* is meant an understanding as to what is to be accomplished with the resources provided, not a legal document or a legal arrangement of some sort. This contract is between the organization and the parties to whom it is accountable including the funding source (s), governing body, or community representatives. For the sake of brevity, these parties will be referred to as the *funding source* but could be any or all of those mentioned. In the case of a clinic or hospital fully supported by patient fees, the contract would be between the organization and the patient or relatives paying the fees.

The need for an understanding of what is to be provided for the resources allocated is so regularly overlooked because the usual answer, "provide some services," seems so obvious. However, it is totally inadequate because it does not clearly specify who is to be served, the amount and nature of the services to be provided, or what is to be accomplished by giving these services.

For the purpose of this chapter, it is not critical how this contract or understanding is developed. It might be entirely at the initiative of one or the other parties involved or it might be jointly determined. Presumably, most administrators would prefer to participate in the determination of this understanding, but it is conceivable that they could be faced with only the decision of whether or not they wish to accept the responsibility for fulfilling a pre-existing contract governing an ongoing program. However, in actual practice, since the contract is so regularly neglected, the administrator will probably have to take the initiative and call his funding source's attention to the need for developing a clearer understanding of what they are trying to accomplish.

The point is that effective evaluation cannot take place without a meshing of values. This means primarily the values of those providing, paying for, and receiving the organization's services. When mental health programs are developed, the discussion usually revolves around the great need for services. Seldom are the values that must be concretized in measures of accomplishment actually spelled out.

The Contract

WHO IS TO BE SERVED: Unless the contract clearly indicates who is to be served, it will be impossible to evaluate whether services are provided to the proper people. It is commonly said that a facility is to serve a given population. However, it is not always obvious whether the entire population is to be considered or only those requesting services. If the former is the case, the program administrator might normally think of including educational and preventive efforts in his program. If the funding source's intent was to serve only those requiring direct services, the administrator's glowing evaluation of the educational and preventative program services might be met with less than enthusiasm.

Further, there might be some unexpressed priorities within the population to be served. For instance, the program might give priority to the treatment of children, whereas the funding source favored the treatment of adults; or a program might aim to serve the relatively few seriously and chronically disturbed, and therefore, not be able to meet the needs of the larger numbers of mildly disturbed individuals seeking services.

With resources limited, there is often barely enough to provide for all those seeking services. However, it is generally assumed there is a large reservoir of individuals needing mental health services who do not seek them out for one reason or another. The administrator who organizes his program to seek out these cases may find himself censured rather than praised if the treatment of these additional cases places additional demands on already strained resources.

WHAT AMOUNT AND KINDS OF SERVICE: The contract should

specify the amount and kinds of services expected from the program. Are all comers to be served or are there some limits on the capacity of the organization? The answer to this question may require a compromise to be reached on the quality and quantity of services to be given. Outpatient facilities have long had to balance the use of the waiting list, while giving extensive care to those admitted, against immediate aid and short-term care for all those applying. With the increasing use of partial hospitalization, state hospitals no longer can use their bed capacity as the upper limit of their service giving capability and must also face this question. Even the relatively simple innovation of providing a range of services within a single work unit or team rather than providing them in separate services may cause misunderstandings between funding sources and program administrators. Because the same services are provided in multiple work units, it may appear that wasteful duplication is taking place. If the program is successful in stressing transitional forms of partial hospitalization rather than keeping everyone an inpatient, the director may find himself penalized for having a low inpatient census. Likewise, if active treatment is stressed rather than custodial care, it looks extravagant on a cost per day of treatment measure, while the cost per case treated is actually less expensive than the custodial program. Unless a clear understanding about the logic of the service delivery can be achieved, the program may be constantly evaluated in terms of the traditional model rather than a model appropriate to the services it is delivering.

WHAT SHOULD THE PROGRAM ACCOMPLISH: Should the program stress returning individuals to the community, or should it give sheltered or custodial care to many or all of its clients? Should it give first aid to the many, or more extensive care to the few? Stressing the return to the community, for instance, would tend to favor the welfare of the individual client involved, with the consequence that this may impose some burden on those in his social group. The emphasis on custodial care would tend to stress the wishes of the client's social group at the expense of his freedom of movement. Studies (Polak, 1970; Anderson, Polak, Grace, and Lee, 1965) have shown marked differences in treatment goals held by patients, their families, and treatment staff. Ideally, the contract should indicate what the balance among these potentially conflicting values should be.

FOCUS OF PERFORMANCE EVALUATION: Note that the specifications in the contract may be capable of only general statement at this point. The next section will give examples of how the questions might be answered. At this point, however, it is important to understand that the function of the contract is to spell out general performance characteristics and not to provide the blueprint for attaining these ends. The development of the program blueprint is the responsibility of the program manager. Once the goals are agreed upon, he and his staff should design the kind of program that will meet these goals most effectively. He should also know what level of resources he will have to work with, because this can be an important consideration in the kind of program he will design.

The contract should also specify the amount of latitude the program administrator has in changing the program plan to better attain the goals specified. In most instances, it would seem to the advantage of the funding source to allow the manager freedom in operating his program and to evaluate performance on goal attainment rather than the degree of adherence to the original program plan. If, however, it is the policy of the funding source to control any deviation from plans, then the evaluation would consist primarily of the degree to which the program plan was preserved and only secondarily would goal attainment be considered. This introduces, incidentally, an entirely different approach to program evaluation not at all uncommon among publicly funded programs. The program may be evaluated almost entirely on whether it spent the budget in exactly the manner originally allocated, with the attainment of program goals entirely secondary or essentially ignored. In such an instance, the program administrator may find himself in direct conflict with this method of evaluation if he attempts to manipulate his program to maximize goal attainment. He must give one criterion primacy over the other; it is not logically defensible to weight both these measures equally. The contract should determine the primary focus of the evaluation.

The Need for Specified Measures

Even with a contract indicating (1) the population to be served, (2) the amount of service expected, and (3) what the program is to accomplish, a considerable amount of additional specificity must be added to the contract before the program can actually be evaluated. Up to this point, the contract only spells out the broad mission and goals of the program. Without further specificity, the number of questions that might be asked and the amount of data that might potentially be needed is still far beyond the capacity of even a well endowed program. Part of the work needed in order to make program evaluation possible includes identifying a finite number of measures that will serve as the primary indicators of program performance.

In a field as relatively new in developing program indicators as mental health, it is clear that the intent and the expectation is that these will not be binding indefinitely on either program managers or their funding sources. The intent of seeking a contract and a commitment as to what should be done and how it should be evaluated is to make an initial attempt at evaluation possible. Without such a prior agreement, it is quite likely that the parties will find it exceedingly difficult to communicate and to agree on what has happened and what it means.

The expectation is that each will understand both the mission and the indicators more completely with each successive experience and that both the concept of mission and the operations defining the goal measures will be refined in the light of this increasing experience. This means that the contract and the related indicators should be renegotiated periodically.

This method of developing the statement of program mission and its related indicators combines the purely logical with the empirical, experiential approach. As any program administrator who has tried to develop a statement of the missions, goals, and indicators of performance for his organization knows, this is no easy task.

If the administrator accepts the premise that the purpose of the program is to help reach some goal and the provision of certain services to certain people are means toward that goal, he realizes that he needs to develop an overall goal or mission statement for the program. If he decides that the program goal is to improve the mental health of the population of the community served, some specific indicators must then be developed that would allow the measurement of progress toward that goal. These might include rates of personal disruption such as suicide, divorce, school dropouts, or battered children. If he assumes the conditions of the physical environment are clearly related to mental health, he might also include the percentage of substandard housing, crowded living conditions, environmental pollution, and sanitation problems in a given population. Crime, delinquency, or unemployment rates might be taken as additional indicators of the state of the mental health of the community. While all these indicators are specific enough to be measured, the administrator may not be able to determine to what extent his program influences changes in any of them. Certainly, they are not trivial or irrelevant indicators of the quality of life but the specific actions of his mental health program may affect them only minimally.

If, on the other hand, the program's goals are limited to the improvement of the mental health of the people directly served, similar measurements can be taken on this sub-population of the community to see if their lives are less disrupted, less involved in criminal behavior, more economically or socially productive than they were before being served by the program. The administrator would have to be careful not to claim that these changes took place only because of the actions of his program or that they could not have taken place in some other way. Nevertheless, if changes did take place, he could indicate the extent of the movement toward or away from the goals sought.

An additional goal might be the reduction of the client's dependency on program supports. Each severely disabled client entering the program risks becoming totally and chronically dependent on the mental health system, as was commonly expected during the custodial era. The degree of program success could be measured by the difference between the amount of resources required to maintain a client in a totally dependent state, such as an inpatient service, and the expense of maintaining him in a less dependent and more functionally autonomous state, such as family care or outpatient service.

In developing a statement of program mission and goals and their measures of success, the administrator may be presented with apparently contradictory advice. One school of thought (Longhurst, 1969; Jarett, 1971) recommends a logical derivative process starting with the most general, abstract statement of program mission and developing successively more concrete statements of program goals and their indicators. Another school of thought argues starting with whatever measures are currently used and successively refining them (Enthoven, 1970). There seems to be a grain of truth and a degree of limitation to both schools of thought. The most constructive resolution seems to be to avoid making an either/or choice and to use the strengths and respect the limitations of each approach.

The strictly logical derivation from an abstract program mission quickly runs into the problem that there never is just one way to translate into concrete measures an abstract concept such as *improving an individual's mental health, improving the quality of his life,* or *improving the mental health of a community.* Some arbitrary decision as to just how these concepts are to be translated must be made in order to make them measurable and it is generally difficult to develop goal measures that fit the abstract concepts exactly.

On the other hand, program measures that are not explicitly related to such abstract concepts tend to lack a directionality that allows one to judge if they are being improved. Thus, a program measure might be improved by making it more predictive to some criterion measure, more reliable, or more internally consistent, but this does not say whether it is more logically related to the program mission. By starting with the best goal measures that can be devised and relating them to the logic of the program's mission and goals, the active interplay of both these approaches can be achieved. It seems unlikely that either one by itself leads to a workable solution.

Thus far the development of specified measures has been discussed as a conceptual problem. Perhaps by this point it is clear that this is a formidable task, to be approached in developmental steps. It is a task that the director cannot avoid if he is to help determine the direction in which the program will move. While no universally acceptable cookbook prescriptions for performing the task can be offered, the next section will illustrate how an organization might attempt to translate its mission into specific program goals and indicators for the attainment of these goals. The section will also illustrate that even with a generous number of indicators suggested, there are still many questions about the program that would be unanswered. However, without the agreement to limit the evaluation of the program to some finite number of indicators, the task is an impossible one.

PART III: A SYSTEMS FRAMEWORK FOR PROGRAM DATA

A framework for organizing the multitude of questions and data that might be considered in evaluating a program helps to provide some coherence to what otherwise might seem like a random collection of facts and observations. A simple systems framework, conceiving of a program as a system with input, processing, and output functions is one such organizing device. This section will suggest some basic questions about each of these aspects of a program's functioning and the data needed to answer them. While certainly not exhaustive, these data would provide a comprehensive picture of the functioning of a mental health program. Variations in either the content or the definitions of the items suggested would allow them to be tailored to a specific program.

The Evaluation of Program Input

In a mental health organization, the input into the system consists primarily of the people being served. In a direct service system this would be the clients receiving direct treatment, although, it might also include the family and others involved with the client. In a program providing consultation or educational services, client input could include teachers, ministers, the police, or other community agencies. It could even include the entire community if a broad preventative effort, e.g. community education on the dangers of drug abuse, is the focus of the program. In a complex organization, different programs will likely have differing input populations. It is crucial to identify the input population accurately because this establishes the target group to be served, and presumably changed in some way by the program.

Direct Service Input

The key question is, "Who is being served?" The organization needs to know if it is serving the intended population. This may necessitate knowing items such as the age, sex, race, or socio-economic characteristics of the incoming population. The same information will be required for the entire service area for comparisons between the incoming and base population.

Another related question could be the geographic origin of the clients. Is one service area much more heavily represented than another? Are there patterns of non-use that suggest transportation problems for parts of the population or enclaves of specific sub-cultures that do not find the services acceptable or do not even know about them?

If the administrator wants to go beyond the sheer volume of various inputs and describe the input mix in terms of the severity of the cases treated, he will need data such as diagnosis, severity and extent of symptoms, degree of social disability, and previous treatment history.

Many mental health systems do not absorb all potential clients. Consequently, as part of their input picture, they should also strive to identify the characteristics of those who were not accepted for treatment, who were referred elsewhere, or who refused treatment after their initial request for help. As nearly as possible, applicants should be identified in the same way as clients accepted for service so that they can be compared to those served, to the base population, or other relevant comparison groups. Data should also indicate the services they were given, why they were not admitted for treatment, where they were referred, and if possible, whether the referral resulted in a successful engagement with another agency or individual.

Questions the administrator may ask of these data include, "It the program differentially turning away certain groups of potential clients?" "Are certain age groups, economic classes, or minority groups not admitted more often than would be expected by chance?" "Is the program refusing the more difficult clients and accepting the easier ones?" Here, the administrator might examine the diagnosis, previous admission history, or severity of symptoms of those not admitted compared to those admitted. Does the program attract fewer than might be expected from various groups, sections of town, or referral sources? For instance, if lower than expected utilization rates are suspected, a study of clients admitted would not reveal that almost all adolescents who apply are admitted and very few who apply are turned down. What seemed like a mild underusage when based on admissions might begin to look like a more serious problem when the non-admission pattern is added to the picture.

Indirect Service Input

If a consultative or education effort is being evaluated, it will be necessary to specify whether changes in the consultees, e.g. clinical staff, teachers, caseworkers, police officers, or the target population with which the consultees deal, are to be assessed. To evaluate changes in consultees, the critical operating characteristics of the consultees to be influenced must be known, such as their level of discomfort in dealing with certain problems; their rate of referral for certain cases; or the range of alternative techniques they employ in their work. If the consultee's target population is to be evaluated, the incidence or prevalence of certain problems or behavior patterns in that population both before and after contact with the program should be known, much like that for the direct service clients.

In all cases, the key characteristics of the input population as well as the volume of cases served must be known. Without the volume, it would be impossible to characterize the input mix, a key variable in interpreting the output of the system.

All this relates to the need to know the input characteristics of the system so that this input can be compared to the stated target populations. Evaluation at this level means evaluation of actions against intent in terms of input. Without knowing this, the interpretation of process and output is greatly hampered. For instance, if the program was intended to serve lower socio-economic minority groups and it turns out that the client population is largely middle class, the fact that the program is getting good results will have to be viewed differently than if the program were serving the intended population. Just what should be done about this discrepancy is then a policy decision to be worked out between the program administrator and his funding source. The example illustrates, however, how output cannot be adequately interpreted without the evaluation of input also.

The Evaluation of System Process

In a mental health organization, the programs represent the process part of the system. This section examines the kinds of information an administrator will need to evaluate the functioning of the programs, i.e. program operating characteristics, and the kinds of information he will need in order to evaluate the soundness of the programs, i.e. program structural characteristics.

Program Operating Characteristics

The evaluation of program operating characteristics can itself be divided into three related groups of questions. The first question is, Are you providing the kinds of services, in the variety, and in the way you said you would? This requires information on the variety of services delivered such as inpatient, day hospital, evening hospital, family care, halfway house, or outpatient. The information required, however, is not just a simple statement of policy or intent that such services are available, but detailed utilization data so that the amount of each of these services and to whom they were delivered can be determined. This would allow an evaluation of the extent to which the spirit as well as the letter of the intent was being fulfilled.

A further level of refinement in the analysis would be information on the amount and kind of actual services being rendered to clients within a given treatment status. That is, what are the amount and kinds of psychotherapies, drugs, psychodrama, vocational training, or recreational therapy delivered to individual clients? While the designation of inpatient, day patient, or out-patient allows some broad inferences as to the services delivered, the actual monitoring of these would give the administrator a more refined tool for evaluating just what activities his programs are performing. An alternative to monitoring these activities continuously would be the periodic time study that would provide estimates of the proportion of staff time devoted to each of these activities. This would not give as refined a picture of the services rendered to a given individual but could be useful for evaluating the functioning of an organization or individual work units within the organization.

Knowledge of the kinds of services delivered and to whom, when linked with the input data, will also allow a further evaluation of the distribution and equity of services delivered to various groups and geographic areas within the organization's total service area. The same information, when linked with output data, will allow an evaluation of the amount and kinds of resources involved in producing certain kinds of outputs.

Another part of the question of what is being done is how it is being done. Especially for administrators of comprehensive community mental health centers, the questions of continuity of care among the various services offered and accessibility to the population served are important ones. Again, evaluation requires detailed utilization data to determine if continuity from one service to another occurs or if patients rarely cross these service boundaries. Accessibility of services might be evaluated by the input data relating to non-admissions, the presence of a waiting list, or the socio-economic or geographic characteristics of clients as compared to the base population of the service area.

Just as with the input data, this information should reflect not only what is being done but also how much of these services are being provided. By knowing the volume of services delivered in relation to costs, the administrator can estimate the costs per each unit of service offered. The volume of services rendered, to the extent that it represents the amount of work done by the organization, may be related to the resources available in order to estimate the workload of the organization. While no norms are available to interpret either of these measures in an absolute way, by plotting trends within his own organization the administrator can evaluate whether these factors are increasing or declining.

The third group of questions related to the operating characteristics of a program are concerned with how these programs are running. Examples of these could be the length of stay of patients, deaths within the program, suicides or suicide attempts by patients, or the readmission rate. Most of these indicators have long been collected by mental health facilities and were sometimes used as though they were output evaluators. By considering them as program operating characteristics this does not deny that they have evaluative implications for the program, but points up the fact that these implications have to be understood within a broader context. For example, length of stay is often taken as an indicator of program effectiveness with the assumption that the shorter the length of stay the more effective the program. If system input mix and system output are taken into account, this is probably a good interpretation of this indicator. Without these considerations, however, it would be difficult to know if a shorter stay is related to an influx of less impaired patients, output of less improved patients, or some other reason. Similar considerations have to be observed in order to safely interpret the other indicators suggested.

It is also important to note that while many of these indicators have been in use a long time, they are commonly calculated in ways that could readily lead to misinterpretations (Morton and Schatz, 1970; Schatz, 1967). For example, length of stay for an agency's program or a specific unit is commonly calculated by taking the number of patients discharged each year, summing their individual lengths of stay and dividing this sum by the number of patients in the group. This might be called the discharge cohort method. Results from this method can be very deceiving for a variety of reasons. If a program is relatively new and it uses this method, it will probably find that each succeeding year's discharges stay a little longer on the average. This may not at all be related to a change in program functioning from year to year, but may easily occur because each succeeding year's discharges include a number of admissions from previous admission cohorts who had not previously been discharged. As each year passes, more and more admissions from earlier years are available for discharge in subsequent years, thereby adding their longer stays to the current discharge cohort's sum. The increases in average length of stay in these cases may be related to these earlier admissions being discharged and not to some change in program functioning during the current year.

A similar artifact may occur if an older program has a reorganization in which many patients who had been chronic for many years are discharged. This may result in an apparent increased average length of stay for an organization at a time when it is actually shortening its length of stay.

These difficulties may be corrected if average length of stay is computed on the basis of all discharges from a given admission year who are discharged by a given point following the admission year. The latter condition is necessary because the more years that have elapsed since a given admission cohort entered the system, the longer stay could have been accumulated. For most practical purposes, the average length of stay for the first year or two after admission is sufficient. Calculation of the median length of stay is also a useful measure and has the advantage of staying the same once it can be calculated, whereas the average must be recalculated with each new time period covered.

The calculation of the readmission rate involves similar problems (Morton, Lantz and Halpern, 1970). Very commonly the readmission rate is computed as a percent of admissions in a given year who are readmissions. This means that if the total number of admissions increases each year while the number of readmissions holds constant, the readmission rate appears to decline. If the reverse occurs, the rate appears to rise. In neither case may these interpretations be correct. A readmission rate calculated in this manner reflects the extent to which an incoming population is saturated with readmissions and may have important implications for program planning and evaluation because of its influence on the input mix. It is not accurate, however, to consider this a readmission rate. It might better be described as the percent of admissions who are readmissions or a readmission saturation index.

A readmission rate should be calculated as a function of the population at risk of being readmitted over a given time period. Thus, for example, in computing a one year readmission rate, the number of patients discharged for a year would be related to the number readmitted from the group within the year. It is important to consider time periods, because the longer the individual has been discharged the greater the opportunity he has for being readmitted. If the information is available, refinements may be made in these calculations by deducting individuals known to have died, moved out of the service area, or otherwise become ineligible for readmission.

The interpretation of readmissions is further complicated by the possibility that readmissions may actually be considered a step forward in the patient's treatment process and not necessarily a sign of failure or relapse (Rutledge and Binner, 1970; McPartland and Richart, 1966). As with length of stay, readmission rates need to be interpreted within the context of the input mix of a service and the output results.

Two general considerations emerge from a review of these common program indicators. First, the administrator must determine that the operations used to compute a given indicator conform to the logic of the interpretation he wished to make of them. He must not assume they do, no matter how long-standing and familiar they may seem. Second, he should be certain that any indicators he wishes to compare are derived from the same set of definitions and operations. Just because two indicators have the same name does not establish this point. While these considerations seem elementary in the extreme, they are often abused.

Program Structural Characteristics

When evaluating programs it is easy to overlook a second major component of the process, the structural soundness of the program. These are primarily considerations of staff variables such as recruiting, retaining and upgrading, the adequacy of staffing, and the proportions of effort devoted to various activities. While input and output indicators might paint a favorable picture of the functioning of an organization, attention to these structural characteristics might warn the administrator of future problems. By the same token, an organization that is not producing favorably might be able to confidently forecast a brighter future if changes in staffing variables suggest the organization has been significantly strengthened.

RECRUITING: All the resources and program plans in the world accomplish nothing until they are translated into action by a skilled and dedicated staff. Consequently, one group of key variables the administrator should consider are those reflecting his recruiting efforts. These might include the average duration a position remains vacant before it can be filled, the level of qualifications of those filling the position, and the level of performance of employees occupying positions. Such information can be developed from the personnel records of most organizations. Linking such data to the output performance of various units can be another factor for the administrator to consider in evaluating the performance of the system.

RETAINING STAFF: Another set of variables reflects the organization's success in retaining staff. These might include the average duration of staff service, the reasons for leaving the organization, or the use of sick leave. Undoubtedly, such a variable must be cautiously interpreted, especially on an individual basis, but as an organizational or group indicator, it might be a valuable evaluative tool for the administrator.

UPGRADING PERSONNEL: An organization rarely obtains staff that are fully trained for their specific jobs or fully developed professionally. Just as an organization draws strength from outside through its recruiting efforts, it can also build strength from within by enhancing the abilities of its employees. Most large and progressive corporations invest extensively in training and travel opportunities, while many publicly funded mental health organizations still regard such activities as optional extras. Unless the organization can provide opportunities for staff growth and improvement within its structure, it will find itself with a staff whose creativity has been exhausted and who then provide the kind of unimaginative bureaucratic services decried by everyone but fostered by the system.

CAPITAL INVESTMENT: Another variable reflecting the structural characteristics of the program is the level of capital investment per employee. Mental health is still largely a handicraft industry, and it may need to remain one in many of its direct service functions. However, the entire organization might well benefit from adequate investments in equipment. This includes dictating and transcribing, printing, data processing, and other equipment. By relating the level of investment (appropriately depreciated) to the output data, the administrator can evaluate whether the capital investment is related to productivity levels as well as monitoring the strength of the organization in material resource terms.

PATTERNS OF TIME UTILIZATION: A final measure of organizational soundness might be the way time and effort are expended within the organization. Time might first be divided into time spent on the direct service mission of the organization and time spent on supportive activities. The time spent on direct services could then be related to the output achieved by these various activities. These might be outputs related to specific service units such as a treatment team or an inpatient service or outputs related to specific services rendered, such as group treatment or consultation.

By splitting off the consideration of direct service time from supportive time, it is not suggested that the maximization of direct service time is necessarily desirable. Rather, the administrator needs to seek the optimal relationship between direct service and supportive activities. This can best be judged by the relationship of the mix of this investment to output rather than by the ratio of the components to one another.

Time devoted to supportive activities may also be divided into time spent to support direct services and time spent to enable the organization to survive within its larger organizational environment. Since the demands for this time come from different sources, it is important to consider them separately.

It is entirely possible, for example, for the organization's overhead related to its direct service activities to decrease, while overhead related to organizational survival increases. Consequently, total organizational overhead might increase. As a result, the funding source may request justification for this result, leading in turn to increased *survival* activity and a further increase in this overhead. This could lead to a cycle of monitorings, questions, and justifications, with each requiring an increasing investment in overhead. With each reading, the funding source may be convinced that not only is it uncovering inefficiency but that this inefficiency is increasing. Moreover, the more it intervenes to correct this inefficiency the more it grows. To those who are familiar with the Byzantine control structures evolved by many publicly funded systems, the possibility of such an occurrence will not seem remote.

Often the justification of expenditures for evaluation is manifested in the improvement of direct services to clients. While this is an entirely legitimate kind of payoff to seek, program evaluation that provides added efficiencies to the administration of mental health organizations may prove to be equally productive. By monitoring these process or program oriented variables, the administrator can judge whether any increases in output variables were achieved at the expense of decreasing the structural soundness of the program or through increases in productivity. Similarly, decreases in output might be related to decreases in productivity or increases in overhead. Without the information contained in these moderating variables, the administrator could not tell what general actions would likely lead to further increases in productivity.

The Evaluation of System Output

The absolutely necessary component of any program evaluation involves measures of the system's output. In a mental health program, the output consists of some kinds of changes in individuals or groups of people. For direct services, this involves changes in patients and sometimes in those people closely associated with the identified patient. In a consultation and education program, it would refer to changes in the consultee or student, or in the consultee's target population. In a program designed to influence the mental health of a community, it would refer to changes in the behavior of the population comprising the community.

Output from Direct Services

In measuring the changes in clients directly served, it is important to consider changes that occur while the patient is in the program, status at the termination of a program, and the level of functioning within the community at some time after termination. It is important to consider and give credit for changes that take place within a program, especially a residential program, because this may be the maximum level of accomplishment possible for some clients. Unless some value is placed on the various levels of functioning within such a program, there would seem to be little justification for providing any services beyond those needed for the survival of the patient. Presumably, additional services are provided to optimize the patient's level of functioning, such as the degree to which he can maintain himself physically, his ability to work productively, his ability to socialize, or his ability to handle various degrees of freedom or responsibility within the bounds of the program.

To the extent that all these activities may require staff time and resources if the patient cannot perform them alone, they represent a positive achievement when the patient can be helped to perform these functions himself. Moreover, it could be asserted that helping an individual realize more of his potential as a human being has an intrinsic value in its own right, whether there are savings of staff time or not. The value might be an arbitrary figure set by the program on the basis of ratings or rankings by panels of judges, or it might be set by the funding source. The manner in which it is set is not as important as the fact that such a value be assigned. If it is not, there is a danger that the value will be treated as though it were close to zero and resources will be assigned accordingly.

With the advances in mental health programs in the past decade, most patients are able to return to the community after a limited period of help. The measure of their response might be as simple as *improved* or *unimproved* or it might involve scales reflecting degrees or kinds of improvement. The latter usually involve areas of functioning such as social behavior, work behavior, ability to function within the law, self-maintenance, and personal comfort. The more specific these scales are, the more explicitly the accomplishments of the programs can be described.

While the status of the patient at termination gives some indication of his functioning, it is not necessarily indicative of how he will function when he returns to his community (Ellsworth, Foster, Childers, Arthur and Kroeker, 1968). Consequently, it is important that this community functioning be assessed in the same terms as those used to describe the patient at the point of termination, to facilitate the comparison of his functioning at these two points. Using the same framework to describe his condition at the time of admission, as part of the input variables, also facilitates a comparison with the patient's level of functioning at the time he entered the system.

Because the patient's functioning in the community may represent the closest approximation of an *ultimate* goal for a mental health program, it is the most valuable kind of output information to have. Unfortunately, it is also the most difficult and expensive to obtain because it occurs after the program ordinarily loses contact with the patient. This means that contact must later be re-established, either through telephone, mail, or personal interview. Certainly, the two former tend to be less expensive and are well worth trying if resources are limited. Mental health clients, as most people, are very mobile. They may have moved several times since leaving the program and may be very difficult to locate. Women who have married and changed their names are difficult to find. Some wish to have nothing further to do with the program, even if they can be located. It is becoming more common to acknowledge the imposition that follow-up contact represents by paying the client for participating. When these usually modest fees are contrasted with the expensive time a professional might spend traveling to the client, they often turn out to be a very efficient use of resources.

Whatever the difficulties, mental health programs can ill afford to continue the common practice of simply ignoring the need for follow-up information. As long as the mental health system allows itself to remain blind to the long-range results of its efforts, it sacrifices a substantial degree of credibility. Perhaps, if a routine six month and one year post-discharge follow-up were considered an extension of the clinical services, it would be easier to allocate the necessary resources for gathering this type of data.

The key question to be answered with data describing a patient's functioning is, "What is being accomplished by the patients in the program?" The most basic kind of evaluation is some kind of assessment of whether or not they improve. A more refined answer relates to the kinds of degrees of change. The data on community functioning give some indication of the change's longevity and whether the patients are moving toward the goals desired.

Value of Program Output

In order for the administrator to assess the worth of the program's results, he must place a value on its outputs. Perhaps the most obvious value of an individual's return to the community is economic productivity. This may be judged by earning capacity, if employed, or by the value of services or unpaid work performed, such as household duties or academic studies. Additional values may be assigned such as the value of the improvement in functioning or reducing previous expenses, such as welfare or other social services, that are no longer incurred because of improved functioning.

Assigning a value to the symptomatic or subjective improvements achieved is largely uncharted ground. Nevertheless, these are often the most important accomplishments of a program and allowing them to be unvalued runs the strong risk of having them treated as though they were of little or no value. The problem is very similar to setting a value on a life or an injury to part of the body, as is regularly done by insurance companies and juries, or setting a value on the largely subjective benefits of some form of entertainment or recreation, as is regularly done by every consumer. Systematic methods for estimating such values have been suggested (Churchman, Ackoff and Arnoff, 1957). The most difficult part of coming to grips with this problem may be breaking the convention of neglect and arriving at a tentative valuation by whatever logic the administrator, the client, and the contract parties can accept. Once the ground is broken and some form of consensus emerges, a steady refinement of these values should develop.

By placing values on the outputs of the program, the administrator is in a position to examine how the value of the achievements compares to the costs involved. To the extent that he can account for both the costs and the values of the results achieved, he can make a cost-benefit analysis of the program. Even if he can only account for part of the costs and part of the benefits, he can begin to estimate the relative productivity of the programs.

As an alternative, the organization can start by specifying the level of functioning to be attained for an individual or groups of individuals. As patients or clients reach the specified goals, the costs involved can be measured. Using this kind of yardstick, the relative costs of reaching the same goals for different people or through different programs can be measured or the relative costs of reaching one level of functioning as compared to another. The administrator strives to achieve the given goals at the lowest possible cost. The level to be achieved is a policy decision to be negotiated in the contract.

Output from Indirect Services

The outputs from consultation and education programs are the changes in the consultee's or student's behavior or changes in the behavior of the consultee's target population. These changes might be internal, such as changes in attitudes toward the mentally ill after exposure to a given educational exeprience, or in the overt behavior of the target population, such as the improved ability to do their jobs or the improved functioning of the client's target population, much in the same way the output from direct services would be evaluated.

It is important to note that the outputs from an educational or consultative effort may result in changes in the process or the output behavior of the target client or agency. For instance, consultation with another social agency may result in changes in the way referrals are made. The success of the consultation may be measured by changes in the number or pattern of referrals made, by changes in the success rate of these referrals, or by changes in the appropriateness of these referrals, i.e., the success rate of the clients who receive the additional services. Each is a different kind of output from indirect services and should not be regarded as interchangeable.

If the indirect services are given to a diffuse target group, such as the community at large, the outputs may take a wide variety of forms, depending on the intent of the service. For instance, an educational effort mounted through the public media might be aimed at increasing the number of clients for mental health services by stressing their accessibility and greater social acceptability. Another educational campaign might seek to reduce the number of clients by trying to improve parent-child relationships. In either case, the knowledge of utilization rates in the target population before and after the educational campaign is crucial.

Even more than in the case of direct services, the outputs of indirect services are often very difficult to establish. Very often, they involve a causal chain with multiple steps, i.e., the change of another caregiver who then influences a client more effectively. They may involve a target population subject to such a wide variety of other known and unknown influences that the relationship of any changes to the indirect services is a very tenuous one.

The decision to support indirect services is often sustained more by faith than by firm evidence that these activities are of value. However, unlike some of the indirect activities of medical care, consultation or education in mental health may have an intrinsic value that serves to justify their existence. For instance, there would seem to be little justification for taking a certain medicine or submitting to an innoculation, if it were not related to preventing disease. In contrast, the provision of constructive educational activities, improved parent-child relationships, or increased social contacts for retired persons may be seen as having some intrinsic value whether or not they reduce delinquency rates or admissions to mental hospitals in the target population. If these values can be quantified, they could give a basis for judging whether or not their attainment can wholly or partially justify their cost.

PART IV: SUMMARY AND CONCLUSIONS

The administrator of a modern mental health program is living in the midst of a revolution in mental health care. Within a single decade, there has been a profound shift from a primarily custodial to a primarily treatment orientation for the care of those with severe mental disorders. With this shift, many of the indicators previously used to monitor and evaluate mental health programs have approached obsolescence. At the same time, the demands for evaluation of programs have increased. Evaluation is one of the core responsibilities of the manager. With few resources and no universally accepted guidelines on how to proceed, he must find ways to discharge this obligation if he is to manage successfully.

To complicate matters further, evaluation can mean many different things. Sometimes it means, "Are you doing what you said you were going to do?" Sometimes the questions become more difficult, like "How much are you accomplishing?" or "Are your accomplishments worth the effort?" These are all legitimate questions and some illustrations were given on how they might be answered. The crucial consideration is that we not confuse the answering of one of these questions with another. It is important to remain clear on what question is being answered when we say the program has been *evaluated*.

Often evaluation is identified with study design considerations that call for comparisons and controlled applications of procedures that are simply beyond the practical capabilities of a service organization. The delivery of services cannot be manipulated, withheld, or controlled to the degree required. It should be possible, however, for the administration to attempt to answer the prior and simpler question of whether or not the clients are moving toward the goals the program was created to achieve. Even without precise knowledge of how much, if anything, the program is contributing, it provides some very useful information for program management.

Because they are well aware of the enormous complexities involved, program administrators and staff are often concerned with the dangers of managing a program on the basis of a necessarily over-simplified evaluation scheme. The administrator is urged to obtain the best evaluative data available. He must strive to use the evaluator fully and wisely, but not to become his captive, for he and not the evaluator must accept the ultimate responsibility for the program. A plan of open scientific discourse among different evaluators is suggested as a system that could serve the administrator well.

In order for productive evaluation to occur, there must be a clear understanding about who is to be served, the amount and kinds of services to be provided, and what these services are to accomplish. Without such a prior understanding, any attempts to evaluate are almost certain to be futile. With such an understanding, it should be possible to provide the basis for an output oriented evaluation related to accomplishments rather than a sterile and essentially self-defeating evaluation of whether or not the original program plans were followed.

Within the framework of a broad understanding between the program and those to whom it is accountable, specific statements of the mission and goals of the program should be described to make measurement of progress possible. It makes a substantial difference in how evaluation can proceed if the mission is conceived of as improving the mental health of all the citizens in the community; improving the mental health of the clients served; or reducing the dependency of the clients served. Both an abstract mission and concrete measures of accomplishment must be developed for the evaluation to succeed.

In order to provide a logical base of organization and to limit the infinite number of possible observations, a simple systems framework for organizing the evaluative data is suggested. Thus, data evaluating the input into the system relates essentially to clients, and those who applied but did not enter. Evaluating the program's adherence to its mission will require knowing something about who these people are, what they are like, what troubles them, where they come from, why they were not admitted, and where they went. Evaluation of the operations or process part of the system requires knowing what is being done with the people admitted, how it is being done, and what some of the operating characteristics of the system are. Evaluation of the soundness of the structure of the program is also essential for properly understanding the program's operating characteristics.

The evaluation of program output consists of monitoring the functioning of clients within the program, at the time they terminate, and the way they function in the community at some time after they leave the program. Methods for placing a value on these levels of functioning and relating these values to program costs will be an increasingly important tool for the program administrator. The outputs of indirect services are the changed behaviors of the consultees or the changed behaviors of the consultee's target population. The relationship between the outputs desired and the indirect services provided is often difficult to demonstrate. The intrinsic values inherent in some of these services might provide some of the justification for their existence.

REFERENCES

Anderson, Mary Lou; Polak, Paul R.; Grace, David and Lee, Aldora: Treatment goals for patients from patients, their families, and staff. *Journal of the Fort Logan Mental Health Center, 3(3)*:101-115, 1965.

Binner, P. R. and Halpern, Joseph: Output value analysis: A model for the evaluation of mental health programs. *Program Evaluation Forum Position Papers.* Program Evaluation Project, Minneapolis, 1971.

Churchman, C. W.; Ackoff, R. L. and Arnoff, E. L.: *Introduction to Operations Research.* New York, Wiley, 1957.

Conley, R. W.; Conwell, M. and Arrill, M. D.: An approach to measuring the cost of mental illness. *Am J Psychiatry, 124(6),* 1967.

Dent, J. K.: *A Bibliographic Index of Evaluation in Mental Health.* Washington, U. S. Department of Health, Education, and Welfare, National Institute of Mental Health, No. 1545, 1966.

Ellsworth, R. B.; Foster, L.; Childers, B.; Arthur, G. and Kroeker, D.: Hospital and community adjustments as perceived by psychiatric patients, their families, and staff. *J Consult Clin Psychol Monograph, 32(5):* 1968.

Enthoven, Alain C.: Measures of the outputs of higher education: Some practical suggestions for their development and use. In Lawrence, B., Weathersby, G., and Patterson, Virginia W. (Eds.): *Outputs of Higher Education, Their Identification, Measurement, and Evaluation.* Boulder, Western Interstate Commisison for Higher Education, 1970.

Fein, R.: *Economics of Mental Illness.* Joint Commission on Mental Illness and Health, Monograph Series, No. 2, New York, Basic Books, 1958.

Fox, P. D.: *Cost-effectiveness of mental health: An evaluation of an experimental rehabilitation program.* Unpublished doctoral thesis, Stanford Univ., 1968.

Jarett, I. M.: Key factor analysis: The logic that relates the hospital to society. *Hospital Financial Management, 24(4),* 1971.

Kuhn, Thomas S.: *The structure of scientific revolutions.* Foundation of the Unity of Science, *II:2,* 2nd ed. Chicago, Univ. of Chicago Press, 1970.

Longhurst, Philip: *Key Factor Analysis, a Systems Approach to Program Evaluation.* Paper delivered at Western Conference on Uses of Mental Health Data, Portland, 1969.

McCaffree, K. M.: The cost of mental health care under changing treatment methods. *Am J Public Health, 56(7),* 1966.

McPartland, S. and Richart, H.: Analysis of readmissions to a community mental health center. *Community Mental Health Journal, 2(1):*22-26, 1966.

Morton, W. Duke; Lantz, Alma and Halpern, J.: Readmissions: Methodology and meaning. *Journal of the Fort Logan Mental Health Center, 6(1):* 1-22, 1970.

Morton, W. Duke and Schatz, Joel: Patient length of stay: How to ask the question. *Journal of the Fort Logan Mental Health Center, 6(2):*67-78, 1970.

Polak, Paul R.: Patterns of discord: Goals of patients, therapists, and community members. *Archives of General Psychiatry, 23(3),* 1970.

Resources for biomedical research and education. *Research in the Nation's Hospitals, State, Local, Voluntary, 1967.* Report No. 19, Part I and II,

Washington, U. S. Department of Health, Education, and Welfare, Public Health Service, National Institute of Health, 1970.

Roberts, L. M.; Greenfield, N. S. and Miller, M. H. (Eds.) : *Comprehensive Mental Health: The Challenge of Evaluation.* Madison, University of Wisconsin Press, 1968.

Rutledge, L. and Binner, P. R.: Readmissions to a community mental health center. *Community Mental Health Journal, 6(2):*136-143, 1970.

Schatz, Joel: *Length of stay patterns of Fort Logan patients, 1961-1966.* Unpublished research report, 1967.

Schulberg, Herbert C.; Sheldon, Alan and Baker, Frank: *Program Evaluation in the Health Fields.* New York, Behavioral Publications, 1969.

Suchman, E. A.: *Evaluative Research.* New York, Russell Sage Foundation, 1967.

AUTHOR INDEX

SUBJECT INDEX

A

Accountability, xi, 30, 39, 44-45, 53, 54, 57, 234, 235
Administration, xii, 67-69, 125, 241, 321, 337
  change (*see* Change, organizational)
  characteristics, xii-xiii, 63-64, 65, 84
  competence in, xi, 36, 37, 40
  criteria of success, 56, 62-64
  definition, xii
  evaluation of, 58-60
  influence of setting, 60-61, 118, 119
  literature, xii
  principles, xii
  role in evaluation (*see* Evaluation)
  training, xii, xiii, 84

B

Board of directors, 33-34, 35, 54, 203, 205
  apathy, 37
  budgetary role, 37-39, 50-51
  community boards, 223-229
  fiscal responsibility, 37
  sub-committees, 33
Budget, 29-55, 115-116
  authorization, 33-34
  control, 29, 30, 42, 44, 45
  definitions, 30
  discretion, 30, 34-35, 40, 44, 51
  efficiency, 51-52
  evaluation (*see* Evaluation)
  execution, 34-35
  executive's role, 36-37
  flexibility, 45, 51
  form and behavior, 43-44
  incremental, 33
  line item, 29
  object, 29-30, 39, 42, 43, 44-45, 53
  policy, 36
  preparation, 31-33, 43
  program (*see* Program budget)
  reasonableness, 32
  survival, 31
  training, 36
Business manager, xi, 36

C

Change, organizational, iv, xxiv, 44, 193, 289-341
  ability, 315-316, 328, 334, 338
  action, 331, 332, 338
  A Victory Model 314, 315, 325-338
  administrator's role, 289
  barriers, 295-296
  case example, 322-325
  circumstances, 318, 329, 334, 338
  evaluation, 336
  forces, 296, 297
  funding, 299
  goal, 330, 336, 338
  guidelines, 325-337
  inevitability, 292
  information, 326, 327, 330, 332, 338
  management of, xxiv, 302-306
  models, 306-314
  need for, 292, 293, 319, 320
  obligation, 326, 327, 331-332, 338
  Pareto Principle, 313
  planned, xxiv, 297-302, 304-305, 307, 310, 335
  publications, 296-297
  rate, 290, 292
  resistance, 287, 290, 293, 294, 320, 321, 330, 334, 335, 336, 338
  resources, 315-316
  rewards, 321
  Scranton Plan, 309
  techniques, xxiv, 297, 298, 299, 305, 307, 308, 317, 318
  technological, xxiv, 337, 338
  timing, 318, 319, 329, 334, 338

planning, 13-15
procedure, 347-349
program, 347-349
role of evaluator, 351-355
staff of work, 58
survival, 51
test of the market, 51

F

Fees (*see* Financing)
Financing, xvii, 21, 22, 25, 86-119
  cmhcs (*see* Community mental health centers)
  current patterns, 91-95
  federal role, xxii, 16, 88, 90, 93, 97-101, 112, 242-243, 245
  fees, 63, 105-109, 110
  government role, 39, 86-94, 97-105
  grants, 99-100
  history, 87-90
  impact on administration, xvii, 113-118
  impact on services, 110-112
  insurance, 89, 105-107
  long range planning, 113-115
  medicare and medicaid, xviii, 87, 90, 93, 107-108
  mental health services, 86-119, 358
  philanthropy, 109-110
  private expenditures for mental health services, 88, 89, 90, 92
  property tax, 103-104
  public expenditures for mental health services, 86, 92-93, 247
  state and local role, xvii, xviii, xxii, 16, 87-88, 93, 94, 101-105, 111, 116, 205, 243
Fund raising, xvii, 231, 232
  for mental health services (*see* Financing)
Funding (*see* Financing)

G

Government, xix, xxi, xxii, 39, 241-287
  consolidation, 257-259
  counties, 254
  federal decision making, xxii, 250, 251, 260-274, 283
  federal system, 248-253
  fragmentation, 253-260

  grants-in-aid, 103, 249-250, 251
  intergovernmental relations, 250-253
  local decision making, 283-285
  municipalities, 255
  Office of Management & Budget 269-271
  Presidency, 267-270
  role in budgeting, 39-40, 43
  role in financing (*see* Financing)
  role in mental health services, 241-248
  role of the governor, 277-282
  special districts, 255-256
  standard metropolitan statistical area, 256-257
  state decision making, 274-283
  townships, 254-255
Grants, 100, 249, 304-305
  construction, 245, 246, 249, 272
  grants-in-aid (*see* Government)
  staffing, 90, 91, 97, 100, 101, 245, 246

H

Hawthorne studies, 139
Human services, xi, xiv, xviii, xxii, 23, 25, 26, 213

I

Indigenous nonprofessional, 67, 203, 205-207
Informal organizations (*see* Organization)
Insurance (*see* Financing)
Interorganizational relations, xviii, xix, 116-117, 149, 150, 167-199, 220
  administrator's role, 168-170, 173, 183, 189, 195-198
  analysis of, 182, 183
  conflict, xix
  contracts, 186, 188
  diagnosis, 197-198
  duplication, 193, 194
  environment, 174-177
  information system, 172-173
  interdependence, 177-179, 190
  interorganizational field, 174-176
  mandated and managed, 190-191
  mandated but unmanaged, 187-190
  need for, 167
  typology, 179-192